Beyond Suffering and Reparation

Timothy James Bowyer

Beyond Suffering and Reparation

The Aftermath of Political Violence in the Peruvian Andes

Springer

Timothy James Bowyer
Swansea, UK

ISBN 978-3-319-98982-2 ISBN 978-3-319-98983-9 (eBook)
https://doi.org/10.1007/978-3-319-98983-9

Library of Congress Control Number: 2018952232

This Springer imprint is published by the registered company Springer Nature Switzerland AG
The registered company address is: Gewerbestrasse 11, 6330 Cham, Switzerland

To
The memory of my mother
and
to all those who suffered
and died in Mauthausen KZ

"To live with the sensation of helplessness:
today, probably this is the moral state under
which, by resisting, we could be faithful to
our times". Imre Kertész

Preface and Acknowledgements

Is it ever possible to properly acknowledge someone else's suffering? If the failure to engage with terrible things is simply the result of detachment and objectivity, what does the adoption of a subjective attitude to suffering really mean? Much of the incentive for this study derives from trying to understand more about the conditions for mutual recognition so that they might be infringed less often and with less devastating consequences. Though the causes and consequences of suffering have been extensively studied, the particular facts with which it is associated have not always been taken into consideration. Instead, the emphasis on impartiality, neutrality, tolerance and pluralism has encouraged the idea that human suffering is "... something that is a mistake...or something to be fixed".[1] To move beyond this situation, the adverse effects of material disadvantage and the effects of insecurity, anxiety and lack of social integration need to be brought into full view. This involves exploring the relationship between the psychological, the historical, the socio-economic and the spiritual by giving emphasis to the importance of such theoretical issues as power, conflict, exploitation and hierarchy. In this way, an attempt can be made to rescue the long-term impact and psychosocial consequences of political violence from acts of closure and the deadening effects of historical amnesia.[2]

By returning to the reality of the lives of the poor and vulnerable, this study aims to bring into consciousness the relevance of history for understanding contemporary problems "...because the present and the future are connected to the past by the continuity of today's institutions. Today's and tomorrow's choices are shaped by the past."[3] To communicate the determining influence of such theoretical issues as

[1] Sontag, S., (2003: 88)

[2] For the purposes of this book, violence is broadly defined as the violation of a person's physical and psychological integrity. However, this study is primarily concerned with structural violence which focuses attention on victims and the harm and humiliation they suffer from forces such as poverty and oppression. In this way, the meaning of violence can be said to overlap with the notion of social injustice. See, for example, Bufacchi, V., (2007, 2009).

[3] North, D. (1990: vii)

power, conflict, exploitation and hierarchy, we need to explore suffering as an organic whole rather than in segmented categories.[4]

From the point of view of the poor and vulnerable, this requires a framework broad enough to ensure that the adoption of a subjective attitude to suffering is the best possible means for making this study relevant to policy-making in complex areas. This is only possible if the criteria for the choice of disciplines to be involved adequately reflect the interconnectedness between specific types of suffering. On these grounds, the adverse effects of material disadvantage and the effects of insecurity, anxiety and lack of social integration can be properly recognised because they are not subject to the conventions of disciplinary boundaries.

To bring the experience of human suffering into full view so as to counter the ".... slow transmutation of suffering and caring into efficiency and cost", an addition of narratives, ethnographies and social histories as a complement to economic indicators is needed.[5] By documenting the vulnerability of lived experience through the psychological, cultural and social origins of responsibility, accountability and decision-making, this study sets out to refigure and analyse human suffering, so that the individual and the specific context in which people live their lives are no longer regarded as redundant or interchangeable.

This effort to better understand what happens to people who suffer and the stand they take towards their situation amounts to an opportunity to challenge modes of political decision-making, professional practice and policy formation. Though resistance to evidence-based policymaking is less pronounced than it used to be, far too many places continue to be dominated by policies and programmes that pay no attention to the importance of a locally informed analysis. In this respect, the need for more empirical research into the long-term consequences of political violence and its impact on the physical and mental suffering of people is clear.

Though this type of analysis is inevitably incomplete and subjective, the insights it provides into the local patterns of suffering and distress might make us better equipped to take on politicians and policy-makers and get them to take action against the circumstances that cause people to live under conditions of so much misery and degradation.[6]

My personal and professional involvement with rural communities in Latin America first began more than 30 years ago. From the very start, I was fortunate enough to be able to build experience in public health policy, social development, administration and rural development. In the early years, this was made possible through my having responsibility for the development and management of primary health-care programmes for rural communities affected by conflict, discrimination and remoteness. In this capacity, I obtained relevant field experience with rural communities from Mexico, Guatemala, El Salvador, Nicaragua, Bolivia, Brazil, Paraguay and Peru. More recently, my work has focused on the social determinants

[4] Kleinman, A. & Kleinman, J., (1997a, b: 8)

[5] Bandura, A., (2001: 1–26)

[6] Kleinman, A., (1995a, b); Das, V., (1994); Das, V., (1997a); Das, V., (1997b)

of health, popular participation, political violence, negotiating power and the development of more effective links between civil society and the state.

The work for this study was supported financially by a major research grant from the British Academy. From the very outset, this study would not have been possible without the loyal and long-lasting support of Armando Gomez Moreno and his wife Clotilde Alfaro Gomez. Both people worked with me throughout this study as well as in earlier fieldwork in the rural Andes dating back to 2001. Their contribution to the study and its eventual outcome has been immeasurable, not just through their local knowledge of the South-Central Andes, but also with their help in introductions, translation work from the Quechua, etc.

The study also owes an immense debt to the other members of my team responsible for the research at community level over a 3-year period. Their dedication to extremely difficult working conditions was exemplary, and the hardships they endured were nobly borne. They are Guillermo Victor Kajatt, Percy Hugo Ochtane, Alegria Julio Cesar Gomez and Victor Amador Bravo Cauna. I would also like to acknowledge the support of the Mother Superior and Sisters of the *Monasterio Carmelitas Descalzas de Borja* for the lease of an office between 2008 and 2011 whilst the fieldwork was being carried out.

In Great Britain, I would like to acknowledge the support and input from Dr. Christopher Barrow and Dr. Jeremy Holland and from Dr. Helen Hintjens, International Institute of Social Studies of Erasmus University, Rotterdam, for their editorial assistance and support in the preparation of the manuscript. I would also like to thank Anita Jo Dunn for her own outstanding support, particularly during the writing up stage. I would also like to acknowledge the support I have received from Honey whose unique brand of cheer and goodwill has been of lasting and inestimable value. Finally, and most importantly of all, I would like to acknowledge my gratitude to all of the people from the five communities who participated in this study and without whose support and cooperation this study would never have been possible. The conditions under which so much hardship and suffering is endured are testimony to an extraordinary capacity for survival against all odds.

Introduction

How can we avoid the tendency to over-objectify human suffering? How can we stop emptying human suffering of its subjective content? From time immemorial human detachment and objectivity have been used to deny the lived experience of other human beings.[1] Instead of adopting an honourable emotional response, the policymaker would routinely ignore the inner world of other people. For the poor and vulnerable victim, this is a violation because it renders the emotional or affective response to their situation null and void.[2] By reducing everyone to "sameness", technocratic, institutionalised and over-objective procedures and ways of thinking were able to transform human suffering into a subject that allowed other people to acknowledge the misery as if nothing in particular had happened. Because it had no regard for the uniqueness of the individual, this objectivist view of the suffering of others removed the human being from the centre of moral concern. Thus, the single lived subjectivity of any one person was replaced by a supra-individual subject that was utterly disconnected from the context in which that person lived.[3] Having no regard for local knowledge, motivation and participation, grassroots organisations and social networks, expression of discontent, moral convictions and responsiveness to the injustices of the past and access to justice, mainstream social inquiry and research would frequently undermine the vulnerable and socially disadvantaged and the meaning and significance they assign to their own situation.[4]

---

[1] How it became possible for the social act of producing knowledge about social life "...as though it was divorced from any enactment of moral value or expression of political preference" is discussed at length in Kleinman, A., & Wilkinson, I., (2016); see also Kleinman, A. & Kleinman, J., (1997: 11–14) in Kleinman, A., Das, V., and Lock, M. (eds.) (1997a, b).

[2] Hoffman, M.L., (2000: 4)

[3] "...To reduce all others to sameness is a politics without ethics which eventually destroys all that does not comply with the reductionist view of other people. It is a perspective that radically universalizes itself and eliminates every non-conforming individual. Whoever does not comply with this approach is ignored as though they did not exist. This is a code of conduct that is without mercy. This strips the individual of dignity and self-respect" Haas, P.J. (1988: 34).

[4] "...The difficulties encountered by models of rehabilitation and peace-building plans proposed for times of war or post-conflict periods are due not only to the complexity of the situations, but

However, a new generation of scholars has emerged in the last two or three decades and begun to fill this gap by exploring such issues as identity, history, violence inequality and cultural transformation. Working in a range of different disciplines, their outputs are helping to bring about a deeper and richer commitment to social justice, social care and humanitarianism.

For instance, the commitment to witness and respond to the root causes of human suffering has received a significant boost from scholars working on community experiences of survival and memories of political violence. In particular, a growing number of studies have been using archival materials and ethnographic fieldwork to explore the historically rooted and locally specific power relations, social conflicts and cultural understandings that shape the lives of ordinary people caught up in political violence.[5] By examining daily life as told by ordinary people who have limited influence or authority, this current generation of scholars is helping to shape a new interpretation of local political culture and memory in relation to local and national power structures over time.

Through this commitment to witness and respond to the root causes of human suffering, the use of archival materials and ethnographic fieldwork is helping to reframe the terms of public debate. By engaging with the lives of ordinary people received, accepted understandings of social issues are being challenged and a new way of thinking about social action and social support is being promoted. Though recognition of the potential contributions of this type of approach is growing, it does not mean that the question of how to respond to human and social suffering is by any means exhausted. Indeed, if this commitment to witness and respond to human suffering is to be effective, it needs to engage with material disadvantage, insecurity, anxiety and lack of social integration in ways that enable researchers to connect critical thought with problem-solving.

Being an ethnographic witness to how life is lived by the poor and vulnerable means that the researcher is able to reconstruct the historically rooted and locally

---

also to their chosen methodological approaches, which overlook cultural and social specificity." See Beneduce, R., (2007: 41ff) in Pouligny, B., Chesterman, S., and Schnabel, A. (eds.) (2007).

[5] Examples of this way of understanding political violence and the impact it has on ordinary people include Lewis Taylor's *Shining Path: Guerrilla War in Peru's Northern Highlands, 1980–1997* (Liverpool University Press, 2006), Olga M. Gonzalez's *Unveiling Secrets of War in the Peruvian Andes* (University of Chicago Press, 2011), Miguel La Serna's *The Corner of the Living* (University of North Carolina Press, 2012), Kimberly Theidon's *Intimate Violence: Violence and Reconciliation in Peru* (University of Pennsylvania Press, 2013). Other examples from other parts of Latin America include Sandy Smith-Nonini's *Healing the Body Politic: El Salvador's Popular Struggle for Health Rights from Civil War to Neoliberal Peace* (Rutgers University Press, 2010), Ellen Moodie's *El Salvador in the Aftermath of Peace: Crime, Uncertainty and the Transition to Democracy* (University of Pennsylvania Press, 2010), Kristi Anne Stølen's *Guatemalans in the Aftermath of Violence: The Refugees' Return* (University of Pennsylvania Press, 2007). Other examples from other parts of the world include Tricia Redeker Hepner's *Soldiers, Martyrs, Traitors, and Exiles: Political Conflict in Eritrea and the Diaspora* (University of Pennsylvania Press, 2011), Azra Hromadžić's *Citizens of an Empty Nation: Youth and State-Making in Postwar Bosnia-Herzegovina* (University of Pennsylvania Press, 2015), and Kristin Conner Doughty's *Remediation in Rwanda: Grassroots Legal Forums* (University of Pennsylvania Press, 2016).

specific power relations, social conflicts and cultural understandings that shape their lives.

However, if the poor and vulnerable are to get the attention they deserve practical knowledge commitments to social justice; humanitarianism and social care by themselves are not enough. What is lacking is the means by which critical thought can be used to more effectively transform the adverse effects of material disadvantage and the effects of insecurity, anxiety and lack of social integration.

The Scope of This Study

From its inception, the fieldwork this study draws upon has focused on the relationship between context and its influence on human nature and responsibility and the failure of the social capital discourse.[6] By returning to the reality of the lives of survivors of the political violence, this study aims to advance understanding of the psychosocial nature of human beings and how they seek to manage and shape the world around them. This way of seeing means that we need to understand the reality of what it is like to live in conditions of low trust, anxiety, high vigilance and insecurity; otherwise, we will not be able to adequately assess the impact of physical and mental suffering.[7] To attain clarity about the forces responsible for this near-total uncertainty of daily life, a locally informed analysis is necessary, for understanding the subjective aspects of individual suffering.[8]

Though this type of analysis is in regular use, its association with research into the long-term consequences of political violence and its impact on the physical and mental suffering of people are less commonplace.[9] To redress this situation, the research for this study sought to provide a longitudinal and comparative analysis of human suffering in five rural communities affected by political violence in the South-Central Andes of Peru.

The overriding objective is to provide a reasoned account of human suffering so that its effects can be sufficiently acknowledged and so that social interactions can be recognised as a step towards improving the lives of rural people and their

[6] For discussions on the social capital discourse see, for example, Coleman, (1989); Putnam et al., (1993). For the importance of context in relation to human suffering, see Kleinman, A., Das, V., and Lock, M., (1997a, b: 207ff) "…There is a profound diversity in the meaning and interpretation of what people mean by suffering that can generate and sustain greatly different responses to suffering"; see also Wilkinson, I., (2005a: 16); Muller, Adam, et al. 2017: Digitized Suffering Reconciliation in Anderson, R.E. (ed) *Alleviating World Suffering,* Springer.

[7] Safety nets or "socioeconomic safety nets" are non-contributory transfer programmes seeking to prevent the poor or those vulnerable to shocks and poverty from falling below a certain poverty level. See Grosh, M, del Ninno, C. & Tesliuc, E. (2008).

[8] Dussaillant, F. & Gonzalez, P. A., (2015: 233–251) Lifetime Suffering and Capabilities in Chile in Anderson, R.E. (ed) *World Suffering & the Quality of Life*, Springer

[9] See Kleinman, (1995a, b, 1996); Das, (1997a); Bourdieu, et al. (1999); Frank (2001); Morgan and Wilkinson, (2001).

communities. While the focus is on rural people in the South-Central Andes, the lessons have far wider application for the understanding of what psychosocial processes and other issues relating to the aftermath of political violence look like from the perspective of victims and survivors.

This effort to better understand what happens to people who suffer and the stand they take towards their situation offers an opportunity to advance ethical and political debate. By making people more alert to the consequences of human suffering, this study aims to challenge established and flawed modes of political decision-making, professional practice and policy formation.

The starting point for such an understanding is to demonstrate that human suffering is powerfully determined by social factors that undermine people's control over their own existence. This study argues that this can only be fully appreciated through an understanding of the various forms of social suffering in the population, which are in turn determined by the legacy of political violence, hunger, deprivation, ill treatment and so forth.[10]

By documenting the psychological, cultural and social origins of responsibility, accountability and decision-making, this study sets out to demonstrate what happens to people who suffer from economic and other hardships. This study explores the roots of the immense difficulties that confront communities affected by political violence.[11]

This is vital because only through a thorough analysis of the relationship between the social context and its influence on human nature and responsibility can the risk of over-objectifying the complexity of human suffering be avoided.

Thinking About Suffering

Because suffering has the capacity to affect every part of our lives, it may be that it is beyond the bounds of language to represent all the ways in which it can afflict people.[12] However, suffering's capacity to be multi-causal (often acting cumulatively) and its power to violate and destroy humans mean that it is supremely important to find ways of researching and representing it effectively. The problem lies with suffering's resistance to conceptualisation.[13]

---

[10] "Social suffering", is a relatively new label for suffering that is produced primarily by social conditions that damage a collectivity's sense of self-worth and heightens powerlessness produced from socially shared traumas. One consequence of social suffering often is the loss of caring for self and others as valued human beings. See Anderson, R. E., (2013: 44); for an extended discussion on the origins of social inquiry and how its original commitment to building knowledge and practices to improve the lives of people who experience social suffering, see Kleinman, A. & Wilkinson, I., (2016).

[11] Hickel, 2017: Addressing the structural causes of Suffering Jason in Anderson, R.E. (ed) *Alleviating World Suffering*, Springer

[12] Kleinman et al. (1997a, b); Wilkinson, I. (2001); Wilkinson, I. (2005a:18)

[13] See Wilkinson, I. (2005a:16ff). For Scarry, "...The fact that suffering cannot be shared means that

Currently the legitimised view of suffering is "...as a commodity and through this cultural representation experience is being remade, thinned out and distorted".[14] In practice, this excludes anything specific about the nature of suffering and replaces it with objectified modes of representation that are both formulaic and standardised.[15] Having removed the actual lived experience of suffering from the realms of public life, researchers have dishonoured the uniqueness of the individual and undermined role and value at the heart of moral concern. This is an unfortunate misconception because it means that the world often attends to suffering without emotional engagement.

By deflecting legitimate moral expectations away from public life, any symbolic representation of suffering can be subsumed under "...issues involving economic factors and the problem of distributing scarce resources to those in need".[16]

For the victim, this failure to properly acknowledge the awfulness of suffering is not just an affirmation of the supreme importance of power, but an indication of how the conventional meaning of dignity and self-respect is invalidated.[17]

By failing to assume a subjective attitude to human suffering, the world undermines and ultimately destroys conventional notions of what is good, trustworthy, beneficial, important, useful, desirable and constructive.[18] Detachment and insensitive over-objectivity deny people proper acknowledgement of their suffering and make it impossible to assume the sort of appropriate responsibilities needed for meaningful dialogue and a shared moral understanding.[19] These over-objective and

---

it confounds representation and defies our capacity to provide an outward expression of the contents of our experience" (Scarry, 1985: 4–5).

[14] Kleinman, A. and Kleinman, J., (1997a, b: 2) in Kleinman, A., Das, V., and Lock, M. (eds.) (1997a, b)

[15] Kleinman, A., (1995a, b, 1996); Das, (1997a); Bourdieu, et al. (1999); Frank (2001); Morgan and Wilkinson, (2001)

[16] Langer (2008: 25–47) in Kleinman, A., Das, V., and Lock, M. (eds.) (1997a, b). See also Farmer, P. (2005) *Never Again? Reflections on Human Values and Human Rights. The Tanner Lectures on Human Values,* University of Utah

[17] In elucidating the implications of this failure to properly engage with the actual awfulness of human suffering, I am indebted to the insights into the human dimension of a situation and the consequences of an objective and detached attitude towards others by Vetlesen: "...Given a detached attitude, there is a danger that I shall remain blind to the human reality of the situation in front of me, that it will awaken no engagement on my part but will instead leave me indifferent. And indifference is a prime threat to morality, even more destructive to it than hatred or resentment, because the intrinsic logic of indifference sets no limits to its spread. What is threatened, often effectively suspended, in indifference is what I term the 'emotional bond' between humans. To miss the human dimension of a situation is also to miss its moral dimension" Vetlesen, A.J., (1994: 10). See also Dussaillant, F. & Gonzalez, P. A., (2015: 233–251) Lifetime Suffering and Capabilities in Chile in Anderson, R.E. (ed) *World Suffering & the Quality of Life*, Springer.

[18] "...Suffering is greatly intensified in relation to the dominant ways in which it is symbolically represented in the realms of public life." Das, V., (2000) in Das, V. Kleinman, A. Ramphele, M. and Reynolds, P. (eds.).

[19] Agamben, G. (1999: 20ff)

reductionist portrayals of what suffering actually is and what might be done to combat the effects it has on people's lives have largely been left unchallenged.[20]

To better understand the ways in which people live in and through their suffering, we need to explore the individual's subjective felt experience.[21] This means giving emphasis to the psychological, cultural and social origins of responsibility, accountability and decision-making.

If we accept that social location profoundly shapes human beliefs and practices, then it is reasonable to expect that suffering is not always going to mean the same thing.[22] However, this does not also mean that the social meaning of suffering is exclusively determined by the local cultural values and power relations associated with that particular social location. This is because the modern world is responsible for a multiple stream of social traditions and practices that compromise and often undermine the authority of local cultural values and power relations. This can alter how people make decisions or act; it can constrain a person's free will; it can also mean that much human suffering is unrecognised.[23]

For people affected by political violence, the emotional consequences are often huge.[24] For example, it may mean that thinking about and experiencing emotional states associated with what happened are perceived not as a symptom of human suffering, but as the expression of a new norm.[25] It is therefore important that particular attention is paid not just to the specific context in which suffering arises, but to its social meaning as well.[26] However, as with the body in pain, it is only when the experience of human suffering is externalised that it is able to offer the best opportunity for being better understood.[27]

---

[20] See Kleinman, (1996); Das, (1997a); Grant, A., (2011)

[21] Turiel, E. (2002: vii)

[22] Bliese, P. D. and Britt, T.W. (2001)

[23] Farmer, P. (2005: 140ff) *Never Again? Reflections on Human Values and Human Rights. The Tanner Lectures on Human Values,* University of Utah

[24] To aid our understanding of the emotional consequences of human suffering, Dominick LaCapra has developed an approach that involves feeling for another without losing sight of the distinction between one person's experience and the experience of the other. He calls this "empathic unsettlement" to denote the desired type of affective involvement and to distinguish it from what he calls "self-sufficient, projective or incorporative identification" LaCapra, D., (2001: 40). See also Silverman, K. (1996).

[25] In this respect, the distinction between the emergence of new post-conflict norms and values and pre-conflict norms and values is consistent with the insights provided by Vetlesen with respect to the performance of our emotional capacities and their relationship with the social setting in which it takes place. This is because "...a faculty such as empathy – giving rise to care, compassion, sympathy – is highly susceptible to changes in the moral subject's social environment, which means that the social environment may help encourage or impede the faculty's actual exercise" Vetlesen, A.J., (1994: 81).

[26] Wilkinson, I., (2005a: 39); Melzack, R., & Wall, P., (1965); Wall, P., (1999); Kleinman A., (1986); Kleinman, A., (1988); Kleinman, A., (1992) in DelVecchio Good, M.J., Brodwin, P.E., Good, B.J., & Kleinman, A. (1992)

[27] Scarry, E., (1985: 52–3)

To break through the detachment and over-objectivity that empties the meaning of human suffering and misery of all subjective content a different approach is needed.[28] It is suggested that "…acts of symbolic violence on the qualitative experience of personal suffering" [29] can be avoided only if the researcher is able and willing to "...engage with how people respond to their feelings in ways that do not simplify them…".[30] In the case of people that lack power, there is no alternative but to begin the investigation into suffering with the testimonies of ordinary people.[31] This allows the researcher to break with the absence of any kind of emotional engagement at both the personal and collective levels and make use of testimony to illustrate what suffering means to the victim.[32] It also provides the researcher with a means to begin to understand the influence of context and social location, as well as the cultural formations and social processes that make up the lived experience of suffering.

To better understand the particular situation as people perceive and cognitively construct it, testimonies provide a means by which we can "...attempt to understand experience and its aftermath, including the role of memory and its lapses in coming to terms with or denying and repressing the past".[33]

This also provides the researcher with the opportunity to better understand the moral and intellectual tensions born in the face of suffering and their influence on cultural innovation, political and practical engagement and to better interpret their implications.

---

[28] The need for a different approach to the representation of suffering is discussed at some length in Langer, L., (2008: 53ff) in Kleinman, et. al., (1997a, b). See also Dussaillant, F. & Gonzalez, P. A., (2015: 233–251) Lifetime Suffering and Capabilities in Chile in Anderson, R.E. (ed) *World Suffering & the Quality of Life*, Springer.

[29] See Bourdieu et al. (1999: 607–26); Frank (2001); Wilkinson, I., (2005a: 27).

[30] LaCapra, D., (2001: 40)

[31] Langer, L., (2008: 55)

[32] "...To testify – to vow to tell, to promise and produce one's own speech as material evidence for truth- is to accomplish a speech act, rather than to simply formulate a statement. As a performative speech act, testimony in effect addresses what history is in action that exceeds any substantialized significance, and what in happenings is impact that dynamically explodes any conceptual reifications and any constative delimitations." See Felman, S. & Laub, D., (1992: 5).

[33] LaCapra, D., (2001: 86–7)

Contents

Glossary of Acronyms

AFAVIP	*Asociación de familias afectadas por la violencia política* (Association for Families who are Victims of Political Violence in Peru)
APAFA	*Asociación de Padres de Familia* (Fathers of Families Association)
APRA	*Alianza Popular Revolucionaria Americana* (American Popular Revolutionary Alliance)
APRODEH	*Asociación Pro Derechos Humanos* (Association for Human Rights in Peru)
CAD	*Comites de auto-defensa* (self-defence committee) – a programme that was made official in 1992 by the Fujimori administration
CBO	Community Based Organization
CCR	*Consejo de Coordinación Regional* (Regional Coordination Council)
CENIA	*Centro Andino de Investigaciones Antropológico Forenses* (Andean Centre for Forensic Anthropology Research)
CEPLAN	*Centro Nacional de Planeamiento Estratégico* "*Plan Bicentenario: El Peru hacia el* 2021" (National Centre for Strategic Planning Bicentenary Plan: Peru Towards 2021)
CMAN	*Comisión Multisectorial de Alto Nivel* (High-Level Multisectoral Commission)
CONACAMI	*Coordinadora Nacional de Comunidades Afectados por la Minería* (National Coordinator for Communities affected by Mining)
CONOI	*Concejo Educativo Institucional* (Institutional Education Council)
CORAVIP	*Coordinadora Regional de Afectados por la Violencia Política* (Regional Coordinating Committee for Victims of Political Violence)
CPR	Civil and Political Rights

CRECER	The national "Grow" strategy, led by the Ministry for Development and Social Inclusion (MIDIS) started in 2007
CVR	*Comisión de la Verdad y Reconciliación* (Truth and Reconciliation Commission) installed in 2001, final report delivered in 2003
DEVIDA	*Comisión Nacional para el Desarrollo y Vida sin Drogas (Encuesta Nacional de Prevención y Consumo de Droga)* (National Commission for Life and Development without Drugs)
DIGESA	*La Dirección General de Salud Ambiental* (General Directorate of Environmental Health)
DIRCOTE	*Dirección Contra el Terrorismo* (Group Counter-Terrorist Directorate) is the branch of the National Police of Peru that is responsible for Peru's anti-terrorist law enforcement efforts
DIRESA	*Dirección Regional de Salud* (Regional Health Directorate)
DNI	(National ID)
DNS	National Sanitation Direction
ELITES	*Equipos Locales Itinerantes de Trabajo Extramural* (Itinerant Local Extramural Teams)
EMZ	Ayacucho Emergency Zone
EPAF	*Equipo Peruano de Antropología Forense* (Peruvian Forensic Anthropology Team)
EPS	Health Provider Entities
ESCR	Economic, Social and Cultural Rights
EsSalud	*El Seguro Social de Salud del Perú* (National Insurance coverage)
FFAA	*Fuerzas Armadas* (Armed Forces)
FGD	Focus Group Discussion
FONB	*Funciones Obstétricas Básicas* (Basic Obstetric Functions)
FONCODES	*Fondo de Compensacion Social* (Social Fund for Social Compensation)
FONCOMÚN	*El Fondo de Compensación Municipal* (a national fund to promote investment in isolated and neglected municipalities throughout Peru)
ICTJ	International Center for Transitional Justice
INEI	*El Instituto Nacional de Estadísticañ e Informática* (National Institute for Statistics and Information)
GAD	Generalized Anxiety Disorder
GEIN	*Grupo Especial de Inteligencia* (Special Intelligence Group)
GPIR	*Grupo sobre el Plan Integral de Reparaciones (*Integral Reparations Plan Group)
GRO	Grass Roots Organization
HW	Health worker
INEI	*Instituto Nacional de Estadística e Informática* (National Institute for Statistics and Information)

IPAZ	*Instituto de Investigacion y Promocion del Desarrollo y Paz de Ayacucho* (Institute for the Promotion of Development and Peace in Ayacucho)
JAAS	*Junta Administradora de Servicios de Saneamiento* (Sanitation Services Management Board)
JUNTOS	*Together* (A conditional cash transfer (CCT) programme started in 2005)
MEF	*Ministerio de Economia y Finaciamento* (Ministry of Finance and the Economy)
MIMDES	*Ministerio de la Mujer y Desarrollo Social* (Ministry of Women and Social Development)
MINSA	*Ministerio de Salud* (Ministry of Health)
MINEDU	*Ministerio de Educación* (Ministry of Education)
MRTA	*Movimiento Revolucionario Túpac Amaru* (Túpac Amaru Revolutionary Movement)
NURAJ	*Nucleo Rural de Administracion de Justicia* (Rural Nuclei for the Administration of Justice)
NGO	Non-Governmental Organization
PAR	*Programa Nacional de Apoyo a la Repoblacion* (Programme to support the Re-Population) or *Programa de Apoyo al Retorno de los Desplazados* (Programme to Support the Return of the Displaced People) created in 1993 by the Fujimori administration)
PARSALUD	*Programa de Apoyo a la Reforma del Sector Salud* (Programme of Support for Health Sector Reform)
PCP-SL	*Partido Comunista Peruano-Sendero Luminoso* (Peruvian Communist Party-Shining Path)
PIR	*Plan Integral de Reparaciones* (Comprehensive Reparations Program)
PNP	*Policia Nacional del Peru* (National Police Force Peru)
PRONAA	*Programa Nacional de Apoyo Alimentario* (National Food Assistance Programme)
PRONAMACHCS	*Programa Nacional de Manejo de Cuencas Hidrograficas y Conservacion de Suelos* (National Programme of Watershed Management and Soil Conservation)
PRONAMA	*Programa Nacional de Movilización para la Alfabetización* (National Mobilization Against Illiteracy)
PRONASAR	*Programa Nacional de Agua y Saneamiento Rural* (National Programme for Rural Water and Sanitation)
PRONEI	*Programa no escolarizado de Educación Inicial* (Programme for early childhood education out of school)
PTSD	Post Traumatic Stress Disorder
RENIEC	*Registro Nacional de Identificación y Estado Civil* (National Registry of Identification and Civil Status)
RUV	*Registro Unico de Victimas* (National Register of Victims)

SEPS *Superintendencia Entidades Prestadoras Salud* (Supervisory Authority Providers Health)
SERUM *Servicio Rural y Urbano Marginal de Salud* (Rural and Marginalized Urban Health Service)
SFT Specialized Forensic Team
SIS *Seguro Integral de Salud* (Comprehensive Health Insurance)
SL *Sendero Luminoso* (Shining Path)
SUNASS *Superintendencia Nacional de Servicios de Saneamiento* (National Superintendence of Sanitation Services)
TBA Traditional Birth Attendant
TRC Truth and Reconciliation Commission
UGEL *Unidades de Gestion Educativa Local* (Local Education Management Units)
UIT *Unidad Impositiva Tributaria* (Tax Unit)
VRAE The VRAE is shorthand for the Valley of the Apurimac and Ene River (Spanish: *Valle de los Ríos Apurímac y Ene*). It is a major centre of coca production and currently at the centre of terrorist activity in the ongoing internal conflict

Glossary of Spanish Words and Phrases

abigeo	Cattle rustler
agente municipal	Municipal agent (local government official)
alfabetizadotes	Literacy workers
anexo	Nucleated settlement in a district under municipal authority
assistentialismo	Handouts
clubes de madres	Mothers Clubs
campesinos	Peasants – the term has ethnic and class connotations
cholo	Acculturated Indian
comedor popular	Soup kitchen
comité popular	Popular committee used within the SL structure in charge of administering community activities
comunidad	A village as a defined territory
comunero	A member of a legally recognised community
condenado	Soul of a condemned person who having been sinful in life wanders in search of other souls at night to gain salvation
conformismo	Attitude of the person who readily accepts any public or private circumstances, especially when diverse or unfair
Consejo de Coordinacion Regional	Regional Coordination Council
Coordinadora Nacional de Comunidades Afectados por la Minería	National Coordinator for Communities affected by Mining
Curandero	Traditional healer
delincuentes	Young offenders usually associated with drugs
desaparecido	Disappeared or missing person

Dirección Nacional de Saneamiento	National Sanitation Direction.
empresa communal	Community workshop
Encomienda	From the Spanish *encomendar*, "to entrust" (dependency relation system used by the Spanish throughout Latin America until it's formal abolition in 1730)
faenas	Obligatory *c*ommunity tasks/chores
hacendado	Owner of a hacienda
hacienda	Land estate, originally part of the *encomienda* system
individualismo	Individualism/selfishness
juez de paz	Justice of the peace
junta directive communal	Communal Executive Board responsible for the management of the community's lands
latifundio	Traditional large estates
Ley Orgánica de Gobiernos Regionales	Organic Law of Regional Governments
mestizo	A person of mixed Spanish-Indian ancestry
minifundios	Small plots of land for cultivation
Ministerio de Vivienda, Construcción y Saneamiento	Ministry of Housing, Construction and Sanitation
muchiladores	Human mules for carrying drugs
Oficina Nacional de Procesos Electorales	Peru's National Office of Electoral Processes
pueblo	Village, community or people
Organizacion Comunal	Community Organization
Regidor	Third ranking member of the *varayoqkuna* authority system
rondas campesinas	Armed peasant patrol started in Ayacucho during the political violence
Senderistas	Members of Shining Path
Sinchis:	Special US-trained "counterterrorist" police battalion
Sinverguenza	Shameless
Subversivos	Terrorists and subversives
teniente gobernador	Lieutenant governor (of a community)
terrucos	Slang for terrorist
turco	Terrorist
Vaso de Leche	Glass of Milk (government programme)
Varayocc	Indigenous mayor (of a community)
Vecino	Neighbour

Glossary of Quechua Words and Phrases

Ayllu	A localised group or work party
Ayni	Reciprocal labour exchange, designed to establish solidarity, hierarchy and indebtedness
Cawananchicaman micushun. Upushun	As long as we have life, let's eat. Let's drink
ćhacra suwa	The poor peasant who steals out of need
chakra	A plot of agricultural land or small farm
ichu	Straw
Juc shungulla cawashun	Let's live with just one heart
llakis	Suffering associated with loss and memories
lloqalla	This refers to all unmarried persons, who are assumed to be dependent and not allowed to take on communal duties and responsibilities
manchay tiempo	Times of fear
minka	A request for labour; a collective work party
mishti yarpay suwa	A thief who steals or rapes out of anger or greed
mishtiyasha	Used to refer to those who turn their back on their heritage
puna	A neotropical ecoregion and one of the eight Natural Regions of Peru; the Puna region comprises high plateaus and cliffs
runa	This refers to all married persons who own land and take on communal duties and responsibilities

sasachakuy tiempo	The difficult time used by Quechua speakers to refer to the political violence
sinchi	A highly specialized counterinsurgency police battalion
suwa	*A* thief
varayoq	A community leader entitled to hold a staff of office
washa rima	To steal a person's reputation by gossip

List of Maps

List of Maps

Chapter 1
The Complexities of Human Suffering

1.1 Defining Suffering

The discussion about suffering presented here cannot reflect the full complexity and variability of human life. It can only accurately apply to those types of human suffering relevant to people in rural Andean communities affected by political violence.[1]

The study is especially focused on the destruction of deeply held commitments and ideals; and on the suffering that arises from the legacies of the past including chronic states, conflict and post-conflict traumas.[2] Also important is the suffering that arises from routine misery and inappropriate policies and programmes, bureaucratic practices and cultural forces.[3] However, it is helpful to start with some broad-ranging characterizations of suffering before moving on to those aspects of suffering most relevant to this study.

To begin, what do we mean by suffering? How does a better understanding of what suffering means improve our insights into the varied experiences of human communities? First and foremost, suffering is a universal human experience that can be described as a negative basic feeling or emotion that involves a subjective character of unpleasantness, aversion, harm or threat of harm to body or mind.[4] Cassell

[1] See also Anderson, R. E., (2013): "...From the data presented on global suffering...it is evident that most suffering, especially in non-affluent countries, results from illness, injuries, disability and poverty, especially poverty-related scarcities. The scarcities are forces largely under human control through social institutions."

[2] See for example: Regel, S. and Joseph, S. (2010: 75); Zoellner, L.A. and Bittenger, J.N., (2004) in Rosen, G.M. (2004) (ed.).

[3] See also Cohen, S. (2001: 227ff); Montoya Vivanco, Y. (2012: 159ff) in Almqvist, J. and Esposito, C. (eds). (2012).

[4] Spelman, E.V., (1997); Cassell, E.J. (1982); (1991); (2004); Hudson, (2012); Kleinman, A., Das, V., Lock, M.M., (1997b); Das, V., (2007); Brady, D. & Burton, L.M., (2016); Fassin, D., (2007); Fassin, D., (2009); Bourgois, P., (2009); Brehm, S.S., Kassin, S & Fein, S.(1996); Levinas, E., (2006).

T. J. Bowyer, *Beyond Suffering and Reparation*,
https://doi.org/10.1007/978-3-319-98983-9_1

(1982) defines suffering as "...a state of severe distress associated with events that threaten the intactness of the person."[5] As he emphasizes elsewhere "...what is threatened or injured in suffering is the intactness of the person as a person."[6] More recently, Hudson, (2012) defined suffering as "...an experience of unpleasantness and aversion associated with the perception of harm or threat of harm in an individual."[7] Cassell (1982) draws our attention to the close relationship between suffering and pain.

He has described this as a sense of impending disintegration, distinct from pain or distress taken alone, and not immediately translatable into terms appropriate to non-human animals.[8] For the individual victim the reality of suffering is self-evident, but it is far from self-evident to others.

To better understand what happens to people who suffer a somewhat broader use of the term is needed. This is partly because no individual suffers "...in the same way anymore than they live, talk about what is at stake, or respond to serious problems in the same way."[9] It is also because suffering is so closely bound up with the human condition that "...we cannot address the question of what it is to be human without also attending to the question of what it is to suffer, of how suffering is to be understood, and of what suffering calls for by way of response."[10] The fact that suffering is such a personal experience may well be part of the explanation of why commentators find it so difficult to agree on a definition.[11]

In practice this means that the human consequences of extreme poverty and political violence cannot be examined as a one-dimensional issue or a uniform experience.[12] It is of no assistance here to assign the victims of political violence to the category of the dehumanized. Where those in authority commonly refer to the powerless as dehumanised, it is likely that context and culturally reinforced beliefs converge.

---

[5] Cassell, E.J., (1982); (1991); (2004); See also Kleinman, A. & Kleinman, J., (1997a); Wilkinson, (2005); Weicke & Guinote, A., (2008); Kleinman, A., (2009b); Langle, A., (2008); Hewstone, M., Stroebe, W., Stephenson, G.M., (1996); Weicke & Guinote, A., (2008).

[6] Cassell, E., (2004: 274).

[7] Hudson, W., (2012) in Malpas, J & Lickiss, N., (eds.) (2012); see also Kleinman, A. & Wilkinson, I., (2016: 14-16ff).

[8] Cassell, E.J., (1982: 639-645).

[9] Kleinman, A., (1988); Geras, N., (1998); Martin-Baro, I., (1994a, b, c).

[10] Malpas, J., & Lickiss, N., (2012:1).

[11] Illich, I., (1976: 146-8) as cited in Wilkinson, I., (2005a, b: 16).

[12] Kleinman, A., Das, V., and Lock, M., (1997a, b: xxiv).

1.2 The Importance of Understanding Suffering

To make the lived experience of suffering a focal point for social and political concern the multiple ways in which suffering takes place need to be understood and emphasized, and that means from the perspectives of ethnography, social history, medical anthropology, critical humanities (including holocaust studies).[13]

This is confirmed by recent social science reviews that argue for multidisciplinary perspectives on violence to counter the tendency to compartmentalize, with "few links among different … approaches."[14] Building on the idea that the appropriate approach to suffering is one that grounds research in social experience, many authors argue that such an approach can lead to more effective local interventions, better social policy, and social change that addresses the roots of poverty, inequality, and social suffering.[15]

From this perspective we can begin to serve the needs of those whose horrific experiences are capable of "...shattering basic assumptions about the self and the world such as the assumption of personal invulnerability, the perception of the world as a meaningful place, and the perception of the self as positive."[16]

To come to a more complex understanding of the human issues at stake this new perspective has to come from the places where the abuse of power tears people "... from the first places where the first affective relationships, the primordial senses of self and basic belonging, formed by reciprocity and complementarity are fashioned."[17] This is particularly applicable to the aftermath of political violence because it focuses attention on the lived experience of distress and injustice, while exposing the "…often close linkage of personal problems with societal problems."[18]

To avoid unconscious collusion with its over-bearing influence we need to pay considerable attention to the ways in which power has the capacity to shape interactions between individuals within groups and between groups.[19] In these circumstances its principal role is associated with the ability to satisfy core self-and group-serving needs. Having power affects the way in which people resolve human suffering and promote well-being.[20]

For the state the exercise of power is used to set the agenda and determine what issues will be recognised as candidates for discussion or influence. To investigate

---

[13] Kleinman, A., (1995b: 181–191).

[14] See (Bufacchi 2009; Krause 2009; Panter-Brick 2010) (McIlwaine 1999:455) as cited by Rylko-Bauer, B. & Farmer, P., (2016: 47-75) in Brady & Burton, L.M., (2016) (Ed); see also Kleinman, (1988); Kleinman and Kleinman, (1997a, b).

[15] Abadia-Barrero, C.& Castro, C. (2006); Adimora et al. (2009) as cited as cited by Rylko-Bauer, B. & Farmer, P., (2016: 47-75) in Brady & Burton, L.M., (2016) (Eds.)

[16] Gautier, A., & Sabatini Scalmati, A., (2010: 132).

[17] Gautier, A., & Sabatini Scalmati, A., (2010: 32).

[18] Kleinman et al. 1997a, b:ix); See also Das, V., (1997b).

[19] Guinote, A. & Vescio, T.K., (2010: 3).

[20] Kleinman, Das, and Lock (1997a, b:ix).

the main sources and symptoms of human suffering, it is vital to research its interconnectedness with power.

To make possible the resolution of moral issues through rule-based (deontological) moral thinking, it is necessary to have sufficient power in terms of political influence, control of institutions, and access to essential commodities and material resources. This applies, irrespective of whether this has positive or negative effects.[21] However, dominant utilitarian ideas about ordinary people mean that efforts to reduce human suffering lack respect for culture, ethnicity, and political tradition, and for local norms, values and beliefs and other aspects of rural community life.

This leads to the objectification of others, not only in the form of stereotypes as the basis for interaction between ordinary people and the state but also as a means by which the state is able to normalize and justify social and economic inequality.[22] In practice this makes an act right or wrong according to whether or not existing rules and principles have been violated.[23]

It is difficult to evaluate responsibly how much these manifestations of inhumanity bear testimony to emotional insensitivity and how much such behaviour is the result of a system incapable of independent moral reflection.[24] By reducing the poor and vulnerable to a nameless stereotypical and dehumanised mass is it conceivable that the state fails to acknowledge the power of suffering to dominate every aspect of human experience and existence?[25] Does this also mean that policymakers and programme builders are likely to do more harm than good by treating human suffering in purely instrumental terms as a 'problem' to be addressed in terms of 'efficiency and cost'?[26]

The interconnectedness of power with suffering means there is a need for interdisciplinary engagements that involve local people and which bring them into the policy-and-programme-making process. It is also about the low level of power that people in rural communities have over material, human, intellectual and financial resources.

[21] Lammers, J; Stapel, Diederik A. (2009: 279-289).

[22] Fiske, S.T., (1993).

[23] Kleinman, Das, V. & Lock, M., (1997a, b:ix).

[24] Post conflict these communities have become a part of a single national narrative of events, people, institutions, culture and politics, an undertaking of massive simplification that not only distorts the past but threatens to impoverish its future. Neglect, indifference and forgetfulness mean that its past and the denial of that past are rapidly eroding the importance of what happened there. Yesterday's killings are perpetuated in today's oblivion. The urge to remember and commemorate is tightly bound with the need to suppress and forget. See Wilkinson, I., (2004: 113-121).

[25] As Adorno has stressed, stereotypes are not merely opposed to experience but highly resistant to it.

[26] Kleinman, A. and Kleinman, J., (1997a, b:11–15) in Kleinman, A., Das, V., & Lock, M. (eds.) (1997a, b). See also the argument put forward by Sen, A., (1998) for the importance of individual case studies as a means by which we are able to move beyond "cold and often inarticulate statistics of low incomes" and look in detail at the various ways in which agency— "the capabilities of each person"—is constrained.

In the aftermath of political violence, harmony, tradition, social interdependence, caring, responsibility for the welfare of others, and community obligations tend to be severely damaged.[27] This is responsible for survivors' feelings of a lack of control and is associated with a host of adverse outcomes including withdrawal of effort and poor performance on cognitive tasks such as decision-making.[28] Its impact seems to undermine the belief that individuals ought to be responsible for others' welfare, making concern for others increasingly unimportant. In these circumstances socially, responsible behaviour and feelings of hope and certainty are more the exception than the rule.

Definitions of human suffering have their origins in what political, economic and institutional power is capable of doing to people.[29] These same forms of power also influence the responses people have to social problems.[30] By taking strong, forceful actions that inherently impact on other people, political, economic and institutional power can be the cause of significant prolonged stress.[31] For the powerless this is responsible for feelings of lack of control and is linked to a range of adverse outcomes.[32] These feelings lead to suppressed immune function and adverse mental health consequences, including depression, anxiety, and reproductive problems.

---

[27] It has also made it difficult to isolate the legacy of the political violence from the social, psychosocial, physical and economic context in which it occurred.

[28] Guinote, A. & Vescio, T.K., (2010: 158ff).

[29] See Kleinman, A., et al., (1997a, b: ix) Words Associated with Common Types of Suffering include: social exclusion, discrimination, ostracized, persecution, incapacitation, disability, shame (self-ostracized), distrust, relative deprivation, subjugation, atrocity, homelessness, unemployment, social rejection, discrimination, bullied, disability, blindness, deafness, bedridden, hunger, war, civil violence, survival risk factors in Anderson, R. E., (2013:11).

[30] Kleinman et al. (1997a, b: ix); For Wilkinson (2005a, b) social suffering is defined as ".... suffering produced by social forces, rendering the victim without a sense of being human and worthwhile." Kleinman (2009b) also defined social suffering as the suffering caused by social forces, but emphasized social institutions, global systems, and culture as the culprits. For Kleinman, A. & Wilkinson, I., (2016: 14ff) any analysis of "...the social meaning and bounds of suffering requires that we recognise from the outset that we are dealing with a profoundly moral experience. Suffering takes place as an intensely violent and harmful assault on human personhood."

[31] For the purposes of this study the definition of stress is as follows "...[A]n interaction of several variables involving a particular kind of relationship between a person and the environment which is appraised by the person as being taxing or exceeding coping resources and endangering well-being" (Schlebusch 1998: 266). The distinguishing characteristics of this definition of stress are as follows:

- Stress is an ongoing process (interaction) and as such can be said to be dynamic
- There are distinct domains involved in the process:
- The domain of the environment
- The domain of the person
- Awareness and appraisal of stress by the individual(s) in the process (typically exhibited as strain symptoms).

Strain is defined as any "......deviation from the normal state or responses" of an individual. Symptoms of stress/strain could be psychological, physiological or behavioural. See French, J. R. P., Jr., Caplan, R. D., & Harrison, R. V. (1982).

[32] Guinote, A. and Vescio, T., (2010: 97-107).

Powerlessness is therefore not just responsible for stress (and negative moods) but for less attention, less focal effort and less flexibility during what some social psychologists call 'goal striving', or goal-oriented behaviour.[33]

Instead of being based on an acknowledgement of the full complexity and variability of human suffering, interactions between ordinary people and the state are characterised by inappropriate policies and programmes, bureaucratic practices and cultural forces.[34] This creates rigid situations and makes authentic communication more difficult. For ordinary people this demonstration of the supreme importance of power only deepens their sense of solitude, unending oppression and slow annihilation.[35] By keeping any legitimate moral expectations at arms' length the state is able to acknowledge human suffering and avoid any concern for its existential and experiential impact. This lack of emotional reaction to human suffering may not automatically transform people into mindless, predictable victims, but it is likely to cause them to "...suffer in part from a devastating loss of their identity as human beings."[36]

The idea that impoverished people acquire their social identity through existing relationships with powerful, often non-rural people is no longer persuasive. Instead, the lack of direction, the conflict of values, the crumbling and loss of traditional roles, undermines and ultimately destroys conventional notions of what is good, trustworthy, beneficial, desirable and constructive.[37] Failure to confront the existential vacuum in their lives head-on means that for victims, participating in officially organised activities may contribute to further depression, addiction or aggression.[38] It thus becomes even more likely that the powerless will concede to the desires of outsiders, irrespective of the legitimacy of the latter's demands.

1.3 The Causes of Suffering

In recent years the concept of victim has become so ubiquitous that the causes of suffering have come to seem less important than the actual suffering of people.[39] To rectify this, we need to analyse the specific causes of suffering, including informa-

---

[33] Rivers, J.J., & Josephs, R.A., (2010: 97-143) In Guinote, A. and Vescio, T., (2010).

[34] For the state the nature of social suffering is inconsistent with established categories because it simultaneously involves health, welfare, legal, moral and religious issues. For example, trauma and pain give rise to health conditions; even though they are also political and cultural matters. See Kleinman, A., et al. (1997a, b: ix).

[35] Fiske (1993).

[36] Bourdieu, P., (2000); Kleinman, A., et al. (1997a, b); Wilkinson, I. (2005a, b) as cited in Anderson, R. E., (2013:11)

[37] Langle (2008) as cited in Anderson, R. E., (2013); See also Marshall, M and Marshall, E., (2012: 54).

[38] Marshall, M and Marshall, E., (2012: 56).

[39] Dean, C.J., (2010: 181ff).

tion about the individual, the family, the community and the broader national and international context.

However, information from these sources tends to be so compartmentalised that any understanding of the causes of suffering is inevitably fragmented. To engage with what shapes local reality and helps us to understand the actual experience of suffering and the specific factors that give rise to it we need to recognise that "....no genre or discipline 'owns suffering as a problem or can provide definitive boundaries for it"[40]

This means that information about the complexity of local situations and institutions is vital to any understanding of the causes of suffering.[41] However, investigations into the causes of suffering using methods involving interactions that permit analysis of their emergence and evolution are not always available. In practice, this only reinforces the tendency to examine the causes of suffering in de-contextualized ways and without interaction, thereby making any knowledge about the predominant causes of suffering theoretical and speculative.[42] This weak engagement with the human issues at stake helps to underline the need for a broader, more holistic set of interpretations, no matter their disciplinary origin. Such a mismatch between how the causes of suffering are theoretically conceived and how they have been empirically studied might be resolved by other influences: from the modern tendency to reify suffering into pathology and from the rhetoric of social science and its attempts to organize local experience within extra-local categories.

Though no single cause of suffering takes precedence the most important area of discussion concerns the extent to which it is ultimately rooted in the harsh effects of national (and international) political and economic forces. However, the causes of human suffering are borne out of a set of circumstances; they are not an infraction of the rules.

Though it is commonplace to place the burden of responsibility on traditional norms, values and practices, the weight of research indicates that suffering is ultimately explained by the structures of social systems and relationships, and not just cultural formations and social processes.[43] This idea was first put forward by Johan Galtung who defined peace as the absence of not only direct physical violence - including everything from interpersonal to collective violence - but also indirect structural violence, generated by forces such as poverty, marginalization, and

---

[40] LaCapra, D., (2001: 96). In the original text LaCapra was referring to trauma and not suffering, but I have adapted this slightly because the two concepts are so inextricably related and have many of the same tendencies.

[41] Kleinman, A. and Kleinman, J., (1997a, b: 8) in Kleinman, A., Das, V., and Lock, M. (eds.) (1997a, b).

[42] For Geras, "...There is a tendency to objectify human suffering and extreme want, to make them part of an objective as it were natural background, emptying them of their subjective content as the lived experience of other human individuals." Geras, N. (1998: 131).

[43] See for example, Kleinman, A., et al., (1997a, b: ix); Kleinman, Das, V. & Lock, M., (1997a, b:ix); Winter, D. Du Nann & Leighton, D.C., (2001); Singer, M., & Erickson, P.I., (2011); Rylko-Bauer, B. & Farmer, P., (2016)

exploitation.[44] From this idea of positive peace as the "absence of structural violence" Galtung went on to make a direct connection between structural violence and unequal power, especially "the power to decide over the distribution of resources," which results in "unequal life chances."[45]

In parallel with this innovative approach to human suffering, liberation theologians from Latin America were seeking to understand the subjective experience of the oppressed, and in particular, of people traumatised by political violence.[46] From this perspective the impact of widespread, destructive, anti-human forces, such as economic exploitation, social injustice, political oppression, terror, war and violence is responsible for immense suffering, both for individuals and communities.[47] This represents a fundamental challenge to the entire structure of repression, because it seeks to reflect back to people their own knowledge and experience, their history and their suffering. In this respect, it would be inappropriate and simplistic to reduce any explanation of the causal factors associated with suffering to the easily identifiable occurrences that indicate suffering.

To strengthen the analysis, we therefore need to engage not only with factors that accentuate and make more severe the underlying causes of suffering, but also with their structural and underlying causes.

This means that we need to understand the extent to which suffering is causally rooted in such concepts as the state, hierarchy, power, conflict and other issues such as exploitation, because they lay stress not only on the actual lived experience of human suffering but also on how the various causal factors are interconnected.

The relation between suffering and national (and international) political and economic forces directs our attention to the relative position of an individual or group within a social hierarchy. In general, high ranking or dominant individuals tend to hold power over others; whereas, low ranking or subordinate individuals do not.[48]

Findings from various literatures, including basic science research, medical research and public health studies all suggest that "...subordinate individuals experience significant prolonged stress that subsequently leads them to exhibit *blunted* (i.e., flat, unremitting and insufficient) responses to acute stress."[49] Exposure to physical and psychological stressors for individuals and groups occupying a low social rank in the social hierarchy is complex because of the multitude of causal factors.

Ultimately, however, physical and psychological stressors are determined by the amount of control or access people have over basic resources.[50] To secure these

---

[44] Galtung, J. (1969-167–91) as cited by Rylko-Bauer, B. & Farmer, P., (2016: 47-75) in Brady & Burton, L.M., (2016) (Eds.)

[45] Galtung, J. (1969:171) as cited by Rylko-Bauer, B. & Farmer, P., (2016: 47-75) in Brady & Burton, L.M., (2016) (Eds.)

[46] Camara, H., (1971); Guttierez, G., (1973, 1983); Martin-Baro, I., (1994a, b, c, d).

[47] Camara, H., (1971); Guttierez, G., (1973, 1983); Martin-Baro, I., (1994a, b, c, d).

[48] Guinote, A. & Vescio, T.K., (2010: 87); Lewis, R.J., (2002).

[49] Guinote, A. & Vescio, T.K., (2010: 97).

[50] This includes: (1) physical resources such as food, water, shelter, safety (2) economic resources such as money, material goods, employment opportunities (3) social resources, including acceptance, a sense of control, social support and a trusting social environment.

resources people need the capacity to alter the state of another individual by providing rewards or punishments.[51] This brings the discussion back to the issue of power.[52]

To understand the capacity to influence another individual in psychologically meaningful ways it is necessary to highlight the sources of power that shape relationships between individuals within groups and between groups. How much control or access individuals and groups have over basic resources is determined by the social rank they occupy in the social hierarchy.

For individuals and groups occupying a high social rank the ability to secure desired outcomes is greater than it is for individuals and groups occupying a low social rank. Because powerful people are able to "...focus attention on the primary aspects of their situation (needs, goals, expectancies, affordances) they are able to deem information related to these aspects relevant and other information irrelevant."[53] This gives rise to the use of a narrower range of processes that guide the judgement and behaviour of powerless people leading to less situated responses and less variability in judgement and behaviour.

The effect this has on the ways in which individuals and groups occupying a high social rank in the social hierarchy process and ultimately perceive the powerless is to ascribe stereotype-consistent information about human behaviour.[54] This includes class-based stereotypes such as laziness, lack of initiative, devaluation of work, a failure to face up to responsibilities, and a departure from other so-called middle-class norms.

By ignoring people as individuals any emotional capacity to engage with the context in which people live their lives and the subjective experiences of physical and mental suffering is blocked. From the liquidation of their uniqueness as individuals the language of normalization and relativization is able to create a state of indifference between people that made the Holocaust possible. By ascribing good and bad traits to low and high power the state is able to normalize and justify social and economic inequality.[55]

This failure to pick up on important individuating information is responsible for inappropriate policies and programmes, bureaucratic practices and cultural forces that make humiliation more or less inevitable.

Under the guise of the righteous polemic about the necessity of doing something humanitarian the reification of the powerless by the powerful has failed to properly acknowledge people's suffering.[56] Being in a powerless position makes it difficult to

---

[51] Guinote, A. & Vescio, T.K., (2010: 178).

[52] Keltner, D., Gruenfeld, D. H., & Anderson, C. (2003); Fiske, S. T., (1993).

[53] Guinote, A. & Vescio, T.K., (2010: 157).

[54] Fiske, S.T. & Depret, E., (1996) in Hewstone, M., et al., (Eds.), (1996); Weicke, M. & Guinote, A. (2008).

[55] Fiske, S. T., (1993).

[56] Fiske, S. T., (1993).

secure desired resources and outcomes and increases the tendency for people to depend on others. This undermines the individual's capacity for self-respect and leads to a destruction of the social sphere, the active life and the mental life.[57]

Powerlessness is responsible for tormenting anxiety, feelings of inferiority, abrupt changes between hope and desperation, self-preservation and self-abandonment.[58] It destroys the flow of time; in its wake it makes people aggressive, over-assertive, and full of a tormenting fear about the future.[59] This "...can have deleterious effects on neural, immunological, cardiovascular and reproductive health, causing an increased risk of mortality in individuals with low social rank."[60] If the feeling of powerlessness is permanent it will produce changes in the individual psyche; for example, loss of self-confidence, depression and physical problems such as weakening of the immune system.[61] In these circumstances the individual has a problem knowing how to feel safe, with the result that social behaviour patterns based on reliability and trust break down.[62] This undermines conventional coping mechanisms (such as popular mobilization, solidarity and grassroots organizations) and their ability to coordinate social life and move shared goals forwards.[63]

In this context the relation between suffering and powerlessness directs our attention to the debilitating effects of the failure to reconstitute a positive meaning of self and society after the experience of political violence. One of the most devastating consequences of political violence is its capacity to affect everything from health services, education, markets, and farming activities, to families and community support systems, the environment, livelihood, and the stability of populations.[64]

The impact this has on the feelings of individuals and groups affected by traumatic experiences is invariably worsened by forms of structural violence that were already in place prior to the political violence.[65] The aftermath of the political violence in the rural Andes of Peru, for example, has been dominated by inadequate access to basic infrastructure such as roads, transport, water, and health facilities, whilst the lack of basic skills, such as literacy, only increases the sense of

[57] Tracy, J.L., & Robins, R.W., (2003).

[58] Tracy, J.L., & Robins, R.W., (2003).

[59] Keltner, D., Gruenfeld, D.H., & Anderson, C. (2003).

[60] Guinote, A. & Vescio, T.K., (2010: 106).

[61] Furthermore, work has linked low power to feelings of general uncertainty (Anderson and Galinsky 2006), which itself is often aversive (e.g., Weary, G., et al. (1993) in G. Weary, F. Gleicher, & K.L. Marsh (Eds.) (1993).

[62] Van der Kolk, B., (2014: 137).

[63] Lever, J. P., (2008).

[64] Leatherman, T. & Thomas, R. (2008); Rylko-Bauer, B. & Singer, M. (2010); Rylko-Bauer, B., Whiteford, L., & Farmer, P. (2009); Singer, M. & Hodge, G.D. (2010).

[65] See for example, Fassin, D., (2009); Miller, K.E. & Rasmussen, A., (2010); Nordstrom, C., (2009); Panter-Brick, C., (2010); Quesada, J., (2009); Becker, Beyene, & Ken (2000); Das (2007); Johnston 2007, 2011).

powerlessness and vulnerability. Furthermore, the lack of access to basic needs, including civic safety, law enforcement, predictability and self-respect only draws attention to how the political violence has reshaped their particular ways of being by undoing and remaking their lives in new and unpredictable ways.

For people affected by political violence this process of societal and personal transformation is exacerbated by the difficulties of "…taming and rendering harmless such psychological features as victimization, dehumanization and humiliation."[66] In this setting, alongside the escalation in alcoholism, drug abuse and other forms of social delinquency, conflict-affected communities in the rural Andes of Peru have seen a marked increase in social-health and mental health problems, from the threat of endless violence and insecurity to alcoholism, sexually transmitted diseases, psycho-social stress, despair, depression, and suicide.

In these circumstances people are compelled to focus their interests on the necessities of the present. To do otherwise would forfeit the opportunity to secure enough resources for themselves and their dependents. For individuals and groups occupying a low social rank in the social hierarchy this makes for a culture of self-interest, increasing materialism, and growing cynicism. In the aftermath of the political violence this has prompted widespread comment and criticism amongst people from conflict-affected communities in the rural Andes of Peru as a result of its impact on social solidarity.

The impact this has on the sense of responsibility people have for each other and with the rules and conventions that govern the wider aspects of community development bring about changes in what it means to feel and regard oneself as human.[67] In the absence of continuity and solidarity these changes develop through such stratagems as "starting all over again", "struggling through hard times", "fighting for justice", and so on.

Surviving under these conditions encapsulates the lived experience of distress and injustice, while exposing the "…often close linkage of personal problems with societal problems."[68] These difficulties persist because they are "…embedded in ubiquitous social structures [and] normalized by stable institutions and regular experience".[69] The implications are clear: the social relations and arrangements that make up the structures that shape how individuals and groups interact within a social system almost invariably have unintended consequences.[70]

---

[66] Volkan, V. (2018: 10) in Trauma, Trust and Memory, Hamburger, A., (ed) (2018)

[67] Biehl, J., Good, B., & Kleinman, A., (2007a, b) Introduction: Rethinking Subjectivity in Subjectivity: Ethnographic Investigations, Biehl, J., Good, B., & Kleinman (eds) (2007a, b) University of California Press

[68] Kleinman et al. 1997a, b:ix); as cited by Rylko-Bauer, B. & Farmer, P., (2016: 47–75) in Brady & Burton, L.M., (2016) (Eds.).

[69] Winter D. Du Nann & Leighton, D.C., (2001:99).

[70] For the purposes of this book structures are understood as those "…social relations and arrangements - economic, political, legal, religious, or cultural - that shape how individuals and groups interact within a social system. These include broad-scale cultural and political-economic structures such as caste, patriarchy, slavery, apartheid, colonialism, and neoliberalism, as well as poverty and discrimination by race, ethnicity, gender, sexual orientation, and migrant/refugee status.

Individual suffering from overwhelming social forces "…thus becomes the ground on which a long series of historical changes and moral apparatuses coalesce."[71]

In this way the social, emotional and motivational elements that impact on the individual in the aftermath of political violence encourages self-seeking behaviour and may even lead to the "…remaking of the habitual inner sense of endurance and the creation of new forms of desire that go beyond commercial interests to structure new ways of feeling and living, that change the world."[72]

To bring about more effective local interventions, better social policy, and social change that addresses the roots of poverty, inequality and social suffering, we need to pay particular attention to "the complexity and the contradictions of the lives of the poor".[73]

To strengthen the analysis, we need to engage with factors that accentuate and make more severe the ways in which suffering is causally rooted in such concepts as the state, hierarchy, power, conflict and other issues such as exploitation.[74] This is because they lay stress not only on the actual lived experience of human suffering but also on how the various causal factors are interconnected.[75]

Building on the recommendations of Rylko-Bauer & Farmer (2016) we need to document how structural violence "operates in real lives"[76]and how it is expressed "physically and psychically in everyday social suffering;"[77] by analysing how past and present oppression and discrimination are inscribed in public policy and discourse, and on bodies and biographies;[78] and by fleshing out the subjective aspects - emotions, meanings, perceptions - of social suffering and exploring the interconnections of structure and agency,[79] as well as examining how structural forces are mediated by cultural understandings.[80]

For the government the injustices of the past belong to the past; they do not have implications for the present. Not only does this help legitimize past suffering and injustice, it also encourages cosmetic changes, selective forms of reparation and

---

These structures are violent because they result in avoidable deaths, illness, and injury; and they reproduce violence by marginalizing people and communities, constraining their capabilities and agency, assaulting their dignity, and sustaining inequalities." Rylko-Bauer, B. & Farmer, P., (2016: 47-75) in Brady & Burton, L.M., (2016) (Eds.).

[71] Biehl, J., Good, B., & Kleinman, A., (eds) (2007a, b: 3).

[72] Biehl, J., Good, B., & Kleinman, A., (eds) (2007a, b: 4).

[73] Green, L., (2004:319-20).

[74] See for example, Abadía-Barrero, César & Arachu Castro. (2006); Adimora, A. A., Schoenbach, V.J., & Floris-Moore, M.A., (2009). Towle, M.S. & Lende, D., (2008); Whiteford, L. & Whiteford, S., (2005).

[75] Hickel, J., (2017).

[76] Bourgois, P. & Scheper-Hughes, N., (2004: 318).

[77] Walter, N., Bourgois, P., & H. Margarita Loinaz (2004: 1167).

[78] Fassin, D., (2007); (2009).

[79] Biehl, J. & Moran-Thomas, A., (2009).

[80] Rylko-Bauer, B. & Farmer, P., (2016: 47).

impunity. From the perspective of the state, justice is concerned with society's criteria for allocating resources (distributive justice) and punishments (criminal justice).[81] It is not concerned with responsibility, complicity, guilt, shame and psychosocial deformation of the culture at large. Instead its preference is for the conventional use of the distribution of resources according to merit.

This disregard for vulnerable and socially disadvantaged groups makes the psychological implications of human suffering inconsistent with the priorities of the state. By failing to help people work through past suffering and obtain some form of integration the government has effectively violated and betrayed the victims' own sense of dignity. In the aftermath of political violence this constitutes an infringement of the conditions of mutual recognition and results in a loss of meaning that diminishes the identity of the victim. In these circumstances it is possible to refuse empathy and compassion on the grounds that neither makes a structural contribution to justice, in spite of their congruence with justice principles and their capacity to provide the motive to rectify violations of justice.[82]

This devalues the past (and the future) to such an extent that it subverts traditional habits and behaviour, for example making people's attitude to time erratic and unpredictable. For the powerless, past injustices have less value than what will be tomorrow, no matter how terrible the memories. In this respect their time sense has been twisted around so as to give the precepts of rationality and self-preservation precedence.

By using this interpretation of the past, the government is able to adopt a forward-looking strategy based around the idea of nation-building. Part of this strategy consists of initiatives designed to make way for societal recognition of what was done to ordinary people and promote reconciliation. However, the idea that Truth Commissions, reparations schemes and other such initiatives can somehow heal victims of violence and defuse opposing groups undermines the authentic meaning of suffering.

Formal cut-off points may help facilitate the state's commitment to a better future, but they are less likely to reassure the victims of political violence that the importance of what happened is properly acknowledged, and that appropriate responsibilities are assumed.

This has far-reaching psychological implications because it prevents the actual experience of suffering from being processed and blocks opportunities for healing. To feel that no one is interested in allowing the victims of political violence to make sense of their situation undermines meaningful human interaction and leads to an adaptation of and reduction in the old values of solidarity. The feeling that the social

[81] There are three principles of distributive justice: (1) merit-based justice calls for allocating resources according to individual productivity, effort or competence. (2) Need or communitarian justice calls for allocating resources according to need - based on poverty, past grievances and discrimination. (3) Equality – everyone should receive the same amount. See Hoffman, M. L., (2000: 226).

[82] Hoffman, M. L., (2000: 235). See also Alain Badiou who argues that human rights discourse conceals its real contempt for victims under the guise of caring for them. Badiou, A. (2001).

environment will never regain its capacity for sympathy, empathy and understanding leaves the victim with a sense of helplessness. In addition, the frustration of such basic needs as safety, control predictability and self-respect make an abandonment of traditional norms, values and customs unavoidable.[83]

This emotional destruction of the old values of solidarity blocks any recognition of what has gone before – and any capacity to act usefully in the face of what is to come. It also weakens the relationship powerless people have with the attitude they bring to their situation.

Instead of assuming full responsibility for themselves and thinking properly powerless people assume an attitude of acceptance and delude themselves with the feeling that the existing situation is sufficient and that it would be inappropriate to want or expect anything more. By failing to adapt their thinking people have moved into a position where there is no critical engagement and things are accepted at face value.

This weakening of cognitive capacities makes people feel unconnected with their own reality, thereby making them more likely to have a reduced feeling of guilt about the attitude they have adopted. By failing to think for themselves survivors are no longer in a position to bear direct witness to the reality of their own ongoing misery. In spite of the pressures that the present imposes past injustices continue to be a significant influence because events that began in the past continue to unfold in the present.[84] This may contradict the Western interpretation of the past as something absent or distant; for the victims of political violence (and for all of the demands associated with a context of daily survival) the past remains very much alive.[85]

To this end we need to assess how the aftermath of political violence in places such as the rural Andes of Peru has led to the "…creation of contexts of shame, stigma, humiliation, loss of respect, and violation of self-integrity, and how they have in turn affected health, well-being, and interpersonal relations, and sometimes lead to self-destructive behaviour, extra-legal activities, and physical - even collective - violence."[86]

Not only does this enable us to obtain "…a clear understanding of the inequalities that shape inequalities" and the power relations that structure and sustain them;[87] it also provides "…a means by which we can get at cumulative root causes, addressing historical forces and social, economic, and political processes that shape risk and local reality."[88]

---

[83] Staub, E., (1989: 45)

[84] King, Preston (2000: 55).

[85] Ignatieff, M., (1999:13).

[86] Benson, P., (2008); Bourgois, P., (2003); Bufacchi, V., (2007); Gilligan, J., (1997); Metz, B., Mariano, L., & García, J.L., (2010); Uvin, P., (1999) as cited by Rylko-Bauer, B. & Farmer, P., (2016: 47-75) in Brady & Burton, L.M., (2016) (Eds.).

[87] Leatherman, T., (2011: 33).

[88] Peña, D. G. (2011) as cited by Rylko-Bauer, B. & Farmer, P., (2016: 47-75) in Brady & Burton, L.M., (2016) (Eds.).

1.4 The Legacy of Political Violence

In a context of daily survival, the pressures of living make the suppression of the past overwhelmingly necessary.[89] Outrage against past injustices inflicted on the individual is of little avail if the available resources are not enough to meet daily needs.[90] In these circumstances people are compelled to focus their interests exclusively on the necessities of the present, since to do otherwise would forfeit the opportunity to secure enough resources for themselves and their dependents.[91]

This devaluing of the past (and the future) can subvert traditional habits and behaviour, making people's attitude to time erratic and unpredictable. Past injustices about what happened in a context of daily survival have less value than what will be tomorrow, no matter how terrible the memories.[92] In this respect the time sense has been twisted around and the precepts of rationality and self-preservation given precedence.[93]

However, this makes no allowance for the long-term psychological damage that past injustices can inflict if no effort is made to confront them and become reconciled to them.[94] It is a fallacy that 'time heals.' Though detachment from their own past may enable people "...to minimize psychological discomfort and responsibility about actions and thoughts,"[95] it does not prevent anxieties, tensions, doubts and conflicts from building up as symptoms "...forgotten by consciousness but remembered by the body."[96]

By subjugating themselves to the social and biological time-sense people are ignoring matters of moral and practical importance and allowing the psychic injuries associated with these issues to remain unhealed.[97]

The biological healing that time can bring about does not annul the damage done to the individual psyche by past injustices. "Time," Walter Benjamin says, "...does not behave like a mechanical clock. It is not just linear…"[98]

---

[89] "...There are forms of forgetting that are "necessary" for the survival and functioning of the individual subject as well as for groups and communities." Jelin, E., (2002: 29) Cited in Theidon, K., (2013: 30).

[90] See also Buckley-Zistel, S. (2006).

[91] Carlson, N. (2012).

[92] For the individual unburdened by past injustices the natural sense of time is biased toward the future. But as Amery writes: "...Future is obviously a value concept. What will be tomorrow is more valuable than what was yesterday. That is how the natural feeling of time will have it." Amery, J., (1980: 76).

[93] This is not unique to people living in extreme conditions. For Watkins, & Shulman "...all human beings have an enormous capacity to live in states of denial, dissociation, forgetfulness and ideologies of the dominant culture." Watkins, M. & Shulman, H. (2008: 131).

[94] Olick, J.K., (2007: 31).

[95] Watkins, M. & Shulman, H. (2008: 85).

[96] Santner, E. (1990: 157).

[97] Amery, J., (1980:72).

[98] From: Theses on the Philosophy of History, In Arendt, H. (1999: 253-264).

In the aftermath of political violence, the suffering of people affected by scenes of horror and state violence is quite different from the simple experience of "… unpleasantness and aversion associated with the perception of harm or threat of harm in an individual."[99] It is a form of suffering "...that can silence an entire people and can cause profound isolation, depression, panic, and renewed violence in subsequent generations."[100]

In the case of someone affected by traumatic violence all the contempt, hatred and revulsion they fought against are turned inwards. For anyone who has suffered the horrors of persecution, torture, rape and the moral violence of the system for a long enough time there is a complicity with regard to their own suffering. This complicity overwhelms all the efforts the individual might make to work through their experiences because the internalization of abuse has undermined their autonomy of thought and established itself in their minds. In this way, the internalized experience of political violence has "…transformed the abuse that was performed externally into internal abuse."[101]

Having assumed dominion over the entire person the internalised effects of persecution, brutality, atrocities and state violence continue to "…attack it directly and indirectly, in all its parts, social, psychological and physical."[102] In these circumstances the horror and persecution that set out to destroy the victim's beliefs and divest them as individuals of all relationships with themselves, with their ideals, and with their memory is unremitting.[103]

What is terrible is that if the victim is unable to find an appropriate outlet for such debilitating forms of psychic and other forms of degradation "…the emotional working through that a generation does not manage to complete will be passed on to the next generation, with the attendant effects on their identity and emotional range."[104]

This type of invisible (symbolic) violence is associated with Pierre Bourdieu (2000) and refers to how people become complicit in their own subordination through the internalisation and acceptance of those ideas and structures that tend to subordinate them.[105] It is an act of violence precisely because it acts as a constraint on the individual, "…but it is also symbolic in the sense that it is achieved indirectly and without overt and explicit acts of force and coercion."[106]

Its power derives from the sociocultural mechanisms and relations of unequal power and domination that exist within interpersonal relationships and in other aspects of life. It is fully integrated into ordinary daily life, to the extent that both

---

[99] Hudson, W., (2012) in Malpas, J & Lickiss, N., (eds.) (2012); see also Kleinman, A. & Wilkinson, I., (2016: 14-16ff).

[100] Gautier, A., & Sabatini Scalmati, A., (2010: xxii).

[101] Gautier, A., & Sabatini Scalmati, A., (2010: xix).

[102] Weil, S. (2005: 43)

[103] Gautier, A., & Sabatini Scalmati, A., (2010: xv).

[104] See for example, Bourgois, P., (2009); Gautier, A., & Sabatini Scalmati, A., (2010: xix).

[105] Bourdieu, P., (2000).

[106] Connolly, P. & Healy, J., (2004).

perpetrator and victim perceive it as a legitimate and inevitable part of the natural social order.[107] This lack of visibility is what makes invisible (symbolic) violence so powerful because "…it engenders doubts and fears in those exposed to it that ultimately cause them to question themselves".[108] This is responsible for an adaptation and a reaction on the part of the victim to cope with feelings of helplessness and despair from their marginal position in a class-stratified, highly individuated society. Because historical time appears to stand still, social realities, including the experience of suffering, become the normal situation of human beings, "…to the point where destiny is identified with suffering: "you are born to suffer"."[109]

From this perspective the prospects of any alternative to the reality facing the individual are so bleak that it devalues the importance of planning for the future.

The hardships these conditions impose on the individual's identity and sense of dignity mean that people will want to avoid all subjects liable to evoke feelings of pain, suffering, and injustice and despair whenever they possibly can.[110]

In the aftermath of the political violence the "...ability to transform traumatic experiences into positive personal growth experiences" can be so limited that people may find it difficult to retain any hope in the future.[111] Having no one to turn to frequently leads people to think about why this is. In a context of daily survival this often involves revisiting particular structural, contextual and historical aspects of their situation time and time again. More specifically, the survivor tends to focus on the state and its failure to reassure people that their suffering is properly acknowledged and that appropriate responsibilities are assumed.

These feelings are often directed against the thinking that it is possible to forget injustice, suffering, fear and misery and is responsible for feelings of anger and humiliation. In a context of daily survival this keeps people in a state of abjection because victims are unable and unwilling to rid themselves of the sense of shame and loss of dignity and self-respect.[112] In a post-conflict context the use of acts of closure as a formal cut-off point from the haunting past may help to strengthen the state's commitment to a better future but it does not make it any easier for victims and their ability to detach themselves from past suffering and injustice. In this respect the idea that Truth Commissions, reparations schemes and other such

---

[107] Rylko-Bauer, B. & Farmer, P., (2016: 47).

[108] Morgan, K. & Bjorkert, S.T., (2006: 448).

[109] Martin-Baro, I., (1994a, b, c, d: 201).

[110] This kind of detachment from past injustices and dangerous memories is a vital factor in the development of social amnesia. Russell Jacoby as "...society's repression of remembrance of its own past." Jacoby, R., (1975).

[111] Lepore, L.G. & Revenson, T., (2006: 27) in Calhoun, L.G. & Tedeschi, R.G., (2009).

[112] The concept of abjection is a powerful neural network combining cognitive and behavioural components, sensory images of past experience, recollection of strong aversive emotions and over-arousal (Folensbee, 2008). To be in a state of abjection is to feel unworthy, unlovable, and to be in utter despair about the situation ever changing. Implicit memories of helplessness, dread, horror and rejection are activated neurologically and communicated in posture, voice and words. See Kristeva, J., (1982: 1-4).

initiatives can somehow heal victims of violence and reconcile opposing groups throws the authentic meaning of suffering into confusion and doubt.

For the victim, a lack of meaningful dialogue with the state confirms the latter's overriding power and its ability to twist around the actual awfulness of human misery.

By deflecting attention away from its responsibilities for any legitimate moral expectations the state is able to partially bury the realities of what happened to the individual victim. Instead of respecting individuality, this increases insecurity.

Ill-considered initiatives intended to appease past victims of injustice, suffering and misery only keep these feelings alive, by making the denial of dignity permanent and unchanging. In these circumstances resentment is almost as inevitable as forgetting is necessary. For Brudholm resentment is "...the reflex expression of an honourable emotional response to inexpiable wrongs and legitimate moral expectations that have not been properly dealt with."[113] In the aftermath of political violence expressions of resentment help to keep the past alive and reflect people's abiding commitment to certain moral standards as the basis for normal human behaviour.

For people in thrall to resurgence in political violence resentment can provide a means by which the truth about state incompetence, negligence and corruption can be exposed. In post-conflict communities giving voice to past injustices provides a means by which state indifference and objectivity can be challenged. In this respect resentment has "...a constructive and positive role to play in the maintenance of social harmony and human relationships."[114] For Murphy "...the individual who let's go of their resentment for psychological, spiritual or material reasons linked with their own daily survival 'lets' go' of useful anger and has less mental energy to put forward toward obtaining justice. Overcoming resentment may compromise values of genuine importance."[115]

For the survivors and victims of the political violence this is a retrospective grudge which has to contend with the multiplicity of life's demands and the forgetfulness induced by the passage of time.[116] In spite of the atrophying effects of endless struggle and emotional exhaustion on the memory of past injustice, suffering is not easily forgotten. Neither is it easily mollified by a package of judicial and non-judicial responses to human rights violations implemented by government and non-governmental officials.

To examine whether injustice, suffering, fear and misery, so widely asserted by victims and survivors, are responsible for their situation we need to assess how the aftermath of political violence has led to the "…creation of contexts of shame, stigma, humiliation, loss of respect, and violation of self-integrity, and how they have in turn affected health, well-being, and interpersonal relations, and sometimes

[113] Brudholm, T., (2008: 17)
[114] Brudholm, T., (2008: 17).
[115] Murphy, J., 2003: 115).
[116] Zolkos, M. (2007): 23-38.

lead to self-destructive behaviour, extra-legal activities, and physical - even collective - violence."[117]

Not only does this enable us to obtain "...a clear understanding of the inequalities that shape inequalities" and the power relations that structure and sustain them;[118] it also provides "...a means by which we can get at cumulative root causes, addressing historical forces and social, economic, and political processes that shape risk and local reality."[119]

1.5 Towards a Framework for Understanding Consequences of Suffering

Human and social suffering affects different people in different ways. The consequences include depression, anxiety, helplessness, isolation, lack of energy and motivation, intensified feelings of guilt and worthlessness, irritability and lethargy, loss of appetite, sleeplessness and insomnia, difficulty making decisions, lack of concentration and suicidal feelings.[120]

This causes social behaviour patterns based on reliability and trust to break down, making it impossible for conventional coping mechanisms and their ability to coordinate social life and move shared goals forwards.[121]The impact of this on feelings of comfort, comradeship, shared destiny and unquestioned certainty is overwhelming, leaving people increasingly at the mercy of their own individual impulses as they submit themselves to the demands of the immediate present.[122]

In these circumstances the impact of hunger, ill treatment, injustice and poor health make it easier to devalue other groups, make use of scapegoats, join new groups, and adopt new ideas; in addition it also makes people less motivated, less engaged, less passionate and less resilient.[123] In essence, human and social suffering

[117] Benson, P., (2008); Bourgois, P., (2003); Bufacchi, V., (2007); Gilligan, J., (1997); Metz, B., Mariano, L., & García, J.L., (2010); Uvin, P., (1999) as cited by Rylko-Bauer, B. & Farmer, P., (2016: 47-75) in Brady & Burton, L.M., (2016) (Eds.).

[118] Leatherman, T., (2011: 33).

[119] Peña, D. G. (2011) as cited by Rylko-Bauer, B. & Farmer, P., (2016: 47-75) in Brady & Burton, L.M., (2016) (Eds.).

[120] See for example, Guinote, A. & Vescio, T.K. (2010: 94-99); Wilkinson, R.G. (2005a, b: 101ff); Wilkinson, R.G. (1996: 175ff)

[121] Lammers, Joris; Stapel, Diederik A., (2009).

[122] Indeed, not having contingent control over one's environment is associated with severe negative consequences, as documented in research on learned helplessness (e.g., Abramson, Seligman, and Teasdale 1978; Seligman 1975). Furthermore, work has linked low power to feelings of general uncertainty (Anderson and Galinsky 2006), which itself is often aversive (e.g., Weary et al. 1993). Being powerless is also associated with less access to physical (e.g., material wealth) and social rewards compared with being powerful (e.g., recognition) See Buss, D.M. and Malamuth, N., (1996).

[123] Wadsworth, M.E., (2012).

devalues the importance of planning for the future, and undermines accepted boundaries, the stability of people's identities, and respect for traditional values and ideologies, thereby making support for established rules, fixed beliefs and practices increasingly doubtful.[124]

The cumulative effect is to make any explanation for the changes in behaviour, attitudes, opinions, goals, needs and values and all other aspects of the individual's sense of responsibility and attachment highly complex.[125] If we ignore the inner reality of suffering and how it is experienced we ignore the contribution social psychology makes to understanding suffering and its consequences.[126]

To better understand how suffering makes people change the way they think, feel and act we therefore need to engage with the emotional consequences of suffering and the environment within which it is experienced. This is because it enables us to better understand and anticipate the diversity of beliefs and behaviour by engaging with the subjective.[127]

It also provides a means by which the determining influence of context, culture and institutions (and the subjective nature that the individual brings to their situation), can be treated in a manner that is neither generalized nor unfocused.

For people affected by political violence and living in a context of daily survival, the dynamic interplay between subjectivity and the contextual environment is an overwhelmingly powerful influence on the performance of the individual's emotional capacities. To put it briefly, feelings of isolation, instability and danger are likely to be so overwhelming that people will want to avoid all subjects liable to evoke feelings of pain, suffering, and injustice and despair whenever they can. Not only does this discourage the need to honour the duty to remember and the obligation to do justice to the past, it also makes the victim of political violence more amenable to the state's idea of reconciliation and nation-building.

Though the individual may deliberately choose to focus on how to improve things, the feeling that their situation does not contain a good choice may result in them making another choice altogether. If this happens the choice they make is likely to be one that emphasizes self-advancement and rationality, instead of one that has a positive influence on the social environment around them.[128] In this respect it is not poverty and deprivation that shapes human behaviour, but what each individual makes of his/her situation and their attitude towards it.[129]

Highly integrated personalities may focus consciously on positive, meaningful values and goals but in a context of daily survival they are as subject to the same

---

[124] See Guinote, A. & Vescio, T.K. (2010: 432-3).

[125] Davidson, W. B., & Cotter, P. R. (1989).

[126] Current definitions of social psychology are usually similar to the one offered by Brehm, S.S., et al., (1996: 6) which is ".... the scientific study of the way individuals thinks, feel, desire and act in social situations."

[127] LaCapra, D., (2001: 40) See also Silverman, K., (1996); Schwartz W (2002).

[128] In the rural Andes of south-central Peru this is known as *individualismo* and will be discussed in some detail in subsequent chapters.

[129] Frankl, V. (1985: 67ff).

sense of impotence as people with less integrated personalities. It is therefore not the lack of autonomy and independence or an evolved sense of the individual's own identity that ultimately drives them to abandon their own responsibilities.

Instead it is the reaction to the impotence they feel about their social environment that blocks any capacity to focus consciously on positive, meaningful values and goals.

Humiliated, sick at heart, overwhelmed, broken, outmanoeuvred, unloved – these are but some of the emotions familiar to people in situations they feel they can neither change nor control.[130] In a context of poverty and deprivation the actual exercise of any emotional performance has been impeded for so long that feelings of ill treatment, injustice and condescension are ubiquitous. It is a social environment in which the freedom of individuals to choose their reaction and attitude towards things is most severely tested.[131] Their situation is not helped by the multiple factors that make up their social environment and which may be of such complexity that they resist understanding.[132]

1.6 Conclusion

Amidst the struggles for daily survival, survivors and victims of the political violence may simply abandon the idea of there being some choices that are better than others. Even if individuals and communities do not adopt this approach, they may still fail to recognise where they have some freedom to see negative things in positive ways.[133]

However, such acts of apparent individual and collective self-sabotage belie more complex motives that can only be understood from 'within' the local context. Among survivors of the political violence and living under constraints of meeting daily survival needs, the individual inhabits a zone of existence where the psychoanalytic categories of western understandings of everyday life may be out of place. For individuals and groups occupying low social rank in the social hierarchy, their world may appear devoid of meanings compatible with their ordinary life, particularly if they have also been affected by political violence.[134]

The individual's rejection of the idea of choice may even constitute a way they have of bearing witness to the horror of naked life stripped of all meaningful

---

[130] Levinas, E., (2006: 78ff).

[131] Agamben, G., (1999: 105).

[132] "Suffering for Frank, A.W. is "...the unspeakable as opposed to what can be spoken; it is what remains concealed, impossible to reveal.... At the core of suffering is the sense that something is irreparably wrong with our lives, and wrong is the negation of what could not have been right." Frank, A.W (2001: 355).

[133] Frankl, V., (1994).

[134] Rozynko, V. & Dondershine, H.E.(1991).

distinctions. This may prove a turning point, a way in which the individual can start to see negative things in positive ways.

From this perspective, an individual's decision to displace his or her own responsibility onto someone else is less an act of self-abandonment than a means, perhaps futile, to redeem lost notions tied up with traditional beliefs about dignity and self-respect.[135] For survivors of the political violence this act of regressive behaviour can be viewed as an attempt to find meaning in everything that has happened and is still happening.

Perhaps through a more nuanced interpretation of what individuals think and do in the context of their struggle for daily survival, it may become possible to start to understand what an individual can make of their situation, and how they can re-examine their individual and collective attitude towards the complex condition of social suffering.

[135] Staub, E., (1989: 17). In the rural Andes of south-central Peru this is known as *conformismo* and will be discussed in more detail in subsequent chapters.

Chapter 2
Setting the Scene: National and Local Perspectives

The aim of this chapter is to provide the reader with an "…understanding of the inequalities that shape inequalities" and the power relations that structure and sustain them.[1] To examine whether injustice, suffering, fear and misery has led to the creation of contexts of shame, stigma, humiliation, loss of respect, and violation of self-integrity, we need to make an assessment of the historical forces and social, economic, and political processes that shape risk and local reality.

Information about these forces and processes provide the means by which we can get at cumulative root causes. This information can be divided into two kinds: the first group consists of factors and processes at the national level and relate to the general crisis brought about by a combination of a failing economy and the political violence of the 1980s and the 1990s. The second group of causes take place at the local level and relate to the reality of what it is like to live in rural Highland communities in conditions of low trust, anxiety, high vigilance and low levels of support.[2]

The chapter also offers a brief historical analysis of the Shining Path movement, giving particular focus to its authoritarian structure and "…how this appeared to abet the organization's advance."[3] The chapter then examines evidence relating to the official response to the political violence, and to the insights provided by the Truth and Reconciliation Commission into the relationship between context and its influence on human nature and responsibility, and the failure of social capital discourse.

To counter the over-objectification of human suffering and reorganise our practical and theoretical ways of thinking about individual and social suffering, this chapter concludes with a discussion concerning the analytic tools needed to explore the situation as people perceive and cognitively construct it.

---

[1] Leatherman, T., (2011, 33).

[2] Kleinman is particularly keen that the subject should not be restricted to one discipline only Kleinman, A., (1988); Kleinman, A. & Kleinman, J., (1997a, b); Locke, (eds) (1997); Burton, J.W., (1990a, b).

[3] McClintock, C., (1998: 91).

T. J. Bowyer, *Beyond Suffering and Reparation*,
https://doi.org/10.1007/978-3-319-98983-9_2

2.1 Historical Background of Peru

To understand the history of Peru we need to begin with its environment and its ecology. Its diverse terrain includes vast regions of tropical rainforests with countless rivers and streams, sub-tropical desert climates composed of sandy or rocky shores and inland cutting valleys, precipitous intermontane valleys and high, windswept plains. The country has 3 main regions according to the traditional method of dividing the country by altitude: coast, mountains and jungle.

This extraordinary diversity of climates and resources has been at the centre of the socio-political structure of Peru ever since the conquest of the Inca empire. To reward the conquistadors and other officials responsible for colonizing new lands, the Spanish crown instituted a land tenure system in the form of haciendas (large pieces of land). From its inception "…this feudalistic system gave much wealth and, in consequence, political power to a small group of hacienda owners called *hacendado*."[4]

To preserve these privileges, a combination of skin colour, class and culture was used "…to reaffirm what the *hacendados* perceived as their superior 'white' racial origins by clinging to European culture."[5] In addition to vast areas of hacienda land, they also acquired "…quasi-feudal rights over and obligations to the people who lived and worked the haciendas."[6]

This was responsible for immense wealth, prestige, power, and money being channelled into the hands of a small elite at the expense of millions of poor peasants who were forced to give labour, goods, or money to their *hacendados*. Though *hacendados* were under an obligation "…to give their peasants certain rights and protections, the system overall exploited the labour of workers."[7]

This type of labour exploitation was subsequently extended to the operation of the mines, sugar and cotton plantations, guano extraction, alpaca and sheep wool for the export market and the production of arts and crafts. These activities, together with a monopoly over trade, formed the basis of the colonial economy. However, this also gave rise to a form of labour exploitation that only served to exacerbate the cultural, racial and geographic divides and which has continued to dominate the life of the country, in one form or another, ever since.

From here onwards Peruvian politics can be seen as an enduring struggle between those who have sought to defend a traditional highly centralised political and economic structure, and those that seek to bring such a system to an end.[8]

There is another equally important factor linking the history of Peru to its diverse environment and ecology, apart from the extremely unequal land ownership. This concerns the enormous cultural divide that separates the indigenous people located

[4] Klaren, P. (2000: 78).

[5] Poole, D. & Renique, G. (1992: 102).

[6] Klaren, P. (2000: 78).

[7] Klaren, P. (2000: 79).

[8] Poole, D. & Renique, G. (1992: 103).

in the Andean highlands from the Spanish-speaking, mixed-blood *mestizos* and *criollos* located along the coast.[9]

Unlike the wealthy coastal elite, the majority of the population live in parts of the country that are utterly different from its desert coast.

The best known of these is the central high *sierra* (highlands), with its massive peaks, steep canyons, and pre-Columbian archaeological sites. This is the region of the Andes; it includes the *altiplano* plateau and is inhabited by Quechua and Aymara-speaking Indians. The other main area is the *selva* (jungle), a region that surrounds the headwaters of the Amazon beneath the eastern slopes of the Andes. This is inhabited by hunter-gatherer, subsistence farming rainforest Indians from the Ashaninka, Kulina, Kaxinawa Cashibo, Achuar and other language groups.

By 1860, income from guano, cotton and sugar had made Peru less dependent on coerced labour and enslavement of the indigenous Andean and Amazonian population. The country was linked up by a railway network, and during the mandate of President Manuel Pardo, Peru organized its first civilian government. However, none of this affected the traditional exclusionary politics of the coastal elite, which meant that the *mestizo* and Indian majorities continued to remain on the margins of political life, as they had done ever since the Spanish Conquest. This all changed with the disastrous 1879–1883 war with Chile over nitrate fields. Following its defeat by the Chilean army, Peru was thrown into deep economic depression and eventual bankruptcy.

In spite of a succession of initiatives designed to modernise the state, the importance of any social and political reorganisation that would help promote the development of a democratic institutional structure was negligible. Instead, Peru underwent another period of military regimes. This only served to strengthen the sense of difference between the elite and the majority of the country's population. Opposition to the traditional exclusionary politics of the coastal elite began to emerge at this time.

This included land takeovers by the indigenous populations in the South-Central Andes, resistance to exploitative working conditions on coastal plantations by the descendants of former colonial slaves and indentured Chinese workers.

Eventually, Peru returned to civilian rule, although the economy continued to be dominated by the land-owning elite. From the early 1900s onwards, an export-oriented model was imposed, as foreign capital - much of it from Britain, Europe and the US - began to invest in Peruvian highland mining, wool, oil, sugar and cotton. In the early part of the twentieth century, foreign investors were also drawn to Peru's Amazon region, following the explosion in the international demand for rubber. By the first decades of the twentieth century, exports of sugar, cotton, oil and rubber boomed. More railways were built and factories opened. However, the fact that this expansion in capitalist development owed its success to the same pre-existing colonial forms of labour exploitation was inescapable. Instead of making itself open to social reform the institutional infrastructure became increasingly intolerant and reactionary.

[9] Poole, D. & Renique, G. (1992: 101ff).

Opposition to such an authoritarian structure from urban, labour and peasant organisations, Marxist and socialist parties, students and other dissenting groups failed to bring about significant change. Its intellectual roots lay in the critical writings of José Carlos Mariátegui and Victor Raul Haya de la Torre. In a collection of essays published in 1928 as *Seven Interpretative Essays on Peruvian Reality*, Mariátegui developed the idea of '*indigenismo*', a new way of seeing Peruvian reality in terms of class, race and imperialism. This was to become a profound influence on generations of students and intellectuals thereafter.

Victor Raul Haya de la Torre represented another strand of Peruvian intellectual life. In his most influential book, *Anti-Imperialism and APRA*, Haya de la Torre argued that capitalist economic development and nation building would only be possible through the creation of an 'anti-imperialist state' based on corporatist principles. To this end Haya de la Torre founded the APRA party in 1930. From this time onwards, APRA remained "…Peru's strongest party and, for many years, the most serious threat to the oligarchy's waning hold on power."[10]

The project to modernize the country through an expanded state apparatus, left the State heavily in debt and unable to deal with the 1929 crash. By the 1930s demand for Peru's exports slumped and the country had fallen into disarray as the coastal elites' struggle to hold on to power came under increasing threat. To put an end to rising working class and peasant activism the coastal elites installed a series of harsh military regimes intended to protect vested interest and promote further capitalist development.

By the 1950s this had brought an impressive growth in US investment and a massive increase in Peruvian capital investment in national industry. These developments took place alongside sustained opposition from working class activists, local and regional trade unions and peasant movements demanding improved working conditions and greater democratic accountability. In a relatively short period this led to an insurrection in Arequipa and a wave of strikes that ultimately gave way to a new, more open political climate with the election of Manuel Prado as president in 1956.

In this more relaxed environment the Prado administration found itself under growing pressure from an increasingly powerful and more versatile range of working class activists, local and regional trade unions and peasant movements.

This gave rise to strikes by workers from within the industrial sector and beyond, including sugar cane workers, and most especially, from the peasant movement, including share croppers and tenant farmers. The peasant uprisings were of such an order that they set the agenda for the 1962 election.

In 1963 Fernando Belaunde became president of Peru. However, his campaign commitment to tackle agrarian reform soon ran into difficulties, with the result that he turned to other, less controversial, but financially ambitious programmes, such as road construction, rural projects, education, jungle colonisation, industrial development and the creation of a state capitalist sector. The collapse of his agrarian reform proposals meant that community organisations, grassroots activism and self-help

[10] Poole, D. & Renique, G. (1992: 107).

movements remained subject to the traditional power of the coastal elite and the influence of local landowners. This undermined the prospects for political government and democratic governance and is reflected in the fact that no commitment was made to develop channels between state and society through which local demands might be communicated and addressed.

In 1968 the Belaunde government was overthrown by a military coup, led by General Juan Velasco Alvarado. Unusually for a military dictatorship, Velasco introduced a fundamental programme of land reform, dispossessing the large landowners and distributing land among the peasants. The government began with the expropriation of the sugar and cotton plantations and mills. From there the government began to break up the large and more profitable livestock haciendas of the central highlands, eventually claiming over 15,000 properties and nine million hectares of land.[11] This seized land was then redistributed to landless peasantry, the majority of whom were pressured into joining agricultural cooperatives.[12]

Though subject to abuse and corruption at local level, the new system ultimately provided as many as 3000 families with the opportunity to participate in these cooperatives "...exercising an autonomy and self-determination that they had never before experienced."[13] However, although this programme of agrarian reform succeeded in breaking the land monopolies, it did not solve many of the problems it hoped to address; instead, "...it transferred them from haciendas to the newly redistributed properties.[14]

By 1975 inflation, unemployment and a growing public debt led to another military coup, replacing Velasco with General Francisco Morales Bermudez. The new government nationalized many industries in Peru and reformed agriculture. The country, however, sank into a serious economic catastrophe with very high levels of inflation. This exacerbated social tensions throughout Peru and partly contributed to the rise of violent rebel rural insurgent movements, such as *Sendero Luminoso* (Shining Path) and the MRTA (*Tupac Amaru*).

Democratic regimes came back in the 1980s. In May 1980, elections were held again and Fernando Belaúnde Terry became President. In 1982 Peru made an agreement for a three-year IMF loan in exchange for the usual stabilisation package. However, by 1983 per capita GDP had fallen to 14.1% and the IMF loan was suspended on account of over missed targets. By 1983 400,000 jobs had been lost in the recession.

In 1985 the new government led by Alan Garcia changed tack and headed for a heterodox stabilization programme, known as the *Inti* plan. Garcia raised and then froze prices and wages, devalued the *Inti* before fixing the exchange rate, and imposed import controls. He also publicly defied the banks and the IMF, declaring that Peru would unilaterally impose a ceiling on its debt repayments equivalent to 10% of export income.

---

[11] Mayer, E., (2009: 20).

[12] Mayer, E. (2009: 20–21).

[13] Mayer, E. (2009: 21).

[14] Mayer, E. (2009: 23).

Peru was severely punished, and a virtual international financial boycott was used to turn Peru into a financial pariah. The *Inti* plan produced 2 years of strong growth and rising wages, but then collapsed in a welter of inflation and uncontrollable fiscal deficits. By 1988 economic policy reverted to more orthodox methods, although by 1990, her foreign reserves were almost exhausted. In this context of growing economic instability doubts about the capacity of the traditional coastal elite to rule escalated, paving the way for increasing militarization and growing political violence. By 1990 the macroeconomic situation in Peru had become so serious that reform was indispensable to the country's survival.

In 1990 Peru elected as President the least neo-liberal presidential candidate, Alberto Fujimori, who inherited a deepening recession and inflation at around 8000%. Despite assurances that he would not plunge into restructuring, he immediately launched the *'Fujishock'*. All subsidies were eliminated - the price of petrol went up 3000% overnight - public spending was cut, a tax reform was used to increase tax revenues and a longer structural adjustment programme of trade and privatisation introduced. In line with mainstream neo-liberal policy, structural reform organised the transfer of property and responsibilities from the public to the private sector.

Unlike other Latin American countries that had undergone high levels of inflation Peru did not seek to soften the negative effects of macroeconomic adjustment through the introduction of safety nets. Instead, once stabilization policies had brought hyperinflation under control, social expenditure was allowed to rise, and this was reflected in a sharp increase in the supply of health services, especially in primary health care. However, increases in social spending did not help to consolidate citizen rights, nor did it have any appreciable effect upon the empowerment of the poor. Instead, social policy was used to create clientelist relationships at the local level as a means of building up future political support amongst the poor.

This only helped to reinforce the traditional power structure, along with all of its customary top-down, authoritarian associations. Not only did this restrict the opportunities available for participation still further, it also served to hasten the demise of political parties as mediators between the state and society.

For people worst affected by political violence and living under conditions of extreme poverty, social deprivation and exclusion, democratic ideals are likely to seem less important than more immediate concerns. In this context, faith in the state's capacity to provide even the most limited forms of security was severely eroded, which meant that support for the conventional political parties' system all but disappeared.

In this environment of growing disillusionment antagonism towards both Congress and the legislature increased, with the result that top-down and vertical forms of government began to seem increasingly attractive. On the night of Sunday April 5, 1992, Fujimori appeared on television and announced that he was "temporarily dissolving" the Congress of the Republic and "reorganizing" the Judicial Branch of the government.

Fujimori then issued Decree Law 25,418, which dissolved the Congress, gave the Executive Branch all legislative powers, suspended much of the Constitution, and gave the president the power to enact various reforms, including various draconian anti-terrorism laws. These actions received immediate backing from both the armed forces and the national police; the number of arrests rose dramatically: most notable was the *Sendero Luminoso* leader, Abimael Guzmán, in 1992. Meanwhile public resistance to political violence increased, in the countryside and towns alike.

Following the *autogolpe* (self-imposed *coup d'etat*) and the immediate election of a new Congress, Fujimori brought a halt to the regionalisation process that had been introduced as part of the 1979 Constitution. Not only did this cause political power to become increasingly concentrated, it also meant that any semblance of a parliament composed of members with direct regional, departmental or provincial representation was at an end. One effect of this was for all 1810 districts to be treated as though they were the same, even though some had fewer than 1000 inhabitants, whilst others had more than a million.

Such a burgeoning authoritarian structure meant that local government and the role of popular movements became increasingly affected by the decline in the distributional capacities of the state. Resources to fund any regulatory and enabling role for local government through training and infrastructure development dwindled, whilst initiatives designed to promote public sector service capacity were neglected or left undeveloped, particularly in rural areas. In absolute figures, an additional 2.1 million people are estimated to have joined the ranks of the poor in the period 1997–2000.[15]

In November 2000, Fujimori resigned and went to Japan in self-imposed exile, to avoid prosecution for human rights violations and corruption charges. An interim government was installed under Valentin Paniagua with responsibility for conducting new presidential and congressional elections. The elections were held in April 2001; observers considered them to be free and fair. Alejandro Toledo (who led the opposition against Fujimori) defeated former President Alan Garcia. The newly elected government took office on July 28, 2001.

The Toledo Administration managed to restore some degree of democracy to Peru following the authoritarianism and corruption associated with the Fujimori and García governments. This included retrials in civilian courts for innocent people wrongfully tried by military courts during the war against terrorism (1980–2000).

On August 28, 2003, the Truth and Reconciliation Commission (CVR), which had been charged with studying the roots of the violence of the 1980–2000 period, presented its formal report to the President.

By 2018, Peru had had a succession of democratic regimes having been led by Alejandro Toledo, Alan García, Ollanta Humala Tasso and most recently Pedro Pable

[15] Following the inauguration of Alejandro Toledo in 2001evidence emerged that the figures produced by INEI, the official statistics gathering institution were manipulated by the second Fujimori administration and that most of the deterioration in poverty levels took place in 1999 and 2000. INEI (*Instituto Nacional de Estadística e Informática*) is a semi-autonomous Peruvian government agency which coordinates, compiles, and evaluates statistical information for the country. However, in the last 4 years of the second Fujimori government (1996–2000) it is generally accepted that the number of poverty living below the poverty line increased from 42.7% to 48.4% (See Javier Herrera, July 2001). See also Programa de las Naciones Unidas para el Desarrollo (PNUD) United Nations for Development (2005); Instituto Nacional de Estadisticas e Informatica Evolucion de la pobreza al 2010 Lima: INEI (2011).

Kucznski. In March 2018 Pedro Pable Kucznsk unexpectedly resigned amid allegations of corruption and was replaced by his Vice-President, Martin Vizcarra. Mr. Vizcarra is expected to serve out Pedro Pable Kucznsk's term, which ends in 2021.

2.2 Historical Background of Ayacucho

The department of Ayacucho is located in the central region of the *Cordillera de los Andes* (Andean mountain range), with the department of Junin to the north, that of Arequipa to the east and those of Ica and Huancavelica to the west. The region is divided into 11 Provinces which are composed of 111 Districts.[16] Most of the Department is made up of broken mountain valleys and high plains with an average altitude of over 3500 metres. To the far south-west the country falls towards the coastal plain and in the far north-east towards the tropical jungle on the banks of the River Apurímac.[17]

[16] The provinces, with their capitals in parenthesis, are: (1) Cangallo (Cangallo)) (2) Huamanga (Ayacucho) (3) Huanca Sancos (Huanca Sancos) (4) Huanta (Huanta) (5) La Mar (San Miguel) (6) Lucanas (Puquio) (7) Parinacochas (Coracora) (8) Paucar del Sara Sara (Pausa) (9) Sucre (Querobamba) (10) Victor Fajardo (Huancapi) (11) Vilcas Huaman (Vilcas Huaman).

[17] It has a geographical area of 43,814.8km^2 (16,917.0 sq. mi) and a population density of 14/km^2 (37/sq. mi). According to the 2005 census the total population was 619,338. This represents a population decline of 2.4% equivalent to a negative growth in population of – 147, 624 since the previous census of 1993. The elevation of the capital is 2746 m (9,009 ft), the highest elevation was 3645 m (11,959 ft) and the lowest elevation is 1800 m (5,900 ft). Information from the *Programa de las Naciones Unidas para el Desarrollo* (PNUD) (United Nations for Development) (2005) ranks the Department of Ayacucho 20th out of 24 departments (HDI = 0.5095) in relation to data on basic necessities which shows that 82.8% of households have less than basic standard of necessities. In the last population census (INEI, 2011), the Department of Ayacucho has a population of 619,338 inhabitants, 43% of which are under 18 years. The rate of maternal mortality in Ayacucho is 304.7 per 100,000, almost double the national average (163.9) (MINSA, 2001); only 41.5% of pregnant mothers get 4 prenatal check-ups (UNICEF 2004), with a percentage a bit higher for hospital births (47.2%). With regard to child health, the rate of infant mortality in Ayacucho reached 50 per 1000 live births and the rate of mortality for children under 5 years, 68 per 1000, in both cases higher than the national average (43 and 60 respectively). Child malnutrition is also very high: one in three children less than 5 years old in the region suffer from chronic malnutrition (UNICEF 2004). Information from the *Ministerio de Educación* (MINEDU) (Ministry of Education) indicates that basic educational coverage is almost universal (93% in Ayacucho, compared to 96% at the national level). However, there are many problems particularly in relation to the quality of multi-grade and single teacher schools, and the lack of appropriate curricula. For families and communities in the rural highlands and other areas with high levels of poverty repetition and dropouts are commonplace. As UNICEF (2004) argues75% of students in areas of poverty are older than they should be for the grade (50% in urban, 60% in rural areas). Ministerio de Salud Dirreccion General de Promocion de la Salud Lima Proyecto 2000 (2001); 2004 PRU: Peru-UNICEF Country Programme Evaluation UNICEF NYHQ; Dewey, K.G., & Begum, K., (2011); Comision de la Verdad y Reconciliacion Informe Final [CVR Final Report] Lima (2003); Scott Palmer, D., (1992); Degregori, I., Coronel, J., del Pino. & Starn, O., (1996); Laplante, L.J., (2007); McCann, I.L. & Pearlman, L.A., (1990a, b); Krznaric, R., (2014); Schwartz, W. (2002); Freire, P., (1998); Baron-Cohen, S., (2011); Buss, D.M. & Malamuth, N. (1996); Domhoff, G. W., & Zweigenhaft, R.L., (1998); Operario, D. & Fiske, S.T., (2001).

Because of the high and rugged mountains, the region is difficult to traverse and not very productive agriculturally. This is because the local vegetation of this dry, arid mountainous terrain is made up of scrub grass and cacti. However, the deep fertile valleys and basins that separate these great mountain ranges mean that the region is subject, not just to a great variety of multiple altitudinal floors, but to a huge range of micro climates as well.

To deal with this unique and inhospitable terrain, people have adapted various parts of the Andes to a series of different production zones that specialise in producing goods appropriate according to each ecological zone.[18] The most decisive agricultural practices typically involve a synthesis of traditional and modern techniques. These include such traditional practices as terraces, ridge fields, local irrigation systems and traditional agricultural tools, crops and livestock spread at different altitudes.[19]

To contend with the severe fluctuations in temperature, the unpredictability of the rainy season, and a multitude of pest threats, farmers cultivate a diverse array of species rather than a mono culture to protect their crop. These consist of tubers, roots, cereals, vegetables, and fruits and the raising of livestock such as cattle, sheep, goats, camelids (llamas, alpacas, vicuna and guanaco), pigs, guinea pigs, mules, donkey, horses and chickens. People rely on livestock as a source of protein, fertilizer, draught power, transportation, savings and insurance. The origins of this production system are pre-Colombian, but features remain, including many of the traditional crops such as potatoes, oca,[20] olluco,[21] mashua,[22] tarwi,[23] and quinoa,[24]among others.

The typical Andean community is dominated above all by the needs of subsistence and should therefore be distinguished from the 'open' peasant community found in the low highlands and tropical lowlands.[25] Unlike the 'open' peasant community the typical Andean community has not evolved out of the growing demand

---

[18]These production zones include: (1) above 3600 to 4000 m (Zone 1). This is the harshest zone and known as the puna. This is a zone of pastoralism and used for animals such as llamas, alpacas, cattle, sheep and horses. (2) The suni (Zone 2), 3300 to 4000 m (also often termed puna) supports the cultivation of tubers such as potatoes, ocas, ollucos, and mashuas as well as wheat and barley. (3) The quechua (Zone 3) 2400 to 3300 m is the primary cereal producing zone. This supports the cultivation of maize, wheat, barley, bean and other crops. (4) The lowest zone (Zone 4) or yunga lies below 2400 m. Sucb-tropical crops such as coca, plantains, sweet potatoes, yucca, citrus fruits, peppers, chilli and sugar are grown here. See Watters, R. F., (1994: 35ff).

[19]It is estimated that more than a million hectares of land have been modified for agricultural purposes throughout the Andean region. The land is modified for use as terraces, the *waru-waru* (raised fields) and *qochas* in the *altiplano*. See Rengifo, G., (1987) *La Agricultura Tradicional en los Andes* Editorial Horizontal-Lima.

[20]*Oxalis tuberosa (Oxalidaceae).*

[21]*Ullucus tuberosus.*

[22]*Tropaeolum tuberosum.*

[23]*Lupinus mutabilis.*

[24]*Chenopodium quinoa.*

[25]See Wolf, E., (1955); (1957) as mentioned by Watters, R. F., (1994: 43ff).

for cash crops that accompanied the rise of capitalism. It has no formalised community structure, and no privately-owned land; it lacks a wide range of individual economic activities and choices and has no outlet for the sale of cash crops. By contrast, its organization derives from its historical role in providing labour, goods, or money for the landholding elite, and other forms of exploitation sanctioned by the political structure of the state.[26]

Though the Andes was occupied by human beings long before the Inca conquest, the population was widely dispersed and made up of many tribal groups and small states. However, their ethnic diversity and linguistic distinctions derive from a common ancestral language. This was responsible for a range of dialects spoken by them, until Quechua became the imperial language of the Inca civilisation. Eventually, this came to supplant the multiple dialects spoken amongst indigenous people, although the range of dialects survived. The most common Quechua dialect is Southern Quechua. Ayacucho is a variety of Southern Quechua spoken in the Ayacucho region and the largest variety of Southern Quechua after Cusco Quechua.[27]

In spite of these linguistic differences, people shared an abundance of cultural characteristics, the most important of which was a basic economic system known as the *ayllu*.[28] This is concerned with the organization of shared collective labour (*minga*) and reciprocal exchanges of assistance (*ayni*). It invariably involves a network of extended family groups and is characterised by various types of work exchange.

Though used for a range of purposes the *ayllu* is frequently associated with the resolution of issues involving subsistence agriculture, including food production, barter and trade; it is also used to settle domestic disputes about the education and care of children from within the family group.[29] For generations the *ayllu* has been associated with the sense of responsibility people have for each other, and with the rules and conventions that govern the wider aspects of community development.

The typical Andean community has also been shaped by influences quite separate from their own shared elements of cultures and customs. Beginning with the unification of the life, institutions, languages and religions of the Inca Empire, these outside influences continued to shape the typical Andean community with the new 'conquest culture' introduced by the invading Spanish, only to intensify still further following Peruvian independence. From the Catholic Church, Spanish language, forms of government, the legal system and many more, no outside influence, it is suggested, has had a more powerful and lasting effect than labour exploitation and the establishment of vast new estates. However, this does not mean that the typical Andean community did not always comply without a struggle. In spite of systematic repression of the native population, harsh conditions of exploitation repeatedly led to revolts by the indigenous farmers, which were forcibly suppressed.

[26] Watters, R. F., (1994: 45).

[27] See for example, Hornberger, N. H. & King, K. A., (1998); (2001); (2006). Quechua became Peru's second official language in 1969 under the military regime of Juan Velasco Alvarado.

[28] Gonzales, O. M. (2011: 27).

[29] Demarest, A. A., Conrad, G. W., (1984: 97).

From its use of dependent labour, the hacienda system "...became an institution with a labour force largely removed from its traditional social environment and permanently settled on land belonging to the estate."[30] In this way the hacienda system was able to align itself with commercial agriculture and the mercantile economy operated by the coastal elite. However, this process also contributed to the destruction of the typical Andean community "...and the transformation of its members into an agricultural proletariat."[31]

This led to a loss of ethnic identity and the Quechua language, as well as to the steady migration of people to large cities (especially to Lima), thereby contributing to the acculturation of Hispanic society there.

Nevertheless, as with other regions of Peru, all or most, of the land in the Ayacucho region was appropriated by the Spanish crown and distributed amongst conquistadors and other officials as rewards for their role in colonizing new lands. However, haciendas did not always provide a way to maintain a good living, because they could not always offer high production yields. Instead, what gave the region its wealth and prestige was its location in relation to the economic centres of Cuzco and Lima. Though haciendas were profitable, in areas such as Cuzco or Trujillo, haciendas in Ayacucho retained their importance as status symbols, rather than as sources of income.

From the Spanish Conquest onwards, social class was, to a great extent, determined by land ownership. In this way, the hacienda became the symbol of a family's social position, even when it failed to translate into economic capital. Beginning with the colonial era and intensifying after Peru gained its independence, a process was created through which landowners would use their social prestige as hacienda owners to gain entry into the professions and thereby generate economic capital for themselves and their dependants. This had a major impact on the hacienda system as a functional system of land ownership.

For landowners in the Ayacucho region this process entailed migration to the capital because of the limited opportunities available for such forms of advancement locally. The result was for many local haciendas to become available for purchase.

In this way, wealthier members of the landless peasantry found themselves able to take on the ownership of hacienda land – together with all its attendant social prestige. This arrangement became active many generations before the agrarian reform programme under Velasco had even begun. The upshot of this was for much of the hacienda system to have already been broken up long before the Velasco plan had been introduced. This made the agrarian reform programme hard to apply because it rarely related to local forms of land tenure. It is, perhaps, significant that government support for the implementation of the agrarian reform programme in the Ayacucho region was, for this reason, less than it was elsewhere.

Instead of a form of large landed estate system, land that had once been owned by one family was now owned and cultivated by many former landless peasants.

[30] Watters, R. F., (1994: 59).

[31] Watters, R. F., (1994: 59).

However, this land was no more capable of high productive yields than it had been under the old hacienda system. In many cases the land was exhausted and no longer retained its economic value (from crops, livestock, mining, etc.). Mass privatization may have broken up the old estates, but the low productive yields from the land brought little benefit to its new owners. In many cases the hacienda system had become little more than a renter landlord system. Instead of making wealth accumulation and upward social mobility more widely available, land redistribution (and agrarian reform) had simply replaced one system of land ownership with another.

Though the Velasco plan was intended to destroy the basis of power of Peru's traditional elite and foster a more cooperative society as an alternative to capitalism, this was not to be. Instead, land redistribution (and agrarian reform) created a system in which questions of ownership were what mattered, not the consequences for output or rural incomes.

Moving the country towards a more egalitarian society was going to need more than the elimination of all large private landholdings if it was to bring an end to class conflict, territorial fragmentation and foreign pressures. Even so, if land redistribution had made wealth accumulation, and therefore, upward social mobility more attainable, it is conceivable that the future political violence may not have resulted in quite as much destruction and upheaval.

However, low productive yields make wealth accumulation no more likely than what landowners had found under the old hacienda system; much of the land is exhausted and, for many, there seem little prospect of that ever changing.[32] Even without dependence on mechanisation, chemical fertilisers, pesticides or other technologies of modern agricultural science, nothing alters the fact that agriculture in the rural highlands has always involved a relatively high level of risk, often resulting in seasonal food scarcity. This means that people have not always had "…physical and economic access to sufficient, safe and nutritious food to meet their dietary needs and food preferences for an active and healthy life."[33]

In these circumstances the individual's bodily capacities are affected, including growth, pregnancy, lactation, resistance to illness, and cognitive and physical development. By failing to consume the minimum number of calories necessary for baseline physiological needs, the body's immune system weakens, making undernourished people more susceptible to infectious diseases.

Though many factors may be to blame, those most closely linked with malnutrition levels in rural highland communities include: very low standards of living,

[32] Soil erosion represents 65% of the total cost of agricultural land degradation and soil salinity around 35% in terms of crop yield reductions associated with these damages. See World Bank, (2007) Republic of Peru Environmental Sustainability: A Key to Poverty Reduction in Peru. Country Environmental Analysis.: Environmentally and Socially Sustainable Development Department Latin America and the Caribbean Region Washington DC.

[33] Food and Agriculture Organization (1996) Rome Declaration on Food Security and World Food Summit Plan of Action.

harsh environmental conditions, water scarcity, and the difficulties meeting such basic needs as housing and health care.[34]

For generations the adverse effect of geography has also frustrated communication, market access and the arrival of state services: roads and infrastructure linking the poor highlands with the more prosperous towns and cities have either been in disrepair or non-existent. In all this time crops and other items from rural highland communities have rarely, if ever, been available for trade on national, regional, or even, local markets. This undermines interest in the improvement of farming methods and reinforces the notion that rural agriculture exists only for subsistence, with little surplus stored, and little or no cash economy, just bartering, and exchange for local obligations and no output to markets.

Being shut out of opportunities to participate in public life affects people's awareness and consciousness of potential issues and conflicts. This helps to preserve the unequal power relationship between people and outside organizations and institutions and the belief that government officials are ineffective and uncaring. By 1980, annual per capita income in the Ayacucho region had fallen to $60, whilst three of its provinces were among the poorest in all Peru.[35] In this disconnected, impoverished region the majority indigenous population remained subject to an antiquated socio-economic structure, making them vulnerable to criminal and insurgent influence. This is the environment that spawned *Sendero Luminoso*.

2.3 Shining Path

The modern history of the Andes is dominated by the activities of the Shining Path and its founder, Abimael Guzman. Following his arrival as a philosophy professor at the University of Huamanga in Ayacucho in 1962 Guzman set out to model a party dedicated to establishing a dictatorship of the proletariat. His teachings created the foundation of its militant Maoist doctrine.

In the 18 years that followed Guzman manoeuvred to model a party dedicated solely to his ideals, which depended on two factors. First, that any collaboration with democratic institutions or movements that campaigned for social change within the capitalist system is criminal. Second, that armed struggle must be carefully prepared by a campaign of research, training and political indoctrination.[36]

---

[34] Aguiar, Christine; Rosenfeld, Josh; Stevens, Beth; Thanasombat, Sup; Masud, Harika (2007) An Analysis of Malnutrition Programming and Policies in Peru; Dewey, KG; Begum, K (2011) Long-term consequences of stunting in early life *Matern Child Nutr* **7** (3): 5–18. This is reinforced by the results of a study into the rural-urban disparity in malnutrition, which found that Peru had the greatest rural- urban disparity in stunting rates. See also Van de Poel, E; O'Donnell, O; van Doorslaer, E (2007). "Are Urban Children really healthier? Evidence from 47 developing countries" Tinbergen Institute Discussion Paper TI 2007–035/3.

[35] Wickham-Crowley, T. P, (1992: 245).

[36] Degregori, C. I., (1990).

The Shining Path is an offshoot of the Communist Party of Peru, which in turn broke away from the original Peruvian Communist Party, a derivation of the Peruvian Socialist Party founded by José Carlos Mariátegui in 1928. Its full name is the *Partido Comunista del Perú-Sendero Luminoso* (PCP-SL), commonly known as *Sendero Luminoso* (Shining Path). Discipline was central to Shining Path ideology. This was reflected in the unquestioned authority of President Guzman (Gonzalo-Thought), the application of Marxist-Leninist-Maoist dogma to Peru.[37]

By the mid-1970s, as its power within the University started to wane, Shining Path focused its attention upon the grievances of the Highland Quechua in the Ayacucho highlands.

Poor communications had left indigenous people isolated from markets and open to exploitation; although the land reforms initiated under Velasco had given former *hacienda* lands to co-operatives, their distribution had been both corrupt and chaotic, thereby providing a huge field of resentment for Shining Path to exploit. In spite of the opportunities this provided, infiltration proved less successful amongst less remote rural communities that had access to basic state services such as health, education, and security.

In May 1980 Shining Path started an uprising with the intention of overthrowing the Peruvian state. One of its main guerrilla strategies was to destroy all real and potential rivals for power. An important aspect of this policy was a refusal to tolerate any social action that reduced their efforts to overthrow the capitalist system. Priests, NGOs, state programmes and other left-wing groups were all targeted. In November, they made their first impact on Lima, by which time they were in control of large stretches of the Highlands of Ayacucho, Huancavelica and Junin.

In the period that followed the state's response remained somewhat muted until December 1982 when the Belaunde regime suspended civil law in an 'Emergency Zone' around the Highlands of Ayacucho, Huancavelica and Apurimac. This suspension of the constitutional rights of liberty and freedom of movement in Ayacucho helped encourage a process in which political opponents were demonised and treated as potential subversives.[38] Anyone suspected of political activity or of collaboration, failing to distinguish between the guerrillas and other left-wing groups was invariably raped, tortured or massacred.

In January 1983 the incumbent government adopted a severe counterinsurgency strategy and sent in the army to track down Shining Path sympathizers. This led to a reign of terror from both sides.[39] Many of these events took place in rural areas of Ayacucho. They included massacres and other large scale human rights violations attributed to members of the national police, the infantry of war marine and members of the infantry of the armed forces.[40]

---

[37] Poole, D. & Renique, G. (1992: 40).

[38] Poole, D. & Renique, G. (1992: 59).

[39] Poole, D. & Renique, G., (1992: 40); Tulchin, J. & Bland, G., (1994: 101).

[40] See *Comisión de la Verdad y Reconciliación, Informe Final* [CVR Final Report] (Lima, 2003), www.cverdad.org.pe/ifi nal/index.php. Vol. VIII, conclusion 55 at 323. These violations by the state are highlighted in a report carried out for the International Center for Transitional Justice by

As the civil conflict led by Shining Path spread, the state's low levels of legitimacy and weak sense of shared values with ordinary people became apparent.

Institutions and organisations controlled by the state were destroyed or severely weakened, urban food provision and Highland Quechua subsistence was threatened and rural conditions for ordinary people underwent rapid decline.[41] Forced by the pressure of events, Highland Quechua began to flee from their communities from 1983 onwards, of whom 50,000 moved to Lima.[42]

By 1985 suspicion and mistrust had become commonplace: a series of social and economic initiatives in the Andean region failed because the government refused to collaborate with local peasant federations affiliated to opposition parties.[43] Inflexible behaviour and a general unwillingness to develop an adaptive capacity gave out the impression of an institutional infrastructure resistant to partial change and indifferent to legitimate concerns.[44]

Under such conditions' inefficiency and corruption, incoherent taxation and inadequate enforcement measures became commonplace. The fragmentation of key health programmes, weak information systems, inefficiencies in the management structure, inadequate geographical distribution, skills mix and human resource quality are just some of the issues to have dominated the public sector in those years.[45] Not only did this weaken the functions of state control and supervision, it also encouraged a relationship with civil society that was dominated by personal, informal or clientele criteria. The absence of any formal, static procedures through which civic demands could be communicated meant that the state was perceived as remote and resistant to negotiated agreements.[46]

This intensification of the violence eventually led to the armed conflict spilling over into other areas of the Country, so that by the late 1980s the political violence had acquired a national dimension.

Throughout this period the vast majority of victims of violence were Highland Quechua. In 1989, for instance, an estimated 76% of guerrilla victims were Highland Quechua or poor urban dwellers.[47] By the end of 1989, 80 districts and 4 provinces had no municipal authorities and more than 70% of public works projects in the rural Andes had been abandoned because of the assassination of 95 government engineers.

Cristian Correa who points out that, "...Torture and the commission of sexual violence and rape, for example, were carried out on a massive scale by the armed forces and the vigilante groups it supported. Seventy-five percent of cases of torture received by the CVR and 83 percent of cases of rape were attributed to them (vol. VIII, 64–67). At that time, no investigations or prosecutions of these violations were carried out, and violence spread across the country." Correa, C. (2013:1).

[41] Scott Palmer, D., (1992: 45); Degregori C. I., et al.,(1996: 15).

[42] Poole, D. & Renique, G., (1992: 78).

[43] Scott Palmer, D. et al., (1992). See also, Degregori, C. I., (1990); Degregori, C. I. et al. (1996).

[44] Poole, D. & Renique, G., (1992: 101ff); Tulchin, J. & Bland, G., (1994: 25).

[45] World Bank, (1999: 6).

[46] Tulchin, J & Bland, G., (1994: 35).

[47] Degregori, C. I., (1990).

In 1988 a major mobilization in Lima was ordered by Guzman that set-in motion the most intense period of violence, affecting both urban and rural areas and continuing throughout the general elections of 1990. In Red October, in the run-up to the 1990 elections, more than 360 were killed, including over 40 elected or government officials. More than 260 candidates withdrew before the elections.

Absenteeism in the April 1990 ballot was around 50% in Ayacucho and Junin. Fujimori, the new President, gave total support to the military in their policy of targeting the Shining Path leadership and confronting the organisation in the countryside.[48] In October 1992 Guzman was captured in Lima together with all but one of the Shining Path Central Committee.[49]

Of those killed or disappeared it is estimated that the majority (79%) were inhabitants of rural areas, and 56% were rural peasants. Three quarters are reported to have come from families whose mother tongue was Quechua, or one of the other indigenous languages.[50]

In the 20 years of political violence in Peru (1980–2000), 69,280 Peruvians were killed (this is higher than the number of Peruvians killed in all external and civil wars that have occurred in the 182 years since Independence). Many of those who died lived in rural areas and were Quechua speakers. Of the total, 12.5% were children.[51]

Even before Guzman's capture, Shining Path had begun to lose the initiative in the Highlands.[52] From the early 1980s, the army had been instrumental in compelling rural communities to set up self-defence committees, importing a model used successfully against cattle-ranchers in the northern Andes since the early 1970's. This system of Highland Community rounds was generally poorly armed and incapable of defeating the Shining path.[53] Their significance was in uniting communities in resistance, acting as scouts for the army and in giving communities a sense of responsibility and power over their own fate.

In the aftermath of the political violence the crisis in human, financial, physical and organisational resources helped promote interest in the institutional aspects of collective action and the importance it might have for a reduction in public sector expenditure and an improvement in support for government strategy.[54]

---

[48] Tulchin, J. & Bland, G. (1994: 101).

[49] Oscar Ramirez Durand (Commander Feliciano) remained at large until his capture in the Upper Huallaga Valley in 1999.

[50] Truth and Reconciliation Commission, Final Report, September 2003. Available at: http://www.cvevdad.org/pe/ingles/final/index.php

[51] Truth and Reconciliation Commission, Final Report, September 2003.

[52] Degregori, C. I., et al., (1996).

[53] Starn, O. (1991); (1999).

[54] M. Tanaka, 'The Changing Boundaries between Society and Politics', in J. Crabtree and J. Thomas (eds) *Fujimori's Peru* (1998).

2.4 The Official Response to Political Violence

Under policy changes introduced in early 1992, the Peruvian Presidency acquired more power over the operational intelligence apparatus, particularly in relation to the armed forces. These changes were made possible by the closure of the principal democratic institutions that followed the self-made *coup d'état* of President Fujimori in April 1992. By making these changes the Fujimori administration introduced a form of authoritarian rule that included subversion of the rule of law, widespread corruption, official immunity and the creation of death squads.

In 1995 the Fujimori administration passed Law No 26749 which granted a general amnesty to all of the members of the police and the armed forces that were being investigated or had been convicted for crimes committed during the political violence.

The consequence of this Law was that "...it was practically impossible to investigate and judicialize the cases related to human rights violations perpetrated against state agents."[55] This situation of absolute immunity was brought to an end in 2000 as a result of growing suspicions of corruption inside the upper echelons of government. This included unconstitutional actions on behalf of Fujimori (who was seeking re-election), the continuing use of arbitrary detentions first adopted after the *coup d'etat* and widespread concern about electoral fraud.

Not long after Fujimori's re-election in September 2000 images of the President's Adviser, Vladimiro Montesinos Torres handing over bribes to a congressman were broadcast on national Television. This became the catalyst for a major change in the political affairs of the nation. The most immediate result was for new presidential elections to be called and a transitional government to be appointed, but corruption amongst the president and the highest officials together with corruption involving high officials from the armed forces and the police had longer lasting effects.

To win back state legitimacy and credibility the transitional government led by President Valentin Paniagua set about the dismantling of the authoritarian state created under the Fujimori administration and the reconstitution of those democratic institutions that had been closed or whose authority had been seriously weakened and discredited.[56] In addition the Peruvian Congress was reconstituted.

These actions cleared the way for the independence of the judiciary to be recovered and for judicial and congressional investigations into both corruption and human rights abuses to be initiated. In 2001 the judiciary was able to honour the judgment by the Inter-American Court of Human Rights invalidating the 1995 amnesty laws.

Under the Paniagua administration the Office of the Ombudsman adopted Resolution No 57 DP-2000 recommending "...the creation of a truth and reconcili-

[55] Montoya Vivanco, Y. (2012: 161) Responding to Human Rights Violations committed during the internal armed conflict in Peru: the limits and advances of Peruvian criminal justice. In Almqvist, J. & Esposito, C. (2012).

[56] In office: 22 November 2000–28 July 2001.

ation commission that would clarify the circumstances under which human rights violations had been perpetrated, to assign personal and institutional responsibilities and to grant reparations."[57] The *Comisión de la Verdad y Reconciliación* (CVR), (Truth and Reconciliation Commission) (TRC) was subsequently created by virtue of a Supreme Decree (No 065–2001) and subsequently approved by the transitional government on 4 June 2001.[58] Its purpose was to investigate human rights violations and crimes committed by terrorist organizations and state agents between May 1980 and November 2000.

It was also mandated to determine the conditions that gave rise to the violence, contribute to judicial investigations, draft proposals for reparations, and recommend reforms.[59] By going into the historical, social and economic causes and conditions that led to the political violence the TRC took its investigation into areas hitherto unexplored by previous truth commissions.[60]

Instead of simply documenting specific types of Civil and Political Rights (CPR) violations, the TRC devoted an entire volume of its report into explaining why these abuses occurred. Through its analysis of economic social and cultural (ESCR) inequalities the TRC was able to show how "…the populations most affected by inequalities were the most targeted, first by SL, and later by the armed forces reacting to SL."[61]

Though it did not specifically mention poverty as the main cause of the violence the TRC did refer to it as "...one of the factors that contributed to igniting [this conflict] and as the backdrop against which this drama unfolded."[62]

This is borne out by the fact that 85% of the estimated 70,000 dead and 12,000 disappeared came from mainly rural highland areas of the six poorest regions of

[57] Montoya Vivanco, Y. (2012: 172). The recommendation was reiterated in Resolution no DP-2001, adopted on 24 May 2001.

[58] The decree that established the Commission (065-PCM-2001, Art 2) set out five overriding aims: (1) To analyse the political, social and cultural conditions and patterns of behaviour that, from society and the institutions of the state, contributed to the tragic situation of violence experienced in Peru; (2) To help in the clarification by the competent judicial institutions of the crimes and human rights violations perpetrated by terrorist organisations or agents of the state, seeking to determine the whereabouts and situation of the victims and identifying to the degree possible those presumed responsible; (3) To produce proposals for making reparation and restoring dignity to the victims and their families; (4) To recommend institutional, legal, educational and other reforms as guarantees that such events would never be repeated, these being considered and implemented through legislation and other political and administrative actions; (5) To establish mechanisms for the implementation of the Commission's recommendations. *Comisión de la Verdad y Reconciliación, Informe Final* [CVR Final Report] (Lima, 2003), www.cverdad.org.pe/ifi nal/index.php

[59] *Decreto Supremo de Peru*, N° 065–2001-PCM., Art. 2(a), *available at* http://www.cverdad.org.pe/lacomision/cnormas/normasOl.php

[60] See for example the Truth Commissions held in South Africa and Sierra Leone, as well as other truth commissions from Latin America, including Guatemala, El Salvador, Argentina, Chile.

[61] Laplante, Lisa J. (2007: 14)".

[62] *Hatun Willakuy, Version Abreviada del Informe Final de la Comision de la Verdad Y Reconciliacion* 337 (2004) [hereinafter Willakuy].

Peru inhabited primarily by *campesinos* (subsistence farmers) of indigenous descent.[63] In addition, the TRC found that 75% of the victims spoke a native language other than Spanish, even though native speakers represent only 16% of the general population. The TRC also found that 56% of the victims were dedicated to agriculture activities and that 68% had minimal education. The greatest concentration of the political violence was in the rural highlands of Ayacucho, which accounted for 40% of the overall number of dead and disappeared.

From these findings the TRC reached the conclusion that "...there exists an evident relation between social exclusion and the intensity of the violence. It was not coincidence that the four regions most affected by the internal armed conflict... are the five poorest in the country."[64] This deliberate targeting of "...a sector of the population historically ignored by the State and the urban society"[65] was seen as testimony to the unequal process of modernization, and how sustained economic development has excluded most rural sectors of Peruvian society.[66] It is also a devastating indictment of the attitude of indifference, disparagement, and discrimination towards this population by the powerful elite.

The destruction inflicted by the political violence on the families and communities across the rural highlands is documented by the TRC's chapter *Las secuelas del conflicto* (The Consequences of the Conflict). This includes a comprehensive list of the many ways in which psychosocial, socio-political and socioeconomic damage were inflicted on individuals and their communities and the types of suffering that the political violence has brought about.[67]

However, instead of restricting its analysis to a clarification of, reparation for and punishment for, CPR violations the TRC report adopted a broader more holistic perspective in which the content of the "damage" and "harm" arising out of CPR violations, "could correspond to violations of ESCR."[68]

In this way the TRC report opened up its analysis to include the social and economic root causes of political violence as well as individual episodes of repression and violence.[69] By including information about the damage inflicted on local infrastructure including the destruction of houses, schools, community centres, health posts, roads, bridges, and even entire communities the TRC report brings into full view issues of contextual complexity that are vital to an understanding of how the consequences of what happened causes the past to remain locked in an eternal present. In addition, the TRC report draws attention to ways in which the political vio-

[63] This includes Ayacucho, Junin, Huanuco, Huancavelica, Apurimac, and San Martin. See vol. VIII, *Conclusiones Generales* [General Conclusions], conclusions 4 and 9, at 315–16.

[64] These are Junin, Huanuco, Huancavelica, Apurimac, and San Martin.

[65] *Hatun Willakuy*, *supra* note 66, at 10.

[66] *Hatun Willakuy*, *supra* note 66, at 339.

[67] Hatun Willakuy, supra note 66, at 353–410. For the unabbreviated chapter on the consequences of the conflict, see TRC Final Report, supra note 12, at vol. VIII, pt. 3 as cited in Laplante, L. J. (2007: 17).

[68] Laplante, L. J. (2007: 17).

[69] LaPlante, L. J. (2007: 18).

lence was responsible for loss of income, disruptions in education, loss of production, robberies and forced acquisition of the principal sources of income and subsistence.

The insight this gives into the relationship between context and its influence on human nature and responsibility and the failure of the social capital discourse provides a means by which human suffering can be properly acknowledged, and some reassurance that appropriate responsibilities can be assumed.

By demonstrating how the political violence had significantly worsened already extreme social, economic and cultural conditions enabled the TRC to make wide ranging recommendations for addressing the suffering inflicted on thousands of families and communities across the rural highlands, to whom society and the State owed reparations.[70]

These include criminal trials, institutional reform and the *Plan Integral de Reparaciónes* (PIR) (Comprehensive Reparations Plan).[71]

The plan is made up of components whose purpose is to bring reconciliation to the country and address deep socioeconomic disparities in Peru. In this respect the focus is not just concerned with human rights violations, but with the factors and conditions that led to those violations, particularly in relation to historically marginalized communities across the rural highlands. By making the PIR a means for addressing the root causes of the political violence the TRC was able to emphasize the importance of the social and economic inequalities that contributed to its conception. In effect, the TRC used the PIR to ensure that the ethnic and racial marginalization of communities from across the rural highlands (and the Amazon), together with the scorn and oppression that helped sustain state indifference over countless generations are duly recognized.[72]

To implement the recommendations for victim reparations President Alejandro Toledo[73] established the *Comisión Multisectorial de Alto Nivel*, (CMAN) (High Level Multisectoral Commission).[74] However, its impact did not start to be felt until

---

[70] In its final conclusions the TRC drew attention to the epidemiology of the political violence by saying that "...social exclusion and poverty in Peru has a rural, peasant face;" Hatun Willakuy, *supra* note 66, at 409. The final nine volume report was officially handed to the interim President Alejandro Toledo, 2 years after it began its work, at a ceremony held in Lima on August 28, 2003.

[71] TRC Final Report at Vol. IX, Part 4, Ch. 2 Institutional reform refers generally to a series of recommendations for reforming the state, such as the judicial apparatus, the military and police, the educational system, among others, with an eye towards creating the rule of law and a culture of rights believed necessary for preventing future regression to violence. *See* Hayner, *supra* note 8, at 154–69.

[72] TRC Final Report, *supra* note 12, at Vol. IX, Part 4, Ch. 2.2. at p.140.

[73] In office 28 July 2001–28 July 2006.

[74] Created by *Decreto Supremo* N° 003–2004-JUS Its purpose is to follow up on state actions and policies in the areas of peace, collective reparations, and national reconciliation. It also has the authority to make awards of pecuniary and non-pecuniary measures to victims of human rights violations, such as disappearances, extrajudicial killings, unjust detention, torture and rape.

2005 when the proposed Comprehensive Reparations Plan was finally approved and passed into law.[75]

The Comprehensive Reparations Plan is made up of six components that include the restitution of civil rights, education, health care, collective reparations, symbolic reparations, promotion and access to housing, and also provision for economic reparations and compensation.[76] In this way reparations not only complement traditional justice measures, they also provide a means for improving accountability and making the state responsible for its own past acts and omissions.[77]

The PIR was specifically targeted at the 5697 communities registered by the Reparations Council as having been affected by the conflict (1980–2000); it is also perceived as a means for improving the relationship between rural communities and the state.

The programme was first implemented by the Garcia administration in June 2007 using the preliminary registries of who was affected in each of the conflict-affected communities that had been collected by the *Ministerio de la Mujer y Poblaciónes Vulnerables* (MIMDES) (Ministry for Women and Vulnerable Populations) prior to the creation of the Reparations Council.[78]

Between 2007 and 2011 the collective reparations programme focused on small scale infrastructure projects of up to 100,000 soles (approximately US$ 37,000) per community. By 2011 165 million soles (approximately US$ 63 million) had been allocated for 1672 projects, implemented in 1649 communities.[79] However, efforts to include reparations for ESCR violations within the Reparations Plan have led to public criticism of the government's approach to reparations on the grounds that it had failed to properly distinguish between reparations and development programmes.

The government's response to these criticisms was to implement its poverty subsidy programme, JUNTOS (Together) in areas most affected by the political violence. This has generated programmes that are funded from contributions out of the budgets of various ministries, including health, education, housing, labour. In 2005 the Peruvian Congress approved 10 million Peruvian *soles* (approximately US$ 3,076,923) as additional funding for the implementation of the PIR programmes.

These additional funds have been channelled through the *Fondo Nacional de Cooperación para el Desarrollo* (FONCODES), (National Office of Development

[75] Law 28,592 of 2005; *Decreto* 015–2006-JUS, later modified by *Decreto* 003–2008 JUS.

[76] TRC Final Report, *supra* note 12, at Vol. IX, Part 4, Ch. 2.2.

[77] See Falk, R. (2006: 484–5).

[78] MIMDES *Ministerio de la Mujer y Desarrollo* Social (Ministry for Women and Social Development).

[79] U. N. Human Rights Council, "...National report submitted in accordance with paragraph 5 of the annex to Human Rights Council resolution 16/21 [Universal Periodic Review]: Peru," August 7, 2012. From the start of the Humala administration (2011 to present), the pace of reparations has slowed.

Cooperation). The funding is used for improving infrastructure, such as mending school buildings and health posts.

Efforts to provide economic reparations and compensation to victims of the political violence began in July 2010, but the lack of clarity on how the programme would be implemented has generated criticism from amongst victims' organizations, civil society, human rights organizations, as well as the Ombudsman's Office.[80]

In June 2011 Ollanta Humala was elected President and the new premier, Salomón Lerner Ghitis, announced the implementation of those reparations recommended by the TRC. In spite of delays, changes in policies and competing narratives victims of the political violence began to start receiving economic reparations and compensation, although many payments are still outstanding.

In a report about the implementation of reparations in Peru the International Centre for Transitional Justice (ICTJ) said that the delays in economic reparation and compensation are "...inconsistent with the message that a reparations policy should carry.

The government's inability to comply with legislated reparations demonstrates the difficulty that mainstream Peruvian society and most of its political elite have in acknowledging their share of responsibility for the violations committed during the conflict and in accepting the history of marginalization reported by the TRC. It also shows the low importance that the rest of Peruvian society places on the situation of indigenous people."[81]

In addition to collective reparations and compensation the Comprehensive Reparations Plan (PIR) includes programmes intended to provide repair when individual assessments of harms suffered by each victim is not possible. However, the lack of commitment and political will mean that their implementation and execution has been uneven and slow.

Nevertheless, progress has been made in the restitution of civil rights and documentation. In addition to the programmes to help victims obtain their civil documentation implemented by the *Registro Nacional de Identificación y Estado Civil*, or (RENIEC) (National Registry for Identification and Civil Status) efforts to improve civil registration (especially in rural areas) have also been successful.[82]

Though some measures to provide reparations with regard to education have been implemented by private and public educational institutions, the state's role has been largely restricted to a scholarship programme to a limited number of beneficiaries. Even more striking is the lack of any individualized health services provided to victims or any health programmes targeting their unique needs. This is further exac-

[80] The programme was defined by Decree 051–2011-PCM as follows: (a) Paying a lump sum of 10,000 soles (USD 3700) per victim (without a clear explanation of how it had reached that amount); (b) Prioritizing the elderly as an equivalent of vulnerability; and (c) Closing the registry of beneficiaries of compensation on December 31, 2011.

[81] Correa, C. (2013:1).

[82] Correa, C. (2013:21).

erbated by a lack of progress in the recommendations in the PIR for the construction of community health care networks or specialized services delivered to victims.

Instead reparations in health care have been mostly limited to registering victims for the *Seguro Integral de Salud* (SIS), (Comprehensive Health Insurance), even though most victims are already entitled to SIS coverage, either because of their socioeconomic condition or because they are already registered as persons of low-income.[83]

In spite of the Comprehensive Reparations Programme on Mental Health created by the Ministry of Health the lack of psychosocial support and any significant improvement in health care facilities, particularly in rural areas, is a source of major concern.

Though there have been improvements in the level of generalized mental health services offered to the entire population affected by conflict, this does not mean that service providers are able to respond to the needs of victims for certain specialized services.[84]

In spite of pressure from civil society there is no national policy on memorialisation and the restoration of the dignity of the victims. However, this has not prevented local initiatives from erecting monuments of their own. This has happened throughout the country, some of which are located in rural highland communities most affected by the political violence. Though many victims are still waiting to find and identify their next of kin the search for and identification of remains of victims of enforced disappearances and of the missing has made little progress. However, efforts have improved since the creation of a Specialized Forensic Team (SFT) at the Bureau of Forensic Medicine after the Ombudsman's Office brought together the Office of the Prosecutor, the Bureau of Forensic Medicine, the International Commission of the Red Cross, and the *Equipo Peruano de Antropología Forense* (EPAF) (Peruvian Forensic Anthropology Team), and later the *Centro Andino de Investigaciones Antropológico-Forenses* (CENIA) (Andean Centre for Forensic Anthropology Research) as well as other organizations with experience working on exhumations and identifications.

In spite of the widespread destruction of private property, particularly housing in rural communities, little has been done to compensate victims beyond the benefits provided to families of police and armed forces personnel killed during the conflict.[85]

Efforts to investigate acts committed by state agents in the context of the political violence by securing court-ordered reparations have proceeded very slowly. This is reflected in the slow progress made with the trials of people accused of grave crimes, the failure to attach sufficient importance to the needs of victims, together with a

[83] Correa, C. (2013:23).

[84] See *Defensoría del Pueblo, "Informe Defensorial* No 140 - *Salud Mental y Derechos Humanos. Supervisión de la política pública, la calidad de los servicios y la atención a poblaciones vulnerables,*" 225–54, www.defensoria.gob.pe/informes-publicaciones.php

[85] *Defensoría del Pueblo, "Informe Defensorial* No 139," 89–93.

widespread failure on behalf of the state to respect the demands of the families of the disappeared.

In addition the lack of resources to investigate cases in combination with the protection that the Ministry of Defence has given to members of the armed forces who are being investigated demonstrate the lack of commitment on behalf of the state to comply with its obligation to fight impunity by denying information about the identity of personnel located in areas or units where violations were committed.[86] It also sends a message to victims that their rights are not taken seriously, which undermines the effect of the reparations effort.[87] In these circumstances victims cannot mourn because there is no acknowledgement of their suffering on behalf of the state. This is a situation that not only sustains a culture of silence but also induces defences that prevent people from working through the past.

2.5 Unpacking the Lived Experience of Suffering

In circumstances of extreme poverty and deprivation the very nature, scale and ongoing impact of the situation is such that individuals find it difficult to assume responsibility for their own lives.[88] If basic material and psychological needs are not met people's perception of each other and how they see themselves change.[89]

To experience suffering is to undergo a lived experience and this means that it can only be understood through the subjective content that gives it meaning. For this to be recognised the feelings and perspectives of another person need to be properly acknowledged.[90]

This involves "...making the other person feel valued, enabling them to feel their thoughts and feelings have been heard acknowledged and respected."[91]

To unpack established assumptions about human beliefs and behaviour we therefore need to examine the idea that general personality traits are an adequate means of describing and predicting the behaviour of individuals and groups. This idea assumes that human beliefs and behaviour are predetermined and that the outcome

---

[86] See Correa, C., (2013: 27). Further supporting evidence may be obtained from the *Coordinadora Nacional de Derechos Humanos* http://derechoshumanos.pe/. Additionally, *Defensoría del Pueblo*, "*Informe Defensorial* No 139," 242–45, and *Defensoría del Pueblo*, "*Informe Defensorial* No 128 – *El Estado frente a las víctimas de la violencia ¿Hasta dónde vamos en políticas de reparación y justicia?*," 215–28.

[87] Report: Ten Years after Peru's Truth Commission, International Center for Transitional Justice (2013) 5 Hanover Square. Floor 24, New York, NY USA 10004.

[88] Scott Peck, M., (1983: 214).

[89] McCann, I. L., & Pearlman, L. A. (1990a); Pearlman, L. A., & Saakvitne, K. W. (1995).

[90] The frustration of basic psychological needs by social conditions is one cause of groups turning against other groups (Burton, J. 1990a, b; Kelman, H. C. 1990; Staub, E. 1989); Dussaillant, F. & Gonzalez, P. A., (2015: 233–251).

[91] Baron-Cohen, S. (2011: 13).

of interactions between people and the situations they meet are therefore predictable. However, people respond to a particular situation not in an objective manner, but through a 'filter' of their worldview, the way they perceive and cognitively conceive it, and it is crucial we try and understand, interpret and make sense of this.[92]

To facilitate practices of "...stepping imaginatively into the shoes of another person, understanding their feelings and perspectives, and using that understanding to guide your actions"[93] requires the development of a culture that systematically emphasizes the importance of respect for the other.[94]

This requires engagement not only with the personalities and the many other facets that make up the inner reality of human suffering but also with how it is experienced in a particular situation. This requires a reformulation of social, political and institutional responses to human suffering and social need.[95]

To counter the over-objectification of human suffering analytic tools are needed to explore the situation as people perceive and cognitively construct it.[96]

Finding out about the feelings, opinions and attitudes held by people in relation to their situation and how they have sought to come to terms with it help to reveal the adverse effects of material disadvantage. The use of objective categories with regard to different forms of psychological distress does not improve the emotional capacity of the government to engage with the context in which people live their lives. This is not just because the local understanding of psychological distress is inconsistent with the use of objective categorization normally associated with western societies[97]; it is also because suffering is something much more general and elusive.

To "...identify with what someone else is thinking or feeling and to respond to their thoughts and feelings with an appropriate emotion"[98] requires an altogether different approach. To make the other person feel valued, enable them to feel their thoughts have been heard, acknowledged and respected requires a way of thinking that puts the human being at the centre of moral concern. Because it is easy to lose sight of the meaning of suffering through the medium of academic prose the challenge is to provide as nuanced an interpretation as possible. In this respect the approach needs to be holistic and involve the use of analytic tools suited to the development of a historical, ethnographic and narrative investigation.

---

[92] Staub, E., (1999a, b, c, d, e, f).

[93] Krznaric, R., (2014: x).

[94] Schwartz W (2002); Schwartz W (2013).

[95] For further details of the worldview as people perceive and cognitively construct it see Freire, P., (1998: 73).

[96] The idea that the human significance of suffering can be "trivialized to a point that is morally objectionable must not be forgotten." See Frank (2001); Steiner, (1967). This is particularly important in relation to the ways in which Western diagnostic classifications are applied to diverse non-Western survivor populations. See Summerfield, D., (1997: 150).

[97] Bracken, P. J., Giller, J. E., Summerfield, D., (1995).

[98] Baron-Cohen, S. (2011: 12).

How best to configure human suffering amongst people affected by political violence and living in a context of daily survival? First of all, the one supra-individual quality that encapsulates much of its essential character is its inexhaustible, uninhibited ghastliness. Its harmful influence on interpersonal discourse, self-respect, servility, conformity, and much more is such that it can bring about the physical and mental disintegration of the individual and be responsible for their ultimate emotional and psychological collapse.[99]

For people affected by political violence living in a context of daily survival it is a commonplace to be tormented by feelings of inferiority.[100]

The psychological implications of trauma, malnutrition, depression, post-traumatic stress,[101] fear, insecurity, feelings of shame etc.[102] are such that a proper understanding of what people are living through can only be mediated through intensely private individual histories.[103] To make people more alert to the consequences of human suffering the experiences with which it is associated need to be brought into full view in all the various and intricate processes responsible for its unfolding development.

In this respect the individual subjective felt-experience is invaluable for the "...understanding of experience and its aftermath, including the role of memory and its lapses in coming to terms with or denying and repressing the past."[104] This is then a study about how the need to remember the terrible things that people have been forced to endure at the hands of others can be used to bear witness "...to what we do not yet know of our lived historical relation to events of our times."[105]

---

[99] See for example, Abramson, Seligman, and Teasdale (1978); Seligman (1975). Furthermore, work has linked low power to feelings of general uncertainty (Anderson and Galinsky 2006), which itself is often aversive (e.g., Weary et al. 1993). Being powerless is also associated with less access to both physical (e.g., material wealth) and social rewards compared with being powerful (e.g., recognition; Buss, D.M. & Malamuth, N. 1996; Domhoff, G. W., & Zweigenhaft, R.L. 1998; Operario and Fiske 2001).

[100] See for example the address by Pope Francis to the Apostolate of the Suffering and the Silent Workers of the Cross in the Paul VI Hall. May 18, 2014.

[101] See for example: Regel, S. and Joseph, S., (2010: 75); Zoellner, L. A. and Bittenger, J. N., (2004).

[102] Other sources and symptoms of chronic stress and suffering include anxiety, helplessness, isolation, lack of energy and motivation, intensified feelings of guilt and worthlessness, irritability and lethargy, loss of appetite, sleeplessness and insomnia, difficulty making decisions, lack of concentration and suicidal feelings. See for example, Mills, C. & Zavaleta, D., (2015: 251–269).

[103] Examples of mental suffering: grief, sadness, depression (mood), disgust, irritation, anger, rage, hate, contempt, jealousy, envy, craving, yearning, frustration, heartbreak, anguish, anxiety, angst, fear, panic, horror, righteous indignation, shame, guilt, remorse, regret, resentment, repentance, embarrassment, humiliation, boredom, apathy, confusion, disappointment, hopelessness, doubt, emptiness, homesickness, loneliness, rejection, pity, self-pity.

[104] LaCapra, D., (2001: 86–7); Dussaillant, F. & Gonzalez, P. A., (2015: 233–251).

[105] Felman, S. & Laub, D., (1992: x).

2.6 Conclusions

This chapter has shown that the typical Andean community has been shaped by historical forces and social, economic, and political processes that operate from within and outside its own shared elements of cultures and customs. In spite of its location, national and foreign influences have been as important in the evolution of the typical Andean community as those at the local level. In this respect, the historical trajectory of the overall political economy of Peru has been as significant as the environmental and geographic context in which the typical Andean community is located.

From the preceding account it can be appreciated that by the time Shining Path began to focus its attention upon the grievances of the Highland Quechua in the Ayacucho highlands, local feelings about being shut out of opportunities to participate in public life were well established.

Ever since the break-up of the hacienda system began the process had been engulfed in controversy. Instead of putting an end to class conflict, territorial fragmentation and outside pressures, the arguments and debates it generated only served to raise political awareness. It also served to radicalise people.

This is particularly significant in relation to the level of government support for the implementation of the agrarian reform programme in the Ayacucho region. Because it rarely related to local forms of land tenure, the agrarian reform programme reinforced the belief that government officials were ineffective and uncaring. Irrespective of how much time has passed since the end of political violence, this disconnected, impoverished region continues to be affected by these same forces and processes, both with respect to the lack of commitment and political will regarding collective and individual reparations, and with the lack of psychosocial support and any significant improvement in health care facilities.

Chapter 3
Exploring the Aftermath of Political Violence

To counter the over-objectification of human suffering and reorganise our practical and theoretical ways of thinking about individual and social suffering, this chapter sets out to explore the situation as people perceive and cognitively construct it. To bring this perspective into full view, the chapter begins with an overview of the nature of human suffering in rural Andean communities. The chapter also outlines how the arrangements for the selection and identification of the rural Andean communities included in this study were made. The chapter concludes by looking at the experience of violence from the perspective of rural Andean communities, giving particular attention to the poor and vulnerable, and of survivors and victims of the political violence.

3.1 Human Suffering in Rural Andean Communities

From the time when militant activists first began to appear in the rural districts of Ayacucho in the late 1970s, local people would have been under no illusion that they were against all independent forms of organization and political action. In most cases this led to the forced removal of community leaders and widespread murder, rape, torture, disappearances, etc.

People's houses and their possessions were not spared, any more than their land: crops were destroyed, animals killed, possessions stolen. In this terrifying unrest, traditional values of human life and dignity were abandoned in favour of new forms of behaviour and social interaction.

Before the political violence people were usually aware of the duties attaching to the social role they were responsible for as well as for ensuring that other people were fulfilling their roles. But in the aftermath of the political violence support for

T. J. Bowyer, *Beyond Suffering and Reparation*,
https://doi.org/10.1007/978-3-319-98983-9_3

established rules, fixed beliefs and practices has become increasingly doubtful.[1] This makes it easier for people to devalue others, to victimise scapegoats, to join new groups, and adopt new ideas. These changes are making inroads into accepted boundaries and the stability of people's identities, thereby making traditional values and ideologies increasingly meaningless.

To be socially responsible and free from feelings of hopelessness and uncertainty in these conditions is not normal. It is the overwhelming urgency of the situation that shapes the aftermath of political violence and defines the meaning of normal behaviour, not respect for certain duties.[2]

The struggle to stand up to the difficult social/cultural environment *in which people find themselves* is therefore not just about the actual situation as it presents itself; it is also about coping with the feeling that the experience of the political violence is not the absolute limit of all possible suffering. Inadequate physical, human, social, political and environmental resources reduce people's capacity (biological, social, psychological and economic) to satisfy core self-and group-serving needs.[3]

In addition to chronic hunger and poverty people have to contend with the memory of pain and loss, suffering, grief and death. These concerns are a further stimulus to feelings of anxiety, shame, desperation, fear, confusion, withdrawal and self-loathing. Inextricably interlinked with the uncertainty generated by these feelings is the lack of control that people have over the attainment of their own valued outcomes.[4]

The realization that these feelings do nothing to change real conditions severely damages social trust, cooperation and mutual aid because they call into question the usefulness of the individual's actions and their influence. The inability to reduce the physical effects of difficult life conditions causes people to feel frustrated and threatened.[5] It is a situation in which people are compelled to either adapt effectively or suffer the consequences. Over time this devalues self-confidence to such an extent that it impairs people's willingness to be assertive.

This is responsible for the erosion of trust, the escalation of uncertainty and an increasing disillusionment with the future of shared values and norms of behaviour.[6]

---

[1] See Suarez, E., (2013); Charbonneau, B. and Parent, G., (eds.) (2012); Justino, P., (2009); Srinisvasa Murthy, R and Lakshminayaranah, R., (2006); Brinkerhoff, D. W., (2005); Moser, C., (1996); Moser, C., (1998).

[2] Harvey and Weary, (1981).

[3] Chouliaraki, L., (2017, 49–61); Hickel, J., (2017).

[4] Mills, C. & Zavaleta, D., (2015: 251–269).

[5] The frustration of basic psychological needs by social conditions is one cause of groups turning against another group. See Burton, J., (1990a); (1990b); Kelman, H. C., (1990) in Burton, J.W. (ed.)., (1990a, b); Staub, E., (1989).

[6] McCann, I. L., & Pearlman, L. A. (1990a); (1990b); Pearlman, L. A., & Saakvitne, K. W. (1995); Staub, E., (1999c) in Chorbajian, L. & Shirinian, G., (eds) (1999); Programa de las Naciones Unidas para el Desarrollo (PNUD) United Nations for Development (2005); Degregori, C.I., (1987); Instituto Nacional de Estadistica e Informatica Evolucion de la pobreza al 2010 Lima: INEI (2011).

It also increases the risk of exploitation and conflict and makes humiliation and inhumane treatment by society endemic.[7]

The pressure this exerts on existing norms and values calls into question people's assumptions about the world and their interpretation of reality; it also undermines the importance of planning for thc future. The resulting uncertainty and turmoil enable people to argue themselves away from personal responsibility for their actions, adopting instead a way of thinking that is focused on pragmatism and self-preservation.[8]

In the absence of a voice, influence and independence, certain motives predominate in the aftermath of political violence: the protection of the physical self, the preservation of the psychological self, including self-image, personal worldview and values and the attainment of some control over specific problems and outcomes.[9] This erosion of traditional culture and beliefs may have brought greater independence from other individuals and groups, but it has also brought the kind of fear, envy, violence, hatred and other features of social isolation normally associated with western cultures.[10]

Instability, fear of ambiguity, fear of threat and loss, the lack of order and structure, or any number of forms of terror during the political violence may all have contributed to this collapse in the intrinsic value of mutual respect, liberty and justice; but the long term effect of these various influences are often much conflated by the neglect shown by successive government administrations to a people who have already suffered so much and whose dignity and self-respect have been so thoroughly impugned.[11]

In effect, the study explores the combined impact of these various forms of suffering and results suggest that the effect has been to break the resistance of individuals and the group. It is argued that this has led to levels of disconnectedness that are quite unprecedented in rural Andean communities. An erosion of both ethnic identity and the Quechua language has also been accompanied by steady migration of people out of rural areas to towns and cities, resulting in acculturation of indigenous people to dominant Hispanic society.

3.2 Selection of Indicators and Study Communities

To provide an in-depth analysis into the impact of human and social suffering on individuals and groups, particularly with respect to unequal relationships, a number of indicators were developed to identify rural Andean communities affected by

[7] Mills, C. & Zavaleta, D., (2015: 251–269).

[8] Staub, E. (1989:38ff).

[9] Staub, E., (1989); Staub, E. (1996a, b); Staub, E. (1999) in Summers, C and Markussen, D. (eds.); Staub, E., (1999); Staub, E. (1999) in Chorbajian, L. and Shirinian, G. (eds.) 1999).

[10] Mills, C. & Zavaleta, D., (2015: 251–269).

[11] Hickel, J., (2017). Staub, E., (1999a, b, c, d, e, f).

political violence, discrimination and remoteness. These include: legacy of political violence, decline in agricultural production, increasing out-migration, land disputes, isolation, discrimination, remoteness, a deteriorating environment, limited access to basic services. Following consultation with the research team who were familiar with the local area it was agreed that the study communities should be selected from those rural districts most associated with SL activities during its first phase of operations in the Department of Ayacucho in the South-Central Andes.[12]

More specifically, it was felt that selection should be made from provinces (and districts) in which rural communities predominate. These include the Provinces of Huanta, La Mar (in the Zone of Tambo and San Miguel), Huamanga, Cangallo, and Víctor Fajardo (See Appendix 1: Maps). The author also felt that priority should be given to rural communities from districts which have schools in abundance because teachers and students always formed the core following of SL, particularly in the Department of Ayacucho.[13]

Other issues taken into consideration included the degree to which communities had provided passive support for the uprising, particularly from amongst established smallholders.[14] In the final selection every effort was made to reflect the relationship between context and its influence on human nature and responsibility and the failure to usefully explain the social capital discourse.[15]

In this respect the coverage of different geographical areas was less important than the fact that the research communities are all representative of the combined impact of the 20-year political violence and a harsh physical environment. This means that they are all isolated from the centres of political and economic activity, in terms of distance, culture, and psychological affiliation. The final selection consisted of five indigenous communities located in five rural districts from two separate provinces in the Department of Ayacucho in the South-Central Andes.

To show how it is possible to revise the outsider's view that people from the selected communities are an undifferentiated 'other' emphasis is given to the

---

[12] The Department of Ayacucho is located in the central region of the *Cordillera de los Andes* (Andean mountain range), with the Department of Junin to the north, that of Arequipa to the east and those of Ica and Huancavelica to the west. Most of the Department consists of high plains broken up with mountain valleys and has an average altitude of roughly 3500 metres. To the far south-west the country falls towards the coastal plain and in the far north-east towards the tropical jungle on the banks of the River Apurímac. It has a geographical area of 43,814.8km^2 (16,917.0 square miles) and a population density of 14/km^2 (37/sq. mi). According to the 2005 census (INEI, 2005) the total population was 619,338, 43% of which is under 18 years. This represents a population decline of 2.4% equivalent to a negative growth in population of – 147, 624 since the previous census of 1993. The elevation of the capital, Ayacucho is 2746 m (9,009 ft.), the highest elevation in the Department is 3645 m (11,959 ft.) and the lowest elevation is 1800 m (5,900 ft.). Information from the *Programa de las Naciones Unidas para el Desarrollo* (PNUD) (United Nations for Development) (2005) ranks the Department of Ayacucho 20th out of 24 departments (HDI = 0.5095) in relation to data on basic necessities which shows that 82.8% of households have less than basic standard of necessities.

[13] Degregori, C.I., (1987:41–42); Degregori, C. I., (1990).

[14] Coronel, J., (1996:45).

[15] Muller, Adam, et al. (2017).

dynamic nature of the relationship between social context and its influence on human nature and responsibility.

Insofar as they share the same hereditary, environmental and cultural background these communities have much in common. All of the communities selected for research are characterized by a decline in subsistence agriculture, increasing out-migration, and the use of remittances to help with the survival of the community-based household.

3.3 Basic Characteristics of the Study Communities

The five communities selected for research are identified by *pseudonyms*: Otoronco, Wamani, Yachaya, Qocha and Unay and are all located at an elevation of between 2900 m (9,154 ft.) and 3645 m (11,959 ft.).

The communities have dirt roads linking them to the nearest towns between 10 km and 50 km away, as well as paths to some of the surrounding communities. Transport is normally by car, mini-bus, and mule or on foot.

Depending on the community the journey time to the nearest towns can be between 3 and 14 h by car; the roads are in bad repair. Communications between many communities and towns are largely by footpaths. This means that access to markets and prospects for receiving outside help are not generally very good.[16] The amount of agricultural land held by each community varies from between 22 hectares (54 acres) and 882 hectares (2179 acres). The land is made up of natural pastures, farmland plots and land terracing, of the total agricultural land approximately 80% is permanent pasturage and 20% is arable. The lands are undulating and sometimes located at levels of up to 4000 m.[17]

In general, the land is dry and suited to animal husbandry and the intensive cultivation of Andean crops. Some of the land is owned by the community and worked by the farmers who cultivate *minifundios* (small plots owned by the community) of 250 m^2–300 m^2 per household; some of this land is also used for grazing livestock (sheep, goats, cattle). However, the amount of land still owned by the community has been in steady decline for some time with the result that *minifundios* are no longer practiced as extensively as they used to be. The rest is former *hacienda* (estate) land.

The planting months are September–December; during these months the entire population move to the fields; the community and its dwellings remain closed until their return. Work in the fields is between 6:00 am and 6:00 pm. Harvesting occurs

---

[16] See Appendix Two: Access to Andean communities studied.

[17] This form of exploitation has been given the name of vertical ecology or the Andean Archipelago by John Murra (see bibliography in Billie Jean Isbell's To Defend Ourselves 1968, 1970, 1972 and 1975). Murra argues that pre-Inkaic kingdoms-controlled production and redistribution of diverse zones often over large distances. The *Inka* pattern of agricultural production and distribution followed the same model.

May–July. Produce from the land is mainly for subsistence although a small amount is sold or bartered for essential goods such as sugar, rice, oil, noodles, and so forth in the neighbouring community market.

The majority of heads of households also have plots of approximately 750 m^2 each; however, a small percentage of household heads have much larger plots of land that have either been bought or inherited.

More than 60% of the population of each community studied is engaged in cattle raising, whilst approximately 25% are involved in sheep and llama raising, 5% in breeding small animals and 5% in other activities, including running a craft and weaving centre.

All these rural communities used to have communal land, yet today only one of the five selected communities (Otoronco) still has these.

These are used for the cultivation and distribution of products to members of Otoronco. It is the only resource that the community continues to manage together. This can be demonstrated by the following statement: "Before the violence the community felt closed; people did not leave the community; they did not know about anything that happened, but that has all gone." Author's field research: Interviewee from Yachaya (Marcos).

Before the political violence each community was characterised by groups of one or two room adobe houses with dirt floors, sometimes interspersed with a few two-storey houses belonging to the richer members of the community.[18] Before the violence community life was focused on the main square with its church, meeting house for community assemblies and a few small stores. The current population size of each community varies from between 400 to 4000 inhabitants of whom about 30% are between the ages of 10 and 14 and most of the others between 45 and 59.[19] Each community consists predominantly of Quechua Indians. On average an estimated 70% of each community is a Quechua speaker and 30% are bilingual in Quechua and Castilian.

[18] Most community housing used to be constructed of adobe or of *tapia*. This is an ancient technique consisting of building walls with damp earth, compacted by a "tamper." In Latin America this is known as *tapia* (rammed earth wall) or *tapial* in Spain and the Mediterranean basin. The frame is usually made of wood, but it may also be metal. The process consists of earth being poured into the frame which is then compacted by ramming. The compacted clay is then left to dry in the sun. The destruction of so much community housing during the political violence means that concrete tiles and calamine are increasingly used to replace more traditional roofing materials, although many houses continue to rely on Ichu. In the five research communities studied, dirt floors in people's houses are standard; every household has to rely on candles for lighting because none of the research communities have access to any or any regular supply of electricity.

[19] Results are taken from the survey carried out for this study in 2009.

3.4 Experiences of Violence

To bring all the various intricate processes shaping its development into full view it is important to situate the emotional consequences of suffering within the peak period of political violence from 1980 to 2000.

The number of people's houses destroyed in each community studied varies between 70 and 200; the number of people 'disappeared' by the military is estimated to be between 3 and 10 villagers per community and anything between 3 and 9 villagers killed by SL.

The total official number of people killed in each community ranges between 40 and 70.[20] However, the actual number is likely to be higher and remains a subject of dispute.[21]

One survivor describes his experience of the killing process as follows: "I saw the terrorists killing people. They killed people by rounding them up and after killing them they would bury them in a pit. This is what the terrorists and the army did to us. I felt sad for my village because my village was completely destroyed." Author's field research: interviewee from Qocha (Agustina).

In spite of the impact of the political violence most people continue to identify themselves as members of the community and of Quechua Indian identity. Nevertheless, the political violence has deeply affected the culture and structure that give shape to community life: "Before we lived better, when it appeared those who walk the night (SL) began to kill people and take our animals then we lived hidden behind the hills, sleeping amongst the rocks, then people began to escape to the cities." Author's field research: interviewee from Wamani (Clementina).

Though people have sought to rescue aspects of identity that served them before the political violence, the recovery of their culture and structure and the restoration of a life worth living continue to be troubled by the memory of suffering as the following testimony indicates: "People say that bad people escape among the innocent. Whether people are still scared or not, I don't pay attention to it. My compatriots are now elderly. Whenever they hear something, they stop crying and say 'when will we ever be left alone?' I think those people are still coming back." Author's field research: interviewee from Unay (Santos).

This distrust is especially evident in the relationships between individuals and groups, including those between men and women, parents and their children, traditional leaders and the community, local authorities and the community. A survivor describes the tensions created by this situation: "Among those who lived here during the violence and the returnees there is a division. Those who continued to live here during the violence have been marginalized, for example my elderly mother and I

---

20 Pers. Comm.

21 Between 2008 and 2011 (the period during which the fieldwork for this study was being carried out), a number of mass graves, hitherto unknown and unreported were discovered and subsequently shown to individual members of the study team.

have been alone in those times that people lived and died like dogs." Author's field research: interviewee from Otoronco (Sanchez).

No one has provided an account of what happened because people are still too afraid to talk about it. Villagers detained by the military were held in a military base but no one was willing to provide any solid information about how many people this involved or how many detainees were still missing.

To be locked into such utter helplessness forced the majority of people to stay in a permanent psychological present that makes it all but impossible to address unresolved issues or insufficiently understood problems most often outside the individual's own control.

Feelings of hostility and self-destructive revenge fantasies are normal responses to abusive treatment as the following testimony demonstrates:

"The military came and took people away, they lied and people disappeared. Many families don't know what happened to their missing. After that people began to hate each other, accusing each other of being terrorists and others were saying that they were in the military and killed innocent people." Author's field research: interviewee from Unay (Lidia).

For the five communities studied the political violence began after initial encounters with SL. Although early contacts could be more ideological than violent, later people's houses were destroyed, and the inhabitants fled their village to live in makeshift huts in the countryside. This began in the early 1980s.

A survivor describes how these early encounters with SL began in her community: "This is all about the time of the political violence when strangers came to the community with their political speeches telling us that we will not see poverty again and that we will all be equal. This was how they got us to allow them to come into the community. But because we would not support them they killed a man whilst he was still in bed, then they killed an old couple with a knife. These people were the first victims of the rebels." Author's field research: interviewee from Qocha (Agustina).

In the mid-80s the violence and killing of people– especially leaders – escalated. People found it increasingly difficult to plan their own behaviour because it was impossible to know the rules according to which the world around them was operating. For many the constant fluctuation between hope and despair, faith and doubt, between fooling themselves and resignation became unavoidable.

To escape from the abusive situation survivors were compelled to live in a state of permanent insecurity as the following indicates: "I have lived here since 1987 and have seen terrorist raids, deaths, kidnappings, torture. I was so afraid because I was a community leader and my name was wanted by the *Senderistas* (SL), I lived moving from one place to another because I was one of the community authorities; I was so afraid of the raids." Author's field research: interviewee from Qocha (Valentin).

By the early 1970s the rural elite and the rich peasantry started to leave the Peruvian countryside for the security of the towns and cities. This was the prelude to what became the most intense period of violence, affecting both urban and rural areas and continuing throughout the general elections of 1990.

The emotional state of the community during this time would be dominated by helplessness and terror, panic, fury and despair as the following testimony indicates: "It all started in 1982. I moved from one place to another. In those days, we were not united. When the terrorists came looking for the authorities and killed them, saying that you were informers, they asked who the authorities were. They came talking politics, saying that they would be alright with you, but it was not like that. They tortured the authorities, hanging them in most of the villages round here." Author's field research: interviewee from Wamani (Sabino).

The struggle to withstand such a difficult environment was not just about the situation as it presented itself; it was also about insecurity, anxiety, fear, low self-esteem, social isolation and lack of control over work and home life and weakening social integration and their impact on the internal resources of the individual.[22] It was also about coping with the feeling that the experience of the political violence was not the absolute limit of all possible suffering.

Though the traumatised person does not always retain a clear memory of what happened to them, it is equally likely that they will remember everything in detail, but without emotion, as the following indicates: "Here in our community there were several murders; there was also a clandestine cemetery which the cops used to bring people from different places and at night so we did not know who they were because after the killing the bodies had been originally buried alongside the riverbank….In those years I saw people killed and brought to the edge of the river to the buried creatures and then later on the dogs ate the remains." Author's field research: interviewee from Otoronco (Carlos).

In the period that followed the State's response remained somewhat muted until the government adopted a severe counterinsurgency strategy in January 1983. This coincided with the increase in terrorist activities by SL that was matched by large scale human rights violations and massacres by the police and the armed forces[23] Between 40 and 60 armed incursions were launched on the five communities included in this study. Some incursions were by the military, but most were carried out by SL, the often-arbitrary violence generating a legacy of distrust.

For people overwhelmed by terror and helplessness the normal connections of memory, knowledge and emotion are destroyed, which means that "...the whole apparatus for concerted, coordinated and purposeful activity is smashed,"[24] as the following testimony indicates: "Before I couldn't stop thinking about where my parents were. All I could think about was how I wanted to see them, and I would start crying. I used to have nightmares and couldn't get to sleep, but it's not so bad now. But sometimes when you remember things, you can't hold back. When I see

---

[22] Mills, C. & Zavaleta, D., (2015: 251–269).

[23] See *Comisión de la Verdad y Reconciliación, Informe Final* [CVR Final Report] (Lima, 2003), www.cverdad.org.pe/ifinal/index.php. Vol. VIII, conclusion 55 at 323. These violations by the state are highlighted in a report carried out for the International Center for Transitional Justice. See Correa, C. (2013:1).

[24] Kardiner, A., & Spiegel, H., (1947: 186) cited in Herman, J., (1992: 35).

people I don't know, I wonder what kind of people they are. Maybe they belong to the Shining Path." Author's field research: interviewee from Wamani (Lorgio).

To oppose the insurrection more effectively the military set up bases in some villages. Local people seized on suspicion of subversive activity would be held in these bases for questioning; as yet there is no solid information about the number of detainees or the number people that went missing.

Nearly everyone that agreed to discuss their experiences felt unable to provide an independent account of what had happened to the detainees. However, one person agreed to talk a little about his experience of torture during detention: "When I was detained I was brutally hit until I could take it no longer. Then I got taken to Lima and then they made me disappear. I have a crippled arm, and when I am busy working, it goes to sleep, which makes it hurt all over. When I was taken prisoner they [the military] treated me horribly. They would hang me by my arm attached to a rope, but I was unable to see who was doing it as I had a hood over my head." Author's field research: interviewee from Yachaya (Alejandro).

The army was also responsible for arbitrary arrests and torture, with lasting consequences as the following demonstrates: "That night when they (the army) took me they put me in a corner in an office, I felt the sounds of the typewriter, every time I felt cold, thirsty and asked for a drink they grabbed me by the hair and hit me against the wall, each time I asked they did that, and I fell on the floor to stop them kicking, then from there they took me prisoner. I was a year and six months in prison. There was this fellow that tried to heal me for two years but it damaged the cerebellum." Author's field research: interviewee from Otoronco (Luigi).

In Qocha the military moved into the community in the late 1980s. They stayed for about 12 months, claiming they would help defend the surrounding communities from terrorist attack.

However, many interviewees' testimonies confirm that during their stay the military began to abuse local people almost as badly as SL. Though some of these abuses could have resulted from confusion about people's identities, it is the widespread use of sexual violence, which generally distinguished the military from the SL: "In Qocha kidnappings occurred almost every day while the military were here. Every night they would go about in search of ladies and girls to take to the barracks. The ones who had been kidnapped normally had to stay for two or three days; after violating them they would be released four days later; it was the same thing with other women who they took from other places. Here there were about 50 or 60 kidnappings, especially amongst young women and ladies of good appearance." Author's field research: interviewee from Qocha (Julio).

This kind of violence was justified by the military on the grounds that villagers belonged to subversive groups. However, any complaint about human rights violations risked imprisonment or being 'disappeared'. It was this situation that helped to transform how the individual experienced other people.

Instead of perceiving them as a source of social support, comfort and self-realization other people became a source of anxiety and tension. In the case of Qocha, there were four raids on the community by the military that led to serious abuses of the villagers.

One of the survivors continues to relive what happened as though nothing will ever allow her to break away from what happened: "The army rounded us up so they could watch us and they wouldn't let us leave because the authorities said that if the army left people would disappear…the terrorists would take away our animals at night and the army would do the samc and they would sell our animals even while we were watching. In our village they killed members of my family; you couldn't say anything even if it was your brother. It was better to hide yourself so that your brother would not recognise you because if he recognised you the army would also accuse you of being a terrorist and kill you. They would tell members of my family that they were terrorists and rape and kill them just for the fun of it." Author's field research: interviewee from Qocha (Felisa).

These military raids led to villagers (at least five) going missing and they have never been seen since, including a community leader. In addition, in all these raids, an unspecified number of people were tortured by the military and there were an unknown number of sexual violations of women and teenagers and destruction of livestock.

Similarities between SL and military tactics were often mentioned: "I'm alive because I escaped a lot. The terrorists entered my house and burned it; the terrorists took my animals and ate them; this was what the military did as well. In 1984 I was an authority in the village so I had to hide from both sides; there was much violence; they killed 3 of my brothers, they also executed people working in the fields. The terrorists always looked to the authorities to kill them; thank God I'm alive yet." Author's field research: interviewee from Yachaya (Yufemia).

In Otoronco the military forced people from neighbouring villages to assemble together to prevent people from being confused with SL. Interestingly, this tactic was also used by SL in earlier stages of the political violence. Under the military as with SL, as one interviewee reports, this became a pretext for further displacement and the destruction of more houses: "The houses of those who had problems with the Shining Path were destroyed and they used the wood from the roofs as fuel to cook their meals. They set mine (my parents') on fire and bombed it…. The situation was very tense...if the soldiers noticed that I had a candle lit while I was cooking in the evening, they would yell 'fuckers, turn off the light or I'll shoot you'." Author's field research: interviewee from Qocha (Joaquin).

The feeling of being under attack from both SL and the military quickly became so strong that people chose to abandon the community altogether. Some survivors find it impossible to prevent themselves reliving their traumatic experiences: "They began raping the girls; it started in the afternoon when they went to pick up girls as a kind of scam saying that this girl has some problems that need sorting out so she has to go to the barracks and this was how these people (military) started to abuse the humble people; they also stole our sheep, our chickens, our pigs; any animals found walking on thc street and it was for them. They entered houses by force, by kicking the door down and some people would jump in fright; they were not afraid to mistreat us, not afraid to give a kick to a mother or a village elder and when people started crying or screaming they all responded with such profanity and used their rifle butt to hit the women and the elderly." Author's field research: interviewee from Otoronco (Esteban).

From March 1989 to September 1992 the political violence intensified as its focus became increasingly directed at towns and cities, including the capital Lima.

This period is also associated with the mass exodus of many people from their highland communities, fleeing the region to take refuge in caves and in the mountains; others preferred to make for neighbouring communities and then moving on from there to the towns and cities.

One survivor of this upheaval captures the extreme urgency of those times: "After the military started to physically abuse us they started to rape the women who stayed, and they accused many others of terrorism so we were attacked by both sides. It was then that people began to escape at night, and we all went to different places, to save our lives." Author's field research: Interviewee from Otoronco (Miguel).

In such a situation the feelings, attitudes and behaviour of people are as unpredictable as they are subject to almost indefinite revision. "I used to sleep on the side of the mountain, in the caves along with my children. Every night I slept in different places but they always pursued us." Author's field research: interviewee from Otoronco (Maria).

Following the capture of Abimael Guzman the leader of Shining Path, in 1992 the *rondas campesinas* (autonomous peasant patrols originally set up by rural communities as a protection force against theft) became increasingly active.

In the final phase of the violence (1992–2000) this led to a much closer working relationship with the armed forces including exchange of information, joint patrols and establishment of *comites de autodefensa* (self-defence committees).[25] It is estimated that between 30–40 men from each of the Andean communities studied participated in the *rondas* during this period.

Not all the participation was voluntary, since punishments were notably harsh for those reluctant to take part as the following statement illustrates: "I arrived late for training and as punishment I was put in a dark hole in the ground and the military then urinated on me, then they poured dirty cold water on me; then a dead dog on me; much later after getting me out of the hole hungry and cold they beat me and broke my teeth." Author's field research: interviewee from Unay (Nestor).

Later, upon learning that the violence had started to recede, the people from Otoronco started to return to their communities, "but very discreetly." This was done with the cooperation of the self-defence committee.

For most villagers, the self-defence committees played a vital part in arming villagers to prevent attacks. "Life was impossible during the time of the terrorism; we always had to flee.... At the time I did not live well, I lived scared, I always escaped to the mountain and returned to my house at 5 in the morning, I was afraid of the people because they walked around armed, they killed people for whatever reason. Once we had guns we did not have to escape." Author's field research: interviewee from Otoronco (Evita).

[25] The *comites de autodefensa* are governed by Decreto Supremo No. 077/DE-92 Cap.iii Art.28.

Having re-established under the protection of the self-defence committees, the returnees would resettle under cover of darkness, and start to re-construct houses in areas (hills, valleys, mountains) safe from the military and SL. This made it possible for people to leave the village for the *chakra* to re-start the cultivation of their farms.

Initially this happened in secret and only under the supervision of the self-defence committees as the following testimony explains: "After 1993 we started to return and rebuild the village and start working on the land again; however, this was difficult because the land was overgrown and the state and institutions did not provide any support on how to recover or maintain the land." Author's field research: interviewee from Otoronco (Fidel).

Over time the self-defence committees were able to help create a bridge in the relationship between the displaced/returnees, the military and other state departments and NGOs. Towards the end of the violence, this bridging role helped to bring about the internal regeneration of the communities.

3.5 Conclusions

Nowadays, people in the communities studied are more inclined to fear drug traffickers than SL, although it is often difficult to tell them apart since drug traffickers frequently contract former guerrillas (eg. as 'mules' *muchilleros*).

Like many other people affected by political violence the situation in which the families and communities in this study find themselves mean that they are compelled to internalise their status as survivors. Though the debilitating effects of foreclosed mourning are likely to lead to a pervasive paralysis and deadening of intellectual, mental and emotional life it also takes people beneath what the theologian Paul Tillich called "...the routines of ordinary life."

For the people of the communities studied this has brought them face to face with the limitations of their own way of life and the norms and values that used to direct and control it.

In many cases this has not brought any greater understanding because the suffering that has accompanied these experiences has made people paralysed by their ordeal. Nevertheless, the emotional reaction to this new situation has the potential to give people a more accurate appreciation of what they can and cannot control.

By successfully confronting the painful truth that the old ways are ill-equipped to cope with the new environment people are in a position to forge a new identity out of the recognition that survival demands nothing less. To this end this study focuses on determining the influence of culture, context and institutions (and the subjective nature that the individual brings to their situation) to determine what happens to people who suffer from economic and all the other hardships, including social injustice and political oppression.[26]

[26] Dussaillant, F. & Gonzalez, P. A., (2015: 233–251) Lifetime Suffering and Capabilities in Chile in Anderson, R.E. (ed) *World Suffering & the Quality of Life*, Springer.

Chapter 4
Losing Trust in the World

Before the political violence, shared experiences (including values and grievances), adversarial attributions and the intervention of society at large, defined the boundaries of what the individual could be and do.[1] This intimate connection between the needs and obligations associated with collective based group-mindedness and practical identity means that people were living through their social group.[2] Before the political violence, people would rarely have violated their obligations, compared with what takes place since the violence. This change is best explained if values of solidarity, equilibrium and duality, which strengthen the cultural identity of indigenous people, were less exposed to the influences of the dominant culture, before the violence. Before values were eroded, people still had the capacity to influence one another in psychologically meaningful ways because they seldom encountered situations where a choice had to be made between incompatible obligations. Consequently, people were better-placed to realize their intended goals.[3] The cumulative effect of violence has been that people lack a moral framework to fall back on and emotional support systems to depend on. Having nothing left to lose, and no status to maintain is to live without pride or dignity. This creates a world devoid of meaning and outside of what, by those of us who do not have to endure such conditions, is understood as an ordinary life.

Using the idea of the development of critical engagement and the need for free and open social spaces this chapter presents testimonials from survivors of the political violence.

The purpose is twofold: to take into account the full complexities of the situations in which the traumatized found themselves and to explore the intense psychic pain and confusion that these situations have since been responsible for. To avoid

[1] Simon, B. & Klandermans, B., (2001).

[2] Korsgaard, C., (1996: 101).

[3] These include: 1) physical resources such as food, water, shelter, safety; 2) economic resources such as money, material goods, employment opportunities; 3) social resources, including acceptance, a sense of control, social support and a trusting social environment.

T. J. Bowyer, *Beyond Suffering and Reparation*,
https://doi.org/10.1007/978-3-319-98983-9_4

any unintentional "…trivialization and disrespect"[4] this study explores the experiences of survivors of the violence by gathering many oral testimonies in the belief that this deepens our understanding of human suffering in a way that over-reliance on a mere handful of accounts does not.[5]

4.1 Key Traumatic Events in the Rural Andean Communities Studied

Most rural Andean people have no access to counselling and advice with which they can work through their trauma. This means that memories of the political violence and how people continue to deal with such memories are vitally important.[6] To gauge this loss of older, more positive views of the world and of themselves, rural Andean people affected by the political violence were invited to tell the story of their traumatic experiences.[7] For any assessment of the relationship between the traumatic experiences and the present situation it is necessary to begin by looking at the facts relating to the events of past violence (time, place, duration and those involved). Important information was gathered about: the person's role during the event (as observer or as participant, active or passive); a detailed description of the events; the individual and social dimensions of the experience, and the person's perceptions and feelings at the time of the event. Testimony-based evidence is placed in five categories:

1. *Material deprivation* including lack of shelter, food or water;
2. *Bodily injury* such as beatings or sexual violence;
3. *Forced confinement and coercion* including forced separation from family, and forced labour;
4. *Disappearance, death or injury of loved ones*, including disappearance or kidnapping of spouse; murder, or death due to violence, of son or daughter; or other close relatives, and
5. *Witnessing violence to others* including witness to torture; witness to rape or sexual abuse.[8]

---

[4] Markle, G. E., et al. (1992); see also Berger, R. J. (2011: 11).

[5] See for example Shamai Davidson who suggested that this approach allows for a perspective that are "denied some individual survivors as they were preoccupied by the bitter drama of their own battle for survival." Davidson, S., (1992: 24); see also Berger, R. J. (2011: 11)

[6] Schreuder, B., Kleijn, W. & Rooijmans, H. (2000); Schreuder, B., et all (2001).

[7] Weine, S., et al. (1998); Cienfuegos, A. & Monelli, C. (1983).

[8] The five general categories derive from five of the eight general categories used by the Harvard Trauma Questionnaire (HTQ) and (HSCL-25).

4.2 Material Deprivation

Material deprivation is part of political violence. Its range of influence is immense. Experiences such as lack of food, shelter, sanitation and safe drinking water belie other less visible but equally potent forces including the death or disappearnace of close friends, or family members, exposure to combat and dead bodies, social exclusion. Their ultimate impact is the same - to undermine hope and threaten people's health and well-being.[9] The result is increased risks of chronic disease, injury, stunted infant development, stress, anxiety and depression, and premature death. In these circumstances marginal groups such as women, children, ethnic minorities, and the disabled are especially vulnerable.[10] For people caught up in the political violence the abject images (tattered clothing, dirt, unwashed faces and bodies) are a mere distraction from the emergence of new illnesses, increasing malnutrition and poor health outcomes. It is a situation in which almost anyone would feel devalued, helpless, uncared for, hopeless and isolated.

Material deprivation is not just about the suffering of people driven from their homes; it is also about "…the atrophy of any sense of having a place in a community, and of one's social exclusion and devaluation as a human being."[11]

4.2.1 Lack of Shelter

Following the outbreak of violence people were often forced to flee their homes. Those that chose to hide and wait for the persecution to cease faced the very real threat of being betrayed or tracked down and killed. This story is typical: "In 1983 strangers (SL) entered the community, making speeches about the rich and poor that they are fighting for equality. We listened to these speeches but we were against the recruitment of our young people into the ranks of the strangers. This led to the killing of several villagers; the rest of us fled to sleep in caves, mountains, hills; we did not return home". Author's field research: interviewee from Yachaya (Victor).

These experiences were commonplace prompting many thousands of people from across the Ayacucho Emergency Zone (EMZ)[12] to flee their communities and ultimately seek refuge in the jungle or urban centres, including Lima.[13] A young girl who survived the political violence describes her own traumatic experiences: "They (SL) came one night and kicked people, then they grabbed them, and gathered everyone in the chapel and killed them; at that time, I was a kid and I escaped. I slept

[9] Hinton, D., Ba, Peou, & Um, (2000); Weine, S. M., Becker, D. F., McGlashan, T. H., Laub, D., Lazrove, S., Voivoda, D., Hyman, L., (1995).

[10] Loppie Reading, C., & Wien, F. (2009); Kirk, R.E., (1995); Alcade, M. Cristina, (2010)

[11] Wilkinson R. G. (1996: 215); Desjarlais, R., Eisenberg, L., Good, B., & Kleinman, A. (1995).

[12] The Ayacucho Emergency Zone (EMZ) was established during the government of President Fernando Belaúnde in January 1983. This covered the whole of the south-central region and was responsible for the counter-insurgency war being handed over to the armed forces. Gonzalez, O. M., (2011: 44ff).

[13] La Serna, M., (2012: 198ff).

in caves, ravines, hills. I slept outside for several years." Author's field research: interviewee from Wamani (Gabriel).

For some this was no more than a temporary refuge from which they would plan their migration into the nearest towns and cities. However, it was also a means by which people could remain close to their community, even if this led to them being trapped in zones of conflict, caught in the cross-fire and at risk of further persecution.

The overwhelming majority tended to be those most at risk of physical attack, sexual assault and abduction, including the elderly, women and children.[14] The misery of those times and the kind of life it imposed on the most vulnerable people is recalled in the following: "From the start of the violence, we hid in the mountains, caves and hills, escaping from these strange and unknown things. We spent most of the time in the mountains alongside our animals, and only went down to the village for certain things." Author's field research: interviewee from Yachaya (Lupe).

The element of surprise, the threat of death and destruction made the need for prolonged vigilance as inevitable as much as the feelings of fear, mistrust and isolation. However, such sustained misery is likely to shatter the sense of connection between the individual and their community as the following illustrates: "We slept with our shoes on in case we had to escape in a hurry. We lived on the run going from hill to hill; we fled because the Shining Path could have arrived at any moment. The Shining Path surprised people while they were sleeping and would kill them. They killed my neighbour and took our animals. Because of all this I left my village." Author's field research: interviewee from Wamani (Victoria).

In the early years people fled their homes out of fear of SL, but as the violence escalated this also happened out of fear of the military and through acts of betrayal from neighbours and friends.[15] Intense surprise, humiliation, helplessness and loss of control intensify the need for protective attachments as much as they cause people to lose trust in themselves, in other people, and in their community as the following testimony demonstrates:

"One night they let my husband go and at about midnight he came back to the house. The military had told him: 'leave with all of your family. If you don't leave, I'll kill them all.' At that point we grabbed our children and went into the hills, with the soldiers watching us. When we got into the hills, they started firing bullets, saying that they would kill us, and that it would've been better for him if he had stayed behind. So, then we hid in a cave." Author's field research: interviewee from Otoronco (Fidel).

In most highland communities this situation continued throughout the scorched-earth and no-prisoners policy advocated in 1984 by General Clemente Noel into the early-1990s until the capture of the leader of SL, Abimael Guzman.[16] For the survivors of the political violence that agreed to take part in this study "… the salient characteristic of the traumatic event(s) is its power to inspire helplessness

[14] See Boesten, J., (2014).
[15] Kirk, R., (1995: 354–367) Chaqwa. In Starn, O., Degregori, C. I., Kirk, R., (1995).
[16] See Poole, D. & Renique, G., (1992).

and terror,"[17] as the following testimony illustrates: "I felt bad about both the military and the terrorists because both sides abused us: my children hid in the caves. I could not eat; I was like crazy, desperate." Author's field research: interviewee from Unay (Gracia).

4.2.2 *Lack of Food or Water*

Hunger dominated the lives of people throughout the political violence. Food stocks, livestock and other assets were routinely destroyed by both the military and SL. In addition, food supplies would be regularly diverted from people and used by combatants, particularly the military. One survivor explains how this would happen: "We were living up in the highlands with our animals. After a long time, they made us come down so that they could take our sheep. In the end it was only the military that got to eat them.

If you tried to stop them (the military) you would be kicked and hit. When those things happened, people didn't say anything, they just hid away." Author's field research: interviewee from Qocha (Agustina).

By cutting off sources of food or livelihood people found themselves unable to dissociate from the helplessness with which such actions were associated as the following testimony illustrates: "The terrorists would take away our animals at night and the army would do the same and they would sell our animals even while we were watching." Author's field research: interviewee from Otoronco (Evita). Unable to access the food that they would normally grow themselves meant that people had little option but to leave their homes. The impassive and wordless quality of traumatic memories is captured in the following testimony: "I cried so much when they obliterated my brothers, my stomach hurt so much because there was nothing to eat. My husband felt bad that I cried a lot to see that my children had no water and nothing to eat." Author's field research: interviewee from Unay (Maximo).

Food supplies from outside can ultimately be restored, but the destruction included all aspects of production including water sources rendering traditional pastures and local grazing unviable. The impact of this on people's well-being was exacerbated by the effects of the political instability on their access to local markets and networks. Normally markets and networks would have provided some support during times of scarcity, but the political violence made this unworkable. Unable to obtain outside support meant that people became increasingly nomadic with devastating consequences for themselves and their families as the following testimony demonstrates:

"I moved from one place to another. Then when we got to Wamani; the community cursed us, saying we were terrorists. We fled again. I had no clothes to wear, nothing to eat. Many people lived like this." Author's field research: Interviewee from Qocha (Agustina). Even for those able to secure food for themselves and their

[17] Herman, J. (1992: 34).

families the situation became so difficult that many chose to leave rather than submit to the restrictions of a military occupation of their community.

4.2.3 Ill Health and Inadequate Health Care

The public health impact of hunger, lack of shelter and other consequences of the political violence have various manifestations. The most powerful damage to be inflicted by traumatic experiences is reflected in the way in which survivors are able to recount horrific experiences as if they were ordinary events and of no significance. This sense of alienation and indifference is illustrated in the following testimony: "The army also started to kill us. During these years we lived with nothing to eat hidden in the hills and on the run from the Shining Path. Due to what we went through we are now more vulnerable to illnesses. We saw a lot of corpses, the terrorists burned our house and all our animals were stolen." Author's field research: interviewee from Wamani (Lorgio).

For people in the research communities' outbreaks of nervous attacks, communicable diseases, under-nutrition and eventually malnutrition have been responsible for worsening vulnerability and insecurity, abandonment of their livelihoods and rising poverty levels.[18]

Because post-traumatic symptoms are readily associated with inner deadness and indifference to external life it can mean that health problems relating to physical damage inflicted on people are overlooked, even though they may well continue to persist long after the political violence, as the following testimony illustrates: "We were caught between the two sides, and there was no peace or trust among any of them; the military and the *sinchis* constantly beat us.[19] Many of us died after the beatings, like in the case of the community's president, who died after suffering for some time from a lung ailment. Many of the people they beat are still ill today." Author's field research: interviewee from Otoronco (Paloma). The breakdown of health and social services and the heightened risk of disease transmission are exacerbated by the fact that the health consequences of the political violence have not received adequate attention from the public health sector and its policies as many other causes of illness and death.[20] This is happening in spite of the fact that the indirect consequences of the political violence are still being felt.[21]

---

[18] The local term for the profound exhaustion brought about by the political violence and the suffering of the *sasachakuy tiempo* is *iquyasaqa*. This can be literally translated as "weakness". See Theidon, K., (2013: 47ff).

[19] *Sinchis*: a special US-trained "counterterrorist" police battalion that became notorious in the 1980s for their human rights violations. The word comes from the Inca term for warrior-chief.

[20] For further details see the report: Peru on Health in the Americas (2012 Pan American Health Organization (PAHO)).

[21] Murray, C J L., King, G., Lopez, A. D., Tomijima, N., Krug E G (2002).

4.2.4 Confiscation or Destruction of Personal Property

Initial rural people's support for SL[22] and its message of social change was rapidly lost in the late 70's following its deployment of intimidation, terror, murder, sexual violence and the destruction of anything thought useful to an enemy while advancing through or withdrawing from an area. In the communities studied these practices also extended to theft and killing of livestock, the destruction of crops, the looting and burning of houses. An interviewee said that: "…it was easy to burn our houses as they were only made of *ichu*."[23] Author's field research: interviewee from Unay (Reyes).

For SL the destruction of property was done for strategic/political reasons as well as strategic/operational reasons. In many cases SL simply used the destruction of property as a reprisal against anyone whom they considered unsympathetic to their activities, so that: "The houses of those who had problems with the Shining Path were destroyed and then they used the wood from the roofs as fuel to cook their meals. They set mine (my parents') on fire and bombed it." Author's field research: interviewee from Otoronco (Ricardo).

Those known to cooperate with the government, and even with civilian government employees, for example engineers or medical staff, were often targeted in such attacks on property as the following testimony illustrates: "I used to lodge some engineers that worked on constructing a road and when the terrorists came they used to tell me that because I lodged those black vultures they would burn my things and my house. I had 6 young children and, when they burned my property, we escaped. On seeing this, the engineers brought straw from high up in order to thatch my house again as they felt sorry for us. Having seen this, the terrorists burned my house again, so I went to live in the forest with my family." Author's field research: Interviewee from Unay (Gabie). Incidents such as these were commonplace following the decision by SL to launch its *Plan de Conquistar Bases de Apoyo Revolucionarios* (Plan to Conquer Bases of Revolutionary Support) in the early 1980s. Another similar testimony reported: "I was between 11-12 years old at the time. I remember that at about 8 pm the terrorists entered the houses to burn them down; we escaped up the mountains, when we woke up we returned and they had burned the community assembly house near the main square; they had also killed 10 people." Author's field research: interviewee from Yachaya (Rebecca).

Following the arrival of the military to the area and the unleashing of its own counter-insurgency campaign the confiscation and destruction of personal property became increasingly widespread. For example, opposition to the forcible recruitment of young people in Otoronco, led to reprisals by the military against the entire community that included several murders, widespread theft, destruction and forced

[22] This is a reference to the early stage of the SL uprising when it made use of land scarcity and dissatisfaction with corrupt officials to appeal to the peasant's moral code and so win over people from rural highland communities.

[23] Ichu is a type of grass that grows throughout the Andean *altiplano*. It is used as fodder for livestock, like the llama.

displacement. One of these oppressed reported: "My house was burnt down and demolished because they said that my house was a terrorist's house, and then they ate all my animals. So, in fear, we escaped on foot to live in the hills." Author's field research: informant from Wanani (Rosa). Another said that this would involve the theft of personal possessions (clothing, household items) as well as their livestock, on a large scale: "… They took all the community animals and everything they could which included about 500 livestock (cows, sheep, pigs, goats) and headed for the highlands." Author's field research: interviewee from Yachaya (Tomas).

4.2.5 Forced Evacuation Under Dangerous Conditions

Terrorism, armed violence and military activity frequently compelled people to leave their homes. Sometimes this happened because they were directly threatened or subjected to the actual use of force. One such survivor said that he and his family didn't wait to find out what would happen after the terrorists arrived: "… As soon as they came into the village we gathered all our clothes and everything we owned and left because we were scared of dying." Author's field research: interviewee from Yachaya (Victor). Following their arrival SL encouraged local people from the research communities to participate in meetings intended to instil sympathy for their revolutionary ideology and rally people to their cause.

Another said that SL used these meetings to indoctrinate people: "… they kept on saying that when they got into power, the millionaires, the wealthy, would disappear since it was them who had lied to us and who were exploiting us. They (SL) confirmed that it would be the end of all theft and adultery." Author's field research: interviewee from Otoronco (Ramon). This tactic was employed throughout the area.

Often the very first signs of violence began with the arrival of strangers: "… I don't remember where they came from, but there were lots of women and men that would walk around the villages and up in the mountains. They would indoctrinate people, gathering them all together in the evenings, telling them to follow Comrade Gonzalo's ideology.[24] And that those who did not agree with this ideology would be put on a blacklist." Author's field research: interviewee from Qocha (Agustina). Over time these efforts to attract the sympathy of people were supplemented by recruitment drives. A survivor said that this usually happened at night: "… they (SL) would come to recruit people and the 'unwelcome people' would threaten us in the public square, saying that the party needed our support to become stronger. Knowing all this made us afraid and not wanting to commit (to SL) so we would run away and hide from them in the mountains and farms." Author's field research: interviewee from Yachaya (Eufemia). Despite these developments people would often return to their communities if they felt that it was safe to do so. One returnee said that the first time SL arrived everyone fled to the mountains, but on the following morning they decided to return to their homes: "… the next day we returned to the village and

[24] Comrade Gonzalo is the soubriquet of the leader of Shining Path, Abimael Guzman.

found people lying around the place, all of them dead." Authors field research: interviewee from Wamani (Rosa).

In this context of rising insecurity and violence people came to see the community not so much as a place of safety and security but rather the symbol of a well-founded fear of persecution. Another survivor said that whenever there were rumours of further attacks on their community they would escape to the mountains at night and return to their homes at 5 in the morning: "… I was afraid of those people because they walked around armed; they killed people for whatever reason." Authors field research: interviewee from Otoronco (Sanchez).

However, as the violence escalated the need to escape from their communities intensified. For many the problem was not about the need to escape, but where to. Over time this led to increasing numbers living out in the open or in caves in the mountains. This often led to the partial or even complete abandonment of their former communities: "Few people stayed (in the community) during those violent years (1980–2000). There were barely any people left here. Everybody left, or went missing. They left in the night, abandoning their houses. The place was silent; only one or two people stayed." Author's field research: interviewee from Qocha (Isabel).

Those that chose to stay on found the conditions so frightening that they did not know what would happen from one moment to the next, as one survivor noted: "In those days everyone had to sleep with one eye open, and when I was 12 years old we all had to escape to the hills in the night. We were always on guard, even when we were eating." Author's field research: interviewee from Yachaya (Regina).

For those particularly vulnerable to assault from SL, such as the former community leaders, local officials, etc., this escalation in the violence quickly became a deadly game: "I was afraid because my name was wanted by the *Senderistas*, I lived by moving from one place to another because I used to be part of the local authorities; I was really afraid of the raids." Author's field research: interviewee from Wamani (Herberto). The desire to resume planting was thwarted by the insecurity: "… we were always fleeing from one place to another. I moved about a lot and then went back to my land after things improved a bit, but I was wanted by the terrorists so I went to live in other parts. People were living scattered here and there; all I wanted to do was to go back to my land and begin the sowing." Author's field research: interviewee from Qocha (Pastor).

By the time the armed forces and the police arrived raids by SL on highland communities had become commonplace. However, the reaction to the situation by the armed forces and the police was so brutal that it only made the situation worse. Instead of helping people to restore the prior social order, rebuild trust and help those worst affected, the military took the position that local people themselves were to blame for the assaults. The damaging impact this had on the relationship among locals, and between local people and the armed forces and the police can be demonstrated by the following statements: "At that time I was about eight or nine years old; I was hit and tortured (by the army). Eventually I went into hiding with my mother; we lived in caves. I remember we used to hear the sound of weapons as we lay awake." Author's field research: interviewee from Qocha (Maximino).

Another similar report comes from someone accused of collaborating with SL: "In one raid SL killed 4 people, a married couple and two elders. The day after this the military and police arrived in trucks and helicopters to restore order. They immediately called the authorities and all of the locals to the public square and started commenting on the deaths that had occurred. They accused the population of being to blame: 'you locals are the real perpetrators and you are killing your own people.' They blamed the deaths on us. After this, people became afraid and ran away, hiding in the mountains and amongst the crops." Author's field research: interviewee from Unay (Reyes). This kind of experience of victims being punished for SL attacks was repeated by many interviewees in other areas.

4.3 Bodily Injury

Bodily injury can be defined as the unlawful use of force so as to deliberately inflict on a human being physical harm or death, whether through sexual violence, or other forms of physical harm to someone's bodily integrity, through torture, beating, maiming or mutilation. Bodily injury can result from an aggressive attitude (or impulse) or of instrumental behaviour meant to incapacitate human beings in order to achieve a variety of other ends, from enforcing dominance, to preventing the dominance of others defined as enemies.[25]

For individuals and groups seeking to destroy the existing social order, bodily injury is perceived as a convenient option because of its capacity to bring about rapid and fundamental change in the social order.[26] Fuelled by rage and frustration its influence on traditional norms, values and trust can often be as profound as the impact it has on the social order.[27]

4.3.1 Beating to the Body

Both police and the military (as well as SL) used this extensively throughout the period of political violence. For SL beating provided a means of intimidating their opponents. It played a fundamental role in the revolutionary process and was an important aspect of its overriding commitment to terror and economic sabotage. When SL first launched its internal conflict in 1980 beatings were regularly employed as a means of instilling fear in its opponents and punishing people considered criminal or abusive, such as perceived political opponents, priests, cattle rustlers, thieves or unpopular and corrupt officials. One interviewee describes this form of punishment in some detail: "Approximately one year after it all started strangers would constantly show up in the community. They began by contacting

---

[25] Schmid, A., (2011: 700).

[26] Arendt, H., (1970: 63).

[27] Galtung, J., (1996: 196).

the authorities, who then told us why they had come. The strangers said that they had come to get rid of rustlers, theft, adultery and rape. I remember that they brought everyone together and brought forward a group of rustlers, who they then punished. Then, they marched around the square with red flags, singing different anthems and saying that they were the 'soldiers of the poor'. In the parade, they would act out the deaths of those who were blacklisted. They then brought forward all of the rustlers and gave them 10, 20, 30, 40, or 50 lashes, depending on the crime. They would also force the rustlers and thieves to parade around the square naked and then punish them to make them repent and promise never to commit crimes or misdemeanours again." Author's field research: interviewee from Wamani (Etalpalli).

In the early years of the political violence paramilitary and military actions against people in the research communities was minimal. However, by the end of the 1980s human rights violations, including beatings to the body had risen to devastating levels. One survivor recounted: "In 1985, the military took me and whipped and beat me by confusing me with a terrorist." Author's field research: interviewee from Yachaya (Flavio).

Following the intensification of the armed conflict in the years immediately prior to the capture of Abimael Guzman (the leader of SL) in 1992 reprisals against suspected supporters of SL escalated. Another similar report comes from someone whose father was accused of collaborating with SL: "I don't remember much about those who came here, but I remember the military repeatedly punished my father. I remember that we were looking after my neighbour's animals and that his own family had warned my father about how the military would continually beat them. They took the animals and our sheep and cows to the mountains where they killed them for food. When they beat my father, I left because I didn't want to see them hit him and they said, 'You stay right there.' It was always like that." Author's field research: interviewee from Wamani (Juana).

Sometimes such beatings would re-traumatise those already victimised before: "Crying, I begged them to stop hitting me, but they ordered me to let them know where these *terrucos* could be found. I only took them to one of the fields, saying that occasionally some of the people on the list would go out there to harvest." Author's field research: interviewee from Unay (Juanito).

Though survivors have sought to create new lives and adjust, a part of their own identity remains stuck in the reality of the political violence. To make sense of their suffering survivors need access to shared values, common humanity and shared responsibility, but in a situation of low trust, anxiety, high vigilance and low safety nets these things are not available. Because of their distressing store of memories there is immense frustration and resentment. This is particularly evident with respect to the victims of sexual violence and rape.

4.3.2 Sexual Violence and Rape

The widespread experience of rape among all the research communities is deeply rooted in the strategies adopted by both sides in the political violence.[28] Though survivors in the research communities said that sexual violence was also carried out by SL reference to acts of rape was mainly associated with those perpetrated by the armed forces and the police.[29] A vivid illustration provided by one survivor illustrates the terrifying ordeal inflicted on countless innocent victims:

"I remember what happened when the military summoned all the locals to the square. They forced everyone to the floor, and then went into people's houses to search for and steal clothes, appliances, and whatever else they came across. Then, they raped the women." Author's field research: interviewee from Wamani (Marco).

Though the armed forces and counterinsurgency forces did not respond to the political violence until 2 years after its outbreak, their arrival transformed the conflict by its use of strategies that treated the entire rural population as potential terrorists.

The effect was to alienate local people and destroy much of their community infrastructure. This strategy was made possible by military barracks being set up by the armed forces and located close to the research communities. By the time of the arrival of the armed forces and the police the local authorities had already fled, leaving local people with no alternative but to treat the armed forces as the sole representatives of the Peruvian State.[30]

The opportunities this gave the armed forces to demonstrate their total control over a community are borne out in several statements, for example: "They began raping the girls; it started in the afternoon when they went to pick up girls saying that there were some problems that needed sorting out so the girls were forced to go to the barracks and this was how these people (military) started to abuse the humble people." Author's field research: Interviewee from Qocha (Mario). The following interviewee explains how rape and other forms of sexual violence were used by the armed forces and the police as a war strategy against suspected terrorists: "The colonel told me that as a woman I was at risk. He suggested that I return to Lima and asked me who it was that threatened me so I pointed the soldier out. He told me not to worry and that the lieutenant would soon be gone. I don't know if it was by way of vengeance, but a few months after the colonel left I was attacked and raped. Three soldiers came to my house to take me. I think one of them is now a teacher." Author's field research: interviewee from Otoronco (Gala).

---

[28] See Boesten, J., (2014); Alcalde, Cristina, M., (2010).

[29] For further details see the Commision of Truth and Reconciliation (Peru) *Comisión de la Verdad y Reconciliación (Perú)* which found that although sexual violence was attributed to all involved parties, the majority of acts of rape were perpetrated by the armed forces and the police *Comisión de la Verdad y Reconciliación (Perú)* Vol. VI (2003: 263ff)

[30] Boesten, J. (2007a; 2007b: 5).

Because the entire rural population were perceived as potential terrorists the armed forces failed to identify with local people and consequently failed to provide suitable protection.

In this environment of uncontrolled military power local people were treated as inferior, disrespected and dehumanised. Though much talked about in all the research communities', fear of reprisal, particularly in relation to specific military personnel, often made any discussion about the abuse of power extremely difficult. This is demonstrated by the following statement: "… and then I saw him (my husband) and told them 'There is my husband, why do you have him locked up?' And the soldiers said 'what you saw, you saw.' Afterwards, they told me that I would see my husband again later. After raping me they locked me in the room again. At one in the morning they released me, threatening me saying 'bitch, you're not going to tell anyone. If you do, we're going to kill you, now get out!'" Authors field research; informant from Yachaya (Gaetan).

Feeling powerless undermines social norms and behaviour and generates increased friction and rivalries that obstruct solidarity. This is reflected in high levels of family disintegration and the erosion of understanding, love and support. It also encourages withdrawal of effort, disinterest and poor performance. To avoid presumption about speaking for the victims the following accounts are included as reminders that the subjective experiences of people compel respect. Sometimes the researchers heard stories so traumatic they had not been shared even with close family members, for example: "When the danger appeared, the soldiers appeared, first making my brother-in-law disappear, and then my husband. Three days from that I forcefully demanded that they let my husband go. They told me that they had taken my husband to Huamanga. I told them no, how could they have taken a man like that, I know he's here, and they replied come in then. Then they grabbed me and threw me in. Once they put me in the room, they locked me in.

In the room, I was sitting in a corner facing the soldiers who watched me with angry eyes. Seeing this frightened me and I began to tremble. When this was happening about ten soldiers entered the room, but I couldn't recognise them because it was very dark and I couldn't see anything. Then they started to grab me by the feet, hands and my head, and started to rape me. I haven't told my husband this; I kept quiet, because they would have killed my husband." Author's field research: interviewee from Unay (Olga).

Sexual and gender based violence was so widespread during the political violence that it is all too easy to assume that it was focused mainly on women.[31] Men are identified as major victims of sexual violence as well, even though the numbers involved are thought to be considerably less than women.[32] This is demonstrated by the following: "When I got back to the square I realised a soldier had followed me. He dragged me into the square and began to hit me. None of the soldiers standing guard helped me. I yelled 'help!' several times, and nothing. This man hit me and tore my clothes and threw me about to undress me. At one point I grabbed at the

---

[31] See for example Alcalde, Cristina, M., (2010: 100–104).

[32] Boesten, J., (2014: 148).

ground and threw dirt in his eyes to try to escape but I couldn't. He grabbed me and got on top of me and told me to let him or he would take me back to the barracks to pass around to all the soldiers. Then he raped me but couldn't finish because I was kicking him, but yes, he abused me physically, and my arm was badly injured for more than a month afterwards." Author's field research: interviewee from Qocha (Felipe).

The profound effects of these experiences inflict more than pain and suffering on its victim. It leaves a shattering image on a victim's body and mind about the overwhelming, unrestrained will to power that will continue to impact on the rest of the victim's life. One survivor describes their own state of psychological degradation as follows: "He threw me to the floor trying to rape me, and if it wasn't for the soldiers who heard me yelling, he would have succeeded. Fortunately, I escaped. I even started sleeping in the field because I was terrified. Later after I had escaped to Lima they looted my house and burnt everything. Seeing all this made me feel like a powerless woman. I just wanted to die because I didn't feel worth anything after being beaten up and raped." Author's field research: interviewee from Qocha (Lina).

No one from any of the research communities had any idea how many rapes or cases of sexual violence, there had been in their own community, either by SL or the military.

4.3.3 Torture

Following the arrival of the armed forces and the police the local population from the research communities became increasingly caught 'between two fires.' Because the entire rural population were perceived as potential terrorists the armed forces and the police would often take local people into custody for questioning. One informant, told of how he was mistaken for somebody else with the same name and transferred to the police station along with several other locals. "… we were tied up with rope and led to the police station like sheep. At the police station we were interrogated and questioned about the others.

They commanded us to name names or face the consequences. I told them that I did not know any, and said: '…even if you shoot me or kill me, how could I do it? Only God Himself knows'. When asked why I was on the list then, I said that there was someone else living nearby who had the same full name. I denied every accusation, for I didn't know anything about what had been going on. So, I had nothing to tell. Then they started to hit and beat me all over. After about 2 h of torture, I began to lose consciousness. The rest of what happened to me I only heard later." Author's field research: interviewee from Qocha (Nacho).

Testimonies such as these will never be sufficient to stop this sort of thing from happening, but they can focus attention on what it means to bear responsible witness. For the research team this required empathic listening, the capacity to identify with the suffering of the victim and the effort to recognise that the tortured individual loses trust in the world forever.[33] To the survivor there is only one thing that matters: the intolerable burden of unexpressed rage: "This sort of thing happened a lot," one survivor, stated curtly, "… because they saw me watching the patrols I was arrested for two weeks and taken away (for questioning). They hit me a lot in the back; they also kicked me. They had me tied up all the time I was being beaten. I was mistaken for a terrorist." Author's field research: interviewee from Yachaya (Marcelo). Local testimony suggests that physical beatings, kicking and striking with objects were as random as they were commonplace. One informant said that people were always being taken away for questioning, and that "… in my case the torture lasted for about 2 h, from around 10 pm 'till midnight. They threw me about and pulled me to the door of the police station like a bag.

After it was all over they let me go I asked someone where I was and he told me that we were in the plaza. He helped me take a few steps and then in a stumbling manner I made my way back home. Moving about 500 meters, from the police station to my house, took about 3 h. Sometime later my neighbours came with home remedies to help me recover." Author's field research: interviewee from Yachaya (Tonatzin).

Not all of those taken away for questioning were so lucky. One interviewee said that when his mother was taken away she "…was tortured with a gun smashed over her head. Now she is a widow and blind from the punching she received." Author's field research: interviewee from Otoronco (Gustavo).

Inevitably, torture would sometimes lead to the betrayal of individuals including family friends. An interviewee explained how this happened to him: "… At that point, I was held for questioning. I was asked for the whereabouts of the members of the Shining Path. I said that the *terrucos*[34] they had pointed out were, in fact, locals but that as they were constantly harassed by the police, they were no longer staying there. Initially, when the torture began, I could not confess as I was afraid of giving away the names of the people. Later, however, the confessions just came out. These diverse traumatic events would sometimes include having the victim placed in a very small space". Author's field research: interviewee from Wamani (Ignacio).[35]

Following interrogation, the victim was as likely to be freed as detained or imprisoned for an indefinite period. However, even if the victim is no longer considered to be of any use to the authorities the 'useless suffering' that has been inflicted is shocking and in the aftermath of the political violence not always recognized for the dehumanizing experience that it is.[36]

The following testimony demonstrates this: "That night when they took me they put me in a corner in an office; I felt the sounds of the typewriter, every time I felt cold and thirsty and asked for a drink they grabbed my hair and hit me against the wall, each time I asked they did that, and they kicked me until I fell unconscious;

---

[33] Amery, J., (1980: 40).

[34] *terrucos* Sp. slang for terrorist.

[35] This is what people called a '*bote*' (can). The '*bote*' was a small room which could only fit one person in at a stretch and so they were boxed in.

[36] Levinas, E., (1998: 78ff).

then from there they took me as a prisoner. I was a year and six months in prison; some people tried to help me but for two years my head hurt so much." Author's field research: interviewee from Wamani (Theodore).

Because torture forces the victim to recognize and accept a truth that is not theirs it only stops when the perpetrators are satisfied that the "truth" it has extracted from the victim is consistent with the ideological convictions of the regime they represent. This can be demonstrated by the following statement: "When the military came they would tie up your hands and say that we were terrorists and beat us. My cousins and uncles were detained for 15 days." Author's field research: interviewee from Unay (Gregorio).

For the armed forces torture was a legitimate weapon in its fight against the elusive adversarial forces of SL. Not knowing enough about their identity, location, resources or influence made it essential to turn their suspicions about the loyalties of the local population into truths. This is borne out by the following statement: "Just when I finally started feeling safe again, a group of around 7 people, who looked like soldiers, appeared one early morning, introducing themselves as 'comrades'. The word 'comrade' was used to confuse me. I started to answer them with the word 'sir' (I did this as a strategy, because answering any differently could be life-threatening). I only answered in Quechua, and they proceeded to beat me, calling me a *terruco*. Then they read out a list of names of local community members. I was to tell them where the '*terrucos*' could be found." Author's field research: interviewee from Yachaya (Emilio).

4.4 Forced Confinement and Coercion

Forcing another person to act in an involuntary manner by the use of psychological pressure or physical force or threats is a widespread strategic act of war. Such actions violate the free will of an individual and usually involve the victim in a situation that they cannot escape from without damage to themselves and/or others. Forced confinement and coercion are therefore as much a physical as a psychological violation.[37] This can be demonstrated as follows: "My complaint against the military was filed as an abuse of human rights but after I registered my complaint it was published in the newspaper. After a few days they (the military) kidnapped me in my house and made me disappear for 25 days. They refused to provide information to my family or to the unions even though they looked for me everywhere.

Finally, I got out, they (my family) got me out of a dark cell; there was a visit from the International Red Cross to see the health status of prisoners, nothing more." Author's field research: interviewee from Otoronco (Temotzin).

---

[37] Byman and Waxman (2000) define coercion as "...the use of threatened force, including the limited use of actual force to back up the threat, to induce an adversary to behave differently than it otherwise would." See Byman, D. L, & Waxman, M. C. (2000).

4.4.1 Kidnapping

Kidnapping was a widespread strategic act of war widely used by both SL and the armed forces. In this context the unlawful taking away or transportation of a person against their will, with the intent to use the abduction for ransom or in furtherance of some other crime was regarded as part of warfare and encouraged from above. Those children abducted by SL would often be taken from their schoolroom, with the oldest being between the ages of 10 and 12. Teachers or family members who protested were given the choice to either give up their child or have the entire family killed.[38] No one from the research communities knows how many kidnappings were carried out by SL or the military in their own community. One informant from Qocha (Severo) simply said that "… it happened almost every day during the stay of the military, especially young women and ladies of good appearance." However, the same informant did suggest that the overall number of kidnappings might have been between 50 or 60 from his community.

Kidnapping by the armed forces usually led to the victim being taken to the local military barracks or the local police station. From there they would be forcibly recruited and posted far from their home region. Families of victims taken by the armed forces or the police invariably found that information about their missing relative was unavailable, or that the authorities simply had no knowledge of the whereabouts of the missing person.

In every testimony the abuse of basic trust is overwhelming, as the following example demonstrates: "My son was kidnapped by the police but the police ignored us and would not give any information. Day after day we returned to the police station, but the response was always blunt and aggressive: 'There are no detainees here; his *terruco* comrades probably took him.' This nightmare continued for several months." Author's field research: interviewee from Qocha (Margarita).

Sometimes victims could pay the army for relatives to be released, including in this case with livestock: "During the week we left, many people died; the soldiers killed 6 of my compatriots who had been imprisoned with my husband. My husband was the only one to be freed, and he was only let go because I gave the army captain a fully-grown bull. The bull died in the place of my husband. Two or three days later the rest of the prisoners were taken away by helicopter." Author's field research: interviewee from Yachaya (Teressa).

Some features such as the actual infliction of physical pain/injury or murder to enhance the credibility of a threat is demonstrated by the following account: "I was kidnapped by the *Senderistas* for 4 days in my homeland and then they took me to another district where they took me to a hill where there were 8 other hostages. In an oversight two of us escaped but the remaining 6 were killed." Author's field research: interviewee from Yachaya (Emilio). Other features of forcing another party to act in an involuntary manner by use of intimidation or threats to induce a

[38] APRODEH. (2004). *Violencia Contra Niños y Niñas: Hasta sus Menorcitos ahora Lloran. In Asociación Pro Derechos Humanos (*Ed.*), Selección de textos del Informe Final de la Comisión de la Verdad y Reconciliación*. www.aprodeh.org.pe

desired response include forced labour, forced separation from family members and threats to induce favours.[39]

A survivor of one such experience describes what they endured: "One day a group of armed men appeared. They took eight of us along to the Military Base for questioning. Eventually I was released, but no sooner had I recovered from all the physical and psychological abuse than there was a new attack on my farm by a large group of rebels. I was taken prisoner and accused of turning in one of their comrades to the military. I was driven overnight and left in a cave. There were about four people in the cave and under such circumstances, I thought the worst. Later, I studied where the door was and then managed to escape by jumping onto the rocks below. I walked aimlessly, completely battered, and with the sun rising on the hill I headed for Huamanga." Author's field research: interviewee from Otoronco (Tenyoa).

4.5 Disappearances, Death or Injury of Loved Ones

Making people 'disappear' was used as a strategy of terror throughout the political violence. It has been used in Latin America since the mid-1960s when it was used by the government of Guatemala. In the 1970s "disappearances" were being widely used in countries such as Argentina, Brazil, Uruguay and Chile.

By the time they began in Peru in the 1980s, 'disappearances' had become commonplace throughout El Salvador and Guatemala. Because the abduction and illegal detention of a victim often led to torture and interrogation 'disappearances' often implied murder. In these circumstances the corpse was usually disposed of to escape discovery so that the victim effectively vanished. Its power as a terror tactic was based on its capacity to silence opponents and critics and generate uncertainty and fear amongst the living. More than 40% of the deaths and 'disappearances' reported to the TRC are concentrated in the Department of Ayacucho.[40]

Those responsible for 'disappearances', include SL and the *Sinchis*, the specialized anti-terrorist police.

It is not clear when people from the research communities first began to be 'disappeared' although in an interview with one informant from Qocha (Julio), it would seem that this particular terror tactic started to happen not long after SL first began to arrive: "… I almost never spoke to the terrorists but I did listen to what they were saying: that there were thieves in our village and that they had come to help the

[39] People from the communities studied said that abductions by Shining Path often led to the victim (often children) being indoctrinated and put to work in production camps or recruited as child soldiers for combat and drug-trafficking activities.

[40] On 20 December 2006, the United Nations General Assembly adopted the International Convention for the Protection of All Persons from Enforced Disappearance. It states that enforced disappearances constitute a crime against humanity and entitle victims' families the right to seek reparations, and to demand the truth about the disappearance of their loved ones.

poor. I listened to this and that is why I didn't trust the terrorists. They were there to make us 'disappear' and this is why we slept high in the mountains." In spite of initial support for its punishment and assassination of individual wrongdoers, rich peasants and other local figures, sympathy for SL and its political aims deteriorated as the scale of their increasingly violent assaults on local people became more apparent. Taking advantage of long standing local disputes failed to win support for SL in the longer term. Instead, it simply alienated them.

Looking back on the early years of the political violence one informant from Wamani (Sabino) described how local people became increasingly alienated and frightened the more SL sought to impose itself: "… there were many strangers arriving and I was scared of offending them about anything because they were very rude and nasty. People out walking at night were always being disappeared."

Having established their presence in a community SL used the intelligence it gathered to attack more and more local people, including social and political activists, leaders of grassroots organizations and other community leaders.

One informant from Otoronco (Alvaro) remembered the terrifying effects this had on people: "… they used a list to hunt people. If they found people that were on this list they killed them. Raids mostly took place at night but if people escaped to the mountains, they suffered from hunger and the cold." For some the SL list would lead to the murder or disappearance of their community leaders. One former community leader from Otoronco (Ramon) said that: "… out of all those who were in authority during that time, only I and one other are still alive. The rest were all massacred." The following account describes how people targeted by SL managed to escape in spite of the actions taken by the terrorists to assassinate them: "I had authority (in the community) in the years 1986, 1987, and 1988 and so they tried to kill me. They killed my father. I had 6 brothers to look after and so I had to work. One afternoon, I was working on the road and the terrorists came and gathered up 14 women, and were taking them to the mountains with their hands tied in order to kill them. One of the women escaped and when we went to see what was going on the terrorists ran away but later when they realized that we were unarmed, they returned. That is when they shot me in my chest and my nose. By 1992, I no longer went outside. I was very frightened because I was number 1 on the terrorists' list to be killed. I moved to the jungle and lived alone, defending myself for 5 years." Author's field research: interviewee from Otoronco (Paulino).

The killing of community leaders was part of SL policy. In the early period of the insurgency SL would hold people's trials and give people from the community the opportunity to decide on the fate of the 'enemies of the people.'

However, as the political violence developed this same SL policy was extended to include anyone suspected of 'collaboration' with government forces or for failing to follow *Senderista* ideology. One former community leader describes what it was like to live in continual fear of being killed by both SL and the armed forces: "I'm alive because I escaped a lot. The terrorists entered my house and burned it; the terrorists took my animals and ate them; this was what the military did as well. In 1984 I was an authority in the village so I had to hide from both sides; there was much violence; they killed 3 of my brothers, they also executed people working in the fields. My position in the village led to my being appointed president of the community for 7 months and this also involved me being in a position of command (with the *Rondas*) for six months. The terrorists always looked to the authorities to kill them; thank God I'm alive yet." Author's field research: interviewee from Yachaya (Florentin).

Throughout the later stages of the political violence SL continued to claim or be attributed responsibility for the killing of numerous mayors of different political parties, particularly of small Andean towns, including those from the communities studied. For example: "When my brother became mayor, he got them (the military) to respect us. He became friends with the captains, and there were no more deaths. Things were calmer in 1985. My brother became mayor twice. But the second-time round they killed him. We don't know who did it, but he was killed in Ayacucho when he went there for negotiations. The killers sent an anonymous letter written in red ink." Author's field research: interviewee from Unay (Joviana).

Having alienated many of its early supporters with the killing of local leaders' SL sought to establish control of entire communities, particularly those opposed to further interference from SL. In the process more and more people from the communities studied began to realise that they were not participants in the revolution. It was in this situation that SL began to go beyond the killing of individual wrongdoers, rich peasants and other local figures. One survivor from this change in strategy by SL describes their experiences as follows: "They killed my mum's sister along with her husband and her son because they were hiding in a cave. They were all killed except for one of the children who escaped and when the terrorists found him, they told him this: "your mum and your dad are black vultures and have died for being black vultures". They grabbed the boy's hand and threatened him, saying that if he told someone, he too would die like his father." Author's field research: interviewee from Unay (Galetée).

Increasingly harsh measures intended to force support including more and more attacks on people's homes, more public executions and disappearances only served to heighten the sense of devastation, loss and grief.[41] The following typifies the experience of survivors: "They (SL) killed my mother and killed my father. This was in 1984. I was young but I saw these things, I also saw people killed in the village. They also killed my uncle; we were orphans, we were poor, we were very afraid; my sister is a widow because they killed her husband." Author's field research: interviewee from Qocha (Godofredo). The following statement also testifies to the appalling tragedies inflicted on countless individuals and families from the research communities and beyond:

"There was a graveyard here at that time. 6 of the 10 people that were taken there were killed and 4 went missing and remain so until this day. This was when the terrorists were coming in the mornings and afternoons. "Author's field research: Interviewee from Yachaya (Mora). Another informant explained that: "As soon as the terrorists came into the village, we left because we were scared of dying. One day, when we were moving further up the mountains I was alone with my brother,

[41] Starn, O., Degregori, C. I., Kirk, R., (1995: 340).

but he disappeared. We looked everywhere for him but never found him." Author's field research: interviewee from Yachaya (Luisa).

Though inured to hardship over many generations the treatment meted out to local people and on such a scale was unknown. Anger and resentment at what was taking place continues to generate hostility and loathing for what happened during the years of violence (1980–2000). An informant, Fabricio from Yachaya, commented, "… how would you feel if your neighbour or your children were taken away, killed and made to disappear? It's terrifying, and that's why I'm scared even today." Similar sentiments of outrage and disgust were expressed by one who preferred to leave her home rather than endure the seemingly endless round of killings, disappearances and retribution: "… they did not respect women and beat them when they were carrying their babies. The dead were found in the pampas. There were people hanging. Sometimes I escaped with my children, from the explosions of many bullets. When they found nobody, they burned the houses. Having seen all these things, I moved away with my children." Author's field research: interviewee from Unay (Lucita).

Though many people from the research communities shared in the general condemnation of Peru's political system, the arrival of the armed forces provided a brief moment of hope that peace would be restored. One informant Gildas from Wamani, described how people were rapidly undeceived of this impression in the following words: "… when the soldiers came, we were happy and hoped to God that our faith in them would spur them on. But they started to treat us badly. They just killed innocent people; it was only the innocent they killed. In reality they didn't find a single criminal; they didn't capture one terrorist."

Though paramilitary and military violence against local people had been minimal during the first few years of the political violence by the end of the 1980s human rights abuses had increased to unprecedented levels. Following the decision to cede control of nine provinces in the departments of Ayacucho, Apurimac and Huancavelica to the military in December 1982 efforts were made to improve the government's intelligence capability. However, this did little to counter the rapid escalation in the number of military assassinations and forced disappearances.

By shifting from short-term, occasional incursions to a more continuous presence in the conflict zone the armed forces through their actions only helped to exacerbate the fears of local people and reinforce the feeling of being caught between two lines of fire. The following account by someone who was wrongfully arrested on suspicion of terrorism illustrates graphically the rapidly increasing tempo of the political violence during these years:

"The military summoned us representatives (from the communities) to the plaza. At this meeting, I was mistaken for somebody else with the same name and transferred to the police station along with several other locals. We were tied up with rope and led to the police station like sheep. Later that night, police officials and some locals moved into one of the nearby communities to get those who had not come to the meeting. When they arrived in the community they proceeded to wipe out the population, using axes and other blunt objects. The raid was led by people known to some of us locals. Those of us taken to the police station were interrogated and questioned about the whereabouts of the others; we were commanded to name names." Author's field research: interviewee from Qocha (Tiburcio).

Though their continuous presence in the conflict zone can be seen as part of an overall strategy intended to make the military response to the insurgency more effective the overall shift from outright oppression to a new way of thinking about counter-insurgency progress did not happen overnight. Regarding human rights abuses, when commenting on the behaviour of the armed forces, one informant said that, "…if complaints were made about abuses (by the military) people were either imprisoned or disappeared." Author's field research: interviewee from Qocha (Isolda). The following account testifies to the ongoing ferocity of the armed forces and the danger they continued to pose to local people in the research communities: "When the military came to the village they had a list of 10 people. Nobody knew who made this list. They gathered everyone together and began to call out the names on the list. They tied their hands and feet together and hurled them to the ground. As the military were armed, we could not do anything." Author's field research: interviewee from Otoronco (Marisa).

Such examples of oppression by the armed forces remained in place through most of the 1980s, particularly in those regions considered to be of strategic importance or with a significant history of SL activity. For the people in the communities studied this meant that the kind of treatment meted out to them in the following example became all too familiar: "The army rounded us up so they could watch us and they wouldn't let us leave because the authorities said that if the army left people would disappear." Author's field research: interviewee from Wamani (Ignacio).

Indiscriminate violence in combination with deep frustration about the shortcomings of its own counter-insurgency policies made the behaviour of the armed forces in the communities studied unpredictable and unremittingly violent. A survivor of this unreliable environment testifies to this change: "First they (the military) had my brother-in-law. Then my husband went to the soldiers and asked why they had imprisoned his brother, and the military told him that if he is your brother then you can go in, and they imprisoned him there but he has never been seen since." Author's field research: interviewee from Unay (Lucita).

Indiscriminate terror by the armed forces and police did little to counter the activities of SL. Instead of undermining SL, political violence continued to flourish. By 1986 new regions of terrorist activity had opened up, including the Upper Huallaga and Lima. For people in the communities studied this phase in the political violence was characterized not just by the extreme measures taken by SL against anyone that stood in their way, but by the absence of any alternative. This is because the intensification of attacks against government officials effectively left the research communities utterly vulnerable and undefended.

This is demonstrated by the following statement: "The *senderistas* came into the village in military clothing, claiming that they were coming from the military barracks. That day they gathered together in the main square and separated into two groups. On one side were those who spoke Quechua and on the other those who spoke Castilian. Many of us suspected that they were not actually soldiers and fled, but my father was not able to escape. He tried but they cornered him and took him back to the square. Then at about 8 at night they left. When my father did not appear, I went with my mother to look for him. We didn't believe that he was dead until a neighbour told me that he had been murdered. Then I and my mother began to cry until dawn. We held a wake for my father the next day." Author's field research: interviewee from Qocha (Marisa).

By the mid-1980s the military presence within the EMZ was increased as part of its overall strategy to provide the civilian population with effective protection. However, this brought little reassurance to local people because the behaviour of the armed forces was widely perceived as disrespectful as much as the attitude shown towards the civilian population by SL was regarded as paternalistic.[42] This increased the difficulties for local people as the following statement indicates: "The rebel group consisted of around 7 or 8 people, and some of them were as young as 12 or 13. They carried handguns around with them. People were very afraid, because there were lots of red flags, which made the community appear pro-*senderista* and the military therefore see us as *terrucos*. It was then that we realized that we were caught in the crossfire, that is to say, in a really bad situation." Author's field research: interviewee from Unay (Eurico).

As part of its overall strategy to increase its presence in the EMZ a policy was introduced by the armed forces that required indigenous communities to establish their own self-defence militias. However, the fragile link this subsequently gave local people with the Peruvian state proved highly controversial and brought instant reprisals from SL.[43] Ill-equipped and insufficiently trained these community-based militias, known as *rondas campesinas*[44] were in no position to provide adequate protection for their communities as the following statement indicates: "It was about 6pm. 6 soldiers appeared. I already suspected something was going to happen. The man who brought those men here was from the village. But at a closer look it was clear that these were not soldiers, but terrorists dressed as soldiers. They opened fire in to the air and rounded up the people. At that point some of them began to escape from the main square. The terrorists began to shoot people and 14 people died in total that day." Author's field research: interviewee from Yachaya (Amaranta).

By the late 1980s the military situation had deteriorated to such an extent that the armed forces presence in the EMZ and within rural Andean communities affected by the political violence had become continuous. However, this did not result in any significant change in its counter-insurgency policy, or in its relationship with local people. This is borne out by the following example: "They stole our sheep, our

[42] CVR (2003).

[43] Theidon, K. (2000).

[44] Nuñez-Palomino, G. (1996); Starn, O. (1999); Fumerton, M. (2001).

chickens, our pigs; any animals found walking on the street and it was for them. They entered houses by kicking the door down and some people would jump in fright; they were not afraid to mistreat us, not afraid to give a kick to a mother or a village elder and when people started crying or screaming they all responded with such profanity and used their rifle butt to hit the women and the elderly." Author's field research: interviewee from Unay (Graciano).

Towards the end of the 1980s the armed forces began to move its policies away from the crudities of some of its earlier practices and replace them with ones that were less repressive and more supportive of the rural population. In spite of this new way of thinking its effects were only gradually felt and in many cases, they came too late, as the following statement demonstrates: "In our village they (the military) killed members of my family; you couldn't say anything even if it was your brother. It was better to hide yourself so that your brother would not recognise you because if he recognised you the army would also accuse you of being a terrorist and kill you. They would tell members of my family that they were terrorists and rape and kill them just for the fun of it." Author's field research: interviewee from Wamani (Fabian).

4.6 Witnessing Violence Done to Others

Bearing witness to traumatic experiences gives the impression of being primarily about the conveying of knowledge. It is not. Though information about the actual traumatic experiences is vital to bearing witness, the facts are nothing more than the raw material from which the psychic pain implicit in such experiences can be turned into moral issues. The following account describes some of the apparently meaningless acts of human suffering witnessed by local people, in the first case from those inflicted by SL: "The terrorists entered the village and began to shout and kill people. I was sleeping next to the wheat harvest (in the chakra and on the ground); I listened to the bursting bullets and people screaming; then they started killing people, I escaped. One day later I returned to the village there was a man with his head cut off by an axe but according to this man's mother he had not killed anyone; seeing these things I fled but that night I approached the place where they had killed that man.

I came across a bridge on which I found several dead that had been killed that night in several different places when they were burning the houses." Author's field research: interviewee from Yachaya (Tenyoa).

Another example of witnessing violence regards the military. Again, this is a violence of such barbarity that makes people withdraw into themselves and submit to profound isolation, depression, panic and mute suffering that will only renew itself in generations to come: "Over these years I saw people taken and killed, these creatures (military) buried them on the river bank and the dogs ate them. They brought people with and without children, blindfolded, facing the barracks. After three or four days they took them and started to make them disappear. They buried them all by the river and when I returned from the city people were talking about how the dogs were eating them, and it was true. There was a human head and this horrified me. They also told me that the dogs ate them there because that's where the soldiers killed them." Author's field research: interviewee from Qocha (Lina).

Bearing witness therefore provides a means by which strong feelings of hate, failure and loss can be made known to others. However, this is not enough on its own. It does not represent the inhumanity of what happened. In the aftermath of the political violence people are unable to disentangle their identity from the horror of what happened because they live in a context of daily survival. Forgetting what happened is not so much an option as a prerequisite for life to continue. To heal the scourge of persecution, torture, rape and other symptoms of brute force people need to be able to re-create some kind of link at the point where the breach took place.[45]

However, the mourning process and the reconstruction of memory can only happen under conditions that restore power and control to the victim.[46] For people affected by political violence and living in a context of daily survival this does not happen. In such circumstances any sense of what happened has effectively been shut out of their lives. The hard struggle for satisfying basic daily needs in conjunction with the effects of an outside environment that has long since lost any interest in the past leave people with no alternative but to adapt themselves as best they can. This is responsible for significant alterations in human relations as is demonstrated from the following statement: "There are a lot of things that have changed here. Now the people are not caring, they are selfish, opportunistic, they just want things easy, and nothing is free now." Author's field research: interviewee from Qocha (Tezcacoat).

At an inter-subjective level this is responsible for significant misunderstandings "… in the form of equivocation, paradox, and confusion, which may provoke unknowing compromise."[47] The impact of this traumatic work of destruction is unavoidable as the following statement demonstrates: "After the military left we no longer do anything to help and sometimes we don't want to know anything about the community." Author's field research: interviewee from Unay (Honoré).

In many cases the witness can be almost matter-of-fact in commenting on the wrongdoing and the unjust circumstances surrounding the violence done to others. For instance, one interviewee reports: "My father and mother were killed by SL; we were orphaned at 2 and 5 years old, I was very young I do not remember much; I just remember that they killed my aunt, in spite of these things we have carried on living here right up today." Author's field research: interviewee from Wamani (Susana).

A similar sense of violence as commonplace can be found in this account of the suffering inflicted on a family by SL from Qocha and witnessed by Ramiro, a member of the same family: "… it was some time in 1984 when they came through here one morning at about 6am. We were having breakfast when they called to my father

[45] Gautier, A., & Sabatini Scalmati, A., (2010: xxii).

[46] Herman, J. L., (1992: 159).

[47] Gautier, A., & Sabatini Scalmati, A., (2010: 6).

through a loudspeaker. As my father was a very humble man, he went out to see why they were calling him. They then tied him up and beat him. My mother began to weep. After that they took 10 people and many of our animals, they robbed the people of about 500 livestock, and they took their clothes and their big saucepans."

Nevertheless, the importance of being an eyewitness to the plight of others enables people to overcome feelings of powerlessness associated with a power relation that obtains when a dominant group's experiences, achievements and values are established as the norm for all.[48] That this can play an analogous role in shoring up the emotional attachment to the victim of wrongdoing is borne out by the first-hand experiences of an eyewitness account of a man from Unay being tortured: "… I saw a man who had his hands tied behind his back being tortured. They began to punch him, they placed him in water and told him to speak, speak...... as if people do not know how to speak?" Author's field research: interviewee from Unay (Ponce).

However, the memory of wrongdoing can also become such an overwhelming presence in the life of the witness that it may undermine their capacity to move forwards. This is borne out by the first-hand experiences of an eyewitness account of Hipolito a man from Otoronco: "… I was 7 years old when I saw what happened to a man the military thought was a terrorist that they had found hiding in a cave. The man was shouting and screaming.

I was able to peer in to see what was happening and saw that the man had no tongue or eyes, I looked through a small peep hole and saw everything that happened because the man shouted a lot before he died."

In many cases the witness is not merely an observer of wrongdoing but someone who has themselves experienced suffering first-hand.[49] For example: "One day we had a family event (a birthday party) when we heard shouting in the street; the terrorists were in the square and everybody was trying to escape. I found my godson just before they broke into his house and shot him. They even threw a grenade. My godson shot a terrorist but he ran away, but he died in the highlands above the village, near the lake.

After that, the terrorists came to burn down the houses which, in those days, were made of *ichu*. After that event we did not return to the village." Author's field research: interviewee from Unay (Severiano).

How to melt the hearts of a people whose world has been frozen by hatred, shame, fear and the abuse of power? To be torn from their own primordial sense of self and the basic belonging fashioned out of the *ayllu* and other culturally important forms of reciprocity is a catastrophe that undermines people's trust in the world. One survivor explains how the life of their community was shattered utterly: "The terrorists burned their houses and killed them. There was a lot of blood flowing. I have seen children and the elderly die. The terrorists would come from the front to kill you. If you tried to escape they got rid of you in the same way the military did. They accuse you of terrorism and just kill you.

---

[48] Blustein, J. (2008: 340).

[49] Blustein, J. (2008: 311); Margalit, A., (2002).

Sometimes the terrorists came saying that they were teachers from institutions and that they had come to find out if we were organized or not. They told us to join them and, with that story, they took people away and just killed them." Author's field research: interviewee from Yachaya (Liana).

In the following statement the experience of bearing witness is concerned with the suffering of intimates as well as strangers, individuals as well as communities: "In 1984 the terrorists came dressed like soldiers. They killed my mother and brother. They also killed my uncle. 14 people were killed that day. Because the people realised that they were not the military, they ran off. If they hadn't more people would have been killed. Only those who stayed in the square were murdered." Author's field research: interviewee from Unay (Suniva).

Bearing witness to wrongdoing and the suffering it produces involves more than a simple relating of facts; remembering what happened involves a journey back to a reality that the people studied have either forgotten or repressed. At this point the survivor may give an account that is emotionless, unconnected and repetitious which can undermine the capacity of the traumatic memory to develop or progress over time: "In those days there was much danger, but I lived on the top of the hill; they burned my house and all my animals were taken. I was left alone with my blanket, they took my husband and I never saw him again. After a while they came back again and burned my house, my kitchen, where my husband used to sleep. I also saw the terrorists kill a lady trying to escape and in her panic her son fell into the ravine below the house, the child cried a lot." Author's field research: interviewee from Otoronco (Jacinta).

4.7 Conclusion

It is important to bear in mind that traumatic experiences do not get resolved by the simple presentation of the facts. The victim and the survivor are bearing witness to "… a spectacular failure of the social and the trans-subjective, the collapse of everything that had been taken as given."[50] In this respect the victim and the survivor is dealing with their inability to integrate, process, link and incorporate their traumatic experiences. For people living in a context of daily survival this constitutes a profound sense of impotence that is unrelenting, an experience of disintegration that goes on to affect people's lives without the knowledge that it will ever achieve anything.

Though people from the communities studied have little opportunity to expand their capacity to bear witness this does not mean that they are unable to talk about the horrible traumas they endured. To the contrary: the loss of contact with the internal or subjective side of their emotional experiences can enable people to talk about what happened to them because they "… preserve contact only with abstractions, or

[50] Gautier, A., & Sabatini Scalmati, A., (2010: 34).

abstracted forms of their experiences."[51] The following testimony captures the situation under the military regime: "Life during the political violence was atrocious. The military curfew was applied after six in the afternoon and no one was to be walking on the streets or animals after then. Some people who had not understood correctly and who dared to go to the corner were shot and after that people started to watch out. Seeing all that sort of thing meant that we had to move from five in the morning to six in the evening and you had to do this with everything going on in view, including all of the people who were being persecuted while we were doing our work.

Sometimes we were unaware of what was happening because when we were coming back (from the fields) the military appeared to be following us and were monitoring what we did. For us it was painful, to be living that way." Author's field research: interviewee from Wamani (Nicanor).

By not being in touch with their emotional experiences people are able to externalize their internal world and recount what happened, but without ever putting into words what those horrible events had done to them. For example: "I saw many terrorists: They entered people's houses and cut their throats. They were left naked on the edge of the field and with them my husband who also died; a woman was taken away leaving her babies behind and they never saw her again. I was nearby and had my little child and we were holding hands watching these things, though I always managed to escape." Author's field research: interviewee from Qocha (Tulio).

Unless other people are able to place themselves in the position of those that suffered they cannot be said to feel the full weight of the psychic pain with which these traumatic experiences are associated. In this respect the importance of empathy and the result of an overriding lack of "…psychological processes that make a person have feelings that are more congruent with another's situation than with his own situation" is paramount.[52] This and the issues that it raises will be explored in greater detail in the following chapter.

---

[51] Gautier, A., & Sabatini Scalmati, A., (2010: 44).

[52] Hoffman. M. L., (2000: 30).

Chapter 5
Psychic Wounds of Political Violence

This chapter considers the response of those affected by political violence. Chapter 4 examined what was done to people by the armed forces, the police and SL. We now explore the infraction brought about by these events and how debilitating effects continue to be entangled with survivors and their everyday reality. For people to have survived is "...literally to live through it, that is, to come out the other side of whatever it is one is said to have 'survived.'"[1] In this way the survivors have outlived their beliefs, their relationship with themselves, with their ideals and with their memory.

The trauma people were subject to has crushed them and turned them into unwitting accomplices of the hatred and abuse that sought to destroy them.[2] By overwhelming their capacity to resist the political violence has opened the door to the internal world of the victim and installed itself in their minds. In this way the abuse that was performed externally has been transformed into an internal abuse and come to acquire dominion over the entire person.[3] These are circumstances in which anyone overwhelmed by brute force has to confront and somehow find an appropriate outlet if these experiences are to be emotionally worked through. However, the difficulties this presents for people living in a struggle for daily survival are of such a magnitude that satisfying basic needs makes this process almost impossible to complete in one generation. The harm done to people in these circumstances is "... unquestionably pathological."[4]

If, "...this working through is arrogantly, even triumphantly shunned by their descendants, then persecution looms, and a disturbing spiral comes into being, in which trauma generates other traumas, the past recreating itself in the present where today's anguish is piled upon that of yesterday."[5]

---

[1] Seeburger, F., (2012: 18).

[2] Gautier, A., & Sabatini Scalmati, A., (2010: xix).

[3] Gautier, A., & Sabatini Scalmati, A., (2010: xix).

[4] Gautier, A., & Sabatini Scalmati, A., (2010: xxiii)

[5] Gautier, A., & Sabatini Scalmati, A., (2010: xxiii)

T. J. Bowyer, *Beyond Suffering and Reparation*,
https://doi.org/10.1007/978-3-319-98983-9_5

To face a situation in which what happened gets left untold makes isolation, depression, anxiety and erratic behaviour inevitable; it also increases the likelihood that the thoughts and memories of the survivor and their past will merge with their present thoughts about and attitudes toward their past.[6] The harm done to people by this internalization of brute force prompts the following questions:

- How has political violence affected people who lived through it?
- What are the main elements of their suffering and how have they sought to overcome a total lack of psychological preparation for what happened?

Answers to these questions will largely depend on how people see themselves in the present and how they project themselves into the future.[7] For people in the communities studied this comprises the overwhelming struggle to satisfy the demands of the immediate present and the fact that their present is characterised by conditions in which violence and the fear of violence are ongoing.[8] Having so little control over their environment makes survivors feel that they have no alternative but to normalize the past by separating themselves from it as much as they can. As one survivor put it "There is always tension inside you. And that stays there, which means that it's a little difficult to think that we are one hundred percent normal." Author's field research: interviewee from Qocha (Agustina).

The following statement is typical of present-day attitudes: "My brother left and was then caught, that's all we know to this day. My mother, who is now deceased, told my son that they (the military) killed him. She also told me that my father had been killed and my brother was missing. One of the neighbours said that he had died. The last time we heard that my brother had disappeared they said that if my brother was alive he would not come back to us. The military did in fact bring him here and we saw him from a distance and cried out to him, but it was no good because you just have to keep hurrying along when you hear gunshots. From then on the rest of us did not speak about what happened." Author's field research: interviewee from Unay (Lidia).

From the present perspective this closing down of feelings can be seen as a natural defence against the experience of death and destruction.[9] A survivor provided an excellent example: "Sometimes I get scared. Sometimes I think that they have already come back and that I will suddenly find myself bumping into the people that walk and that they will say that I am a health promoter and kill me. I get upset quickly." Author's field research: interviewee from Qocha (Luna).

---

[6] Laub, D., & Auerhahn, N, (1993: 293).

[7] Volf, M. (2006: 26).

[8] Saona, M., (2014).

[9] Though the organization's numbers have considerably reduced, a militant faction of Shining Path called *Proseguir* (Onward) continues to be active. It is believed that the faction consists of three groups known as the North, or Pangoa, the Centre, or Pucuta, and the South, or Vizcatán. The government claims that *Proseguir* is operating in alliance with drug traffickers. United States Department of State (2005) Country Reports on Human Rights Practices: Peru: (2005)

In the immediate aftermath of violence this helped to protect people and provide them with the means by which they could begin to come to terms with their traumatic experiences.[10] In this respect the refusal to recognise the reality of a traumatic perception provided a useful and valuable process.[11] Jelin describes this as "… forms of forgetting that are 'necessary' for the survival and functioning of the individual subject as well as for groups and communities."[12]

By refusing to think or talk about the emotional reality of their experience of extreme events survivors are able "…to minimize psychological discomfort and responsibility about actions and thoughts that would otherwise be prohibited."[13] The significance of this is that many discard any emotional contact with their past experiences which have a lasting effect that ultimately separates people from their own sufferings.[14] According to Krystal, (1995) it is a process that leads to "…a progressive constriction of cognitive processes, including memory and problem solving until a mere vestige of the self-observing ego is preserved."[15]

This leads unconsciously to the pretence that immersion in the present and the resumption of routine and regular activity are enough to re-connect people with "… the ways of thinking, speaking, acting and relating through which they previously made sense of the world."[16] Though this may enable survivors to withdraw to live as they had done before the violence it is significant that this severance from what they have done or what was done to them is motivated by negative experiences.[17] Though survivors may not always consciously register the impact of this on their lives the psychological effects are powerful and enduring.

By excluding their experiences of the political violence from conscious memory survivors dissociate themselves from the emotional pain of wrongs suffered through such unconscious strategies as disavowal, psychic numbing, splitting of consciousness and doubling. This means that survivors tend to react to subsequent stressful events as if they are in some way linked with what happened to them during the violence.[18]

The response to collective traumas from war, violence, terror, rape, torture has shown that, from Syria to Bosnia and from Rwanda to Southern Sudan, a psychology

[10] Though people from rural highland communities would not normally experience suffering in the same ways and with the same symptomatic outcomes as people from Western cultures the events of the political violence are such that the decision to close down their feelings as a natural defence against the experience of death and destruction is consistent with a universal response to extreme events and not one that is exclusive to the culture of the rural Andes.

[11] Janoff-Bulman, R., (1992: 98).

[12] Jelin, E., (2002: 29), Cited in Theidon, K. (2013: 30).

[13] Watkins, M. & Shulman, H. (2008: 85).

[14] For Carnes, P. J., trauma splitting is defined as the aspect of betrayal bonds that ignores "… traumatic realities by splitting off the experiences and not integrating them into personality or daily life." Carnes, P. J., (1997: 14–17); See also LaCapra, D. (2001:39ff); LaCapra, D. (2004).

[15] Krystal, H., (1995) in C. Caruth (ed.) (pp. 76–99).

[16] Watkins, M. & Shulman, H. (2008: 106).

[17] Volf, M. (2006: 145).

[18] Janoff-Bulman, R., (1992: 103).

that would enable people to make sense of what happened to them and their world remains largely absent, as the following testimony suggests: "In the community everything is dangerous, no one has any security; those most affected by fear are the women and children." Author's field research: interviewee from Yachaya (Imaculada). For people in the communities studied this means that the reasons for symptoms such as tension, anxiety, fear and insecurity are often left unexplained and unexplored. This is demonstrated by the following statement: "We are a people with many anxieties and worries because we don't know what is going to happen next or from what direction it might come. I never stop worrying about this and it has caused me to suffer some health complications." Author's field research: interviewee from Otoronco (Perla).

Some attempt to skirt around the memory of extreme life events "…allows no room for the validating formalization of one's knowledge or, at best, refers it to an extremely restricted social circle."[19] Unless this mechanism is "…supplemented by practices of working through and integration,"[20] its capacity for preventing the experience of extreme life events from continuing to interfere with survivors' lives will be significantly diminished. "There is always this tension inside you and that stays there, which means that it's a little difficult to think that we are one hundred percent normal." Author's field research: interviewee from Wamani (Jaquline). The terrible anxiety which may develop following exposure to any one of a variety of traumatic events, such as threatened death, or serious injury are seen as the biggest cause of concentration deficits and erratic behaviour and can also cause people to worry that the situation may recur.

Typical is the following testimony: "I don't know if it is the fear talking, but I am nervous and afraid to walk in the streets at night. I always feel this way." Author's field research: interviewee from Unay (Amalia).

Though the experience of extreme life events may appear less threatening over time the opportunity survivors have for talking about what happened to other people in the communities studied is limited. In addition, extreme life events resist representation and destroy speech because they are outside the range of normal daily activity. This means that the individual subjective felt-experience is vulnerable to "…the lie of a prevailing discourse that denies, ignores, or disguises essential aspects of reality."[21] To make sense of their situation survivors need their suffering to be properly acknowledged and an assurance that appropriate responsibilities by the authorities will be assumed.[22] In practice this does not happen. Instead, the feeling that no one is interested in allowing them to make sense of their situation causes survivors to believe that nothing can be done and that further misery and suffering are inevitable.[23] This lack of recognition and respect for what suffering does is a

[19] Martin-Baro, I., (1989: 3–20).

[20] Schwab, G., (2010: 20).

[21] Martin-Baro, I., (1986).

[22] Amery, J., (1980: 62ff).

[23] See for example, Jnl. of Community Psychology Special Issue: The Assessment of Power Through Psycho Political Validity March 2008 Volume 36, Issue 2.

breach of normative expectations. For Amery "…the expectation of help, the certainty of help is one of the fundamental experiences of life."[24] If this expectation of help is not properly honoured it keeps the victim entangled in the past and unable to move on. To be able to make sense of pain and loss, suffering, grief and death people need access to shared values, common humanity and shared responsibility.

However, these resources have been shattered by the political violence. Before the violence people lived and died in a relatively contained social environment in which ethical responsibilities were confined to the immediate realm of their own experience.

In the aftermath of the political violence the multiplicity of life's demands means that conventional coping mechanisms including popular mobilization, solidarity and grassroots organizations are ill-equipped to coordinate social life and move shared goals forwards. In this way, as Bowlby, (1988) noted, the "…lack of secure attachment stunts the development of empathy, especially the ability to make the emotional connection with other people's feelings, which is the basis of affective empathy."[25] For survivors in the communities studied this means that any help to confront the emotional legacies of their past is likely to be restricted to the support they receive from those closest to them, including members of their own family.

However, the empirically unpredictable nature of any empathic responsiveness to the suffering of others means that emotional support is often unavailable, or if available, ineffective and unconvincing, even with respect to those closest to the survivors of the political violence. For the children who lost a parent or were orphaned the consequences are particularly severe since the "…child's understandings of relationships can only be from the relationships he's experienced."[26] This is demonstrated by the following statement: "Children who lost their father or mother during the violence are still traumatised. It is for this reason that people aged between 25 and 30 still have many problems. Many are illiterate, as they were unable to study during the violence. Many of their teachers also took to the hills because they were afraid of being in the village. This age group still has health problems because they were unable to eat properly during that time." Author's field research: interviewee from Otoronco (Guido).

The absence of an empathic listener or the presence of "…an 'other' who can hear the anguish of one's memories and thus affirm and recognize their realness"[27] is commonplace amongst people in the communities studied. This lack of empathy and solidarity has devastating consequences for survivors for whom these qualities had been at the centre of their existence for generations. For example, in Yachaya 80% of randomly selected interviewees said that they did not have access to anyone with whom they can discuss and share their experiences of extreme events. Outside of the family support from other people and society in general is mainly restricted to the *Asociación de familias afectadas por la violencia política* (AFAVIP) a

---

[24] Amery, J. (1980: 25, 28, 70, 81) See also the discussion on this point in Zolkos, M. (2011:94); Marcos, (2001); Staub, E., (1999a, b); (2003); Chorbajan, L. & Shirinian, G., (1999).

[25] Bowlby, J., (1988) cited in Krznaric, R., (2014: 15).

[26] Alan Sroufe quoted in Rifkin, J., (2010) cited in Krznaric, R., (2014: 15).

[27] Felman, S. & Laub, D. (1992: 68).

relatively new grassroots organization mandated to help those affected by the political violence. However, AFAVIP's activities are primarily concerned with the exhumation of mass graves, recording the number of deaths, disappearances and torture and the lobbying for a public works budget.[28]

In this respect AFAVIP's role in helping survivors process the emotional legacies of the violence is insignificant, and this has diminished still further as the interval between the extreme events and the present increases. This is shown by the following statement: "Many people from the community do not participate (in AFAVIP) because they do not trust the government and they think it a waste of time." Author's field research: interviewee from Otoronco (Nahuatl). This happens because the government fails to reach out and relate to the emotional experiences of other survivors. Instead rules and institutional procedures to eliminate uncertainty and reduce stress and anxiety in the face of ambiguity and misunderstanding deny them access to the human implications of a situation and its moral significance for misery and suffering.

This has a detrimental effect on the way people perceive and interpret social behaviours and is responsible for their own indifference, apathy and lack of interest as the following statement can testify: "The lack of progress on individual reparations mean that members are unhappy with the association and do not come to the meetings." Author's field research: interviewee from Wamani (Sabas).

Over time the failure to consider the historical and particular conditions under which survivors live their lives is likely to result in the individual preferring to abdicate their condition to a form of reductionism that makes no concession to the available empirical evidence. This is borne out by the following: "I have been President of the Victims of Political Violence for three years. This year marks the end of my period and I will call a general election to find a successor because the members are moving away; they are distancing themselves from the organization. Basically, for me this is because people have become used to state handouts, such as the glass of milk programme, the soup kitchen programme and JUNTOS. These things make people want to stick with these things as the new norms and nothing else. It means that they don't want to come to the AFAVIP to discuss individual reparations or anything else, particularly since collective reparations started." Author's field research: interviewee from Qocha (Valentin).

For people physically weakened by malnutrition and neglect this lack of recognition and respect for their suffering frustrates the basic need for safety, control predictability and self-respect.[29] This encourages survivors to minimize their own

[28] Other support has come from an NGO working with widows from the conflict, but the coverage is limited. In Qocha a mental health project funded by an international NGO was halted only weeks after starting because the project's psychologists did not speak Quechua and lacked training in mental health issues associated with conflict-affected victims. According to one interviewee from Qocha the only government funded support for people with mental health problems is in the city and not the countryside.

[29] See for example, Jnl. of Community Psychology Special Issue: The Assessment of Power Through Psycho Political Validity March 2008 Volume 36, Issue 2

psychological discomfort and responsibility for actions and thoughts that would otherwise interfere with their ongoing struggle for survival.

However, although extreme denial and dissociation may help to protect survivors from the memory of past pain and suffering the idea that large aspects of their experience of death and destruction can be split off and completely disowned is unthinkable.[30] Even though dialogue about the past has been cut off, anxieties, fears and tensions about what happened build up as symptoms that cause survivors to re-experience the political violence through recurrent memories, nightmares, nervousness and tension. For example, only 6 of 35 randomly selected for interview from Wamani said that they were now able to sleep peacefully, whilst others such as Lola admitted to being "...overwhelmed by fear and the return of nightmares" if suddenly awoken by trivial events such as dogs barking.

In Yachaya 28 of 35 randomly selected for interview said that they still get woken up in the night by feelings of panic and fear about what had happened. One recalled: "I live with fear because what happened has never left me. Even when I don't think about it I see it in my dreams. When I hear something I get up, because I react quickly and then cannot sleep because I am alert." Author's field research: interviewee from Unay (Yoyotli). In this example of complex sleep disturbance, the underlying sleep patho-physiology interacts with PTSD and related psychiatric distress. Though these disturbances may become less specific over time the majority of survivors associate sleep disturbance and insomnia with flashbacks of the traumatic incident which often appear without warning. For example: "When I sleep at night into my mind comes those times of violence that we have passed through; sometimes those things occupy every aspect of my sleep and I feel very desperate." Author's field research: interviewee from Wamani (Mariangela).

These symptoms of sleep disturbance overlap with the way intrusive thoughts and images including flashbacks of the traumatic incident appear out of the blue without any triggers or reminders.[31] Being reminded of what happened and the injustice of the event(s) often gives rise to irritability and anger. Though most commonly directed at those thought to be responsible for what happened it is also frequently directed at loved ones, close family, friends or colleagues as the following indicates: "In those years, the danger was too much. It terrified me and I never want to return to those times. Every time I remember it, I feel frightened and ill. I'm only OK if I don't remember, but if I do start to remember, I feel terrible. Sometimes it makes me want to beat my children or mistreat them." Author's field research: interviewee from Otoronco (Eva).

Because the thoughts and memories of the victim and their past merge with their present thoughts about and attitudes toward their past the terrible anxiety of the new and the total lack of any reference point mean that people remain entangled in their traumatic past. This is demonstrated by the following: "We have nightmares when

[30] Psychic splitting tends to be used to suggest "...a sequestering off of a portion of the self so that the split off element ceases to respond to the environment or else is in some way at odds with the remainder of the self." See Lifton, R. J., (1986: 419).

[31] Frankel, F. H. (1994).

we try to remember the things that happened, through conversations, or listening, or some other reason. We remember everything that happened." Author's field research: interviewee from Otoronco (Yolanda). Metz calls these memories of human suffering "dangerous memories" because they "interrupt" how people prefer to think about "the way things are" and "…reveal new and dangerous insights for the present."[32]

For people in the communities studied the emotional intensity of these dangerous insights threatens their refusal to remember their past.

These memories have a subversive power that "…open a crack in history"[33] and "…illuminate for a few moments and with a harsh and steady light the questionable nature of things we have apparently come to terms with."[34] This is demonstrated by the following testimony: "Almost everyone will say the same: it was the worst thing that happened to them and their lives have never been the same again. Everyone lived completely stressed, very sad; they were very difficult times for all people of the community. They did not have enough to eat, and that situation robbed them of the will to live; it was like a nightmare that seemed as though it would never end." Author's field research: interviewee from Wamani (Theodore).

For survivors the obsession with a *tabula rasa*, with new beginnings is anathema. How could it be otherwise? One survivor noted: "When the terrorism started we fled and lived hidden in the mountains and didn't have anything to eat. I saw the terrorists kill my family – they hung them and then cut them up with knives. It was very scary, we thought we would die, we thought we would never survive." Author's field research: interviewee from Wamani (Judit). To understand why memories of human suffering "make demands on us"[35] and "make the present unsafe" we need to recognize that by "break[ing] through the grip of the prevailing consciousness" the events of the past are given a new quality because they radically challenge the present in light of unfulfilled hopes.[36] By keeping these events present in their mind a recollection of what happened can be made known to others and an opportunity for that experience to be processed and worked through becomes possible. By reliving in memory the experiences of that time survivors are reliving the pain as well as the events with which those traumatic memories are associated. This is not something that remains isolated from the rest of the inner life of the individual, but something that spreads and colours all aspects of their interior space.

In the end the memory of pain and loss, suffering, grief and death haunt survivors in a fashion that erodes their consciousness of reality. Of the 35 randomly selected for interview from Unay everyone said that they felt traumatized by what they had lived through.[37] In these circumstances the natural interval between past and present

---

[32] Metz, J. B., (1980: 171).

[33] Marcos, (2001: 209).

[34] Metz, J. B., (1980: 109). See also Iafrate, M. J., (2009).

[35] Metz, J. B. (1980: 109).

[36] Metz, J. B., (1980: 200).

[37] In addition to the shocking events the interviewees said that they associated the political violence with the times when they had nothing to eat, no one to turn to for help, nowhere safe to flee to, of

is obliterated and the domination of the present by the past reduces the significance of everything else. How could it be otherwise? It is not by chance that a kind of incomprehension and bafflement should arise out of the memory of suffering as the following statement indicates: "Sometimes to escape people dropped into the ravines to try and save themselves. Sometimes people hid in the lavatories and then they found them and killed them. How can these people have hated us so much? Some accused you for fun and killed you. They hated you because of the farms you had, because of the property you had; it was all out of jealousy." Author's field research: interviewee from Otoronco (Rufo). Efforts to prevent the memory of what happened from overwhelming their future and present lives increases the weakness of the psyche and the capacity for what was repressed to resurface in flashbacks that are beyond the control of the individual.[38] A survivor reports how a history of extreme experiences has caused them to become hypersensitive to anything that may remind them of their 'dangerous memories' as the following statement indicates: "Yes I am tense and worried; anything can make me think those times could come back; when I remember those times I get as cold as when I climb up in the highlands." Author's field research: Interviewee from Yachaya (Rebecca).

These intrusive recollections and images of the terrible past with which they are associated have brought into being a situation that survivors believe will never end and live on unceasingly until the end of their lives.[39] Author's field research: interviewee from Yachaya (Isandro).

In the longer term this can result in further problems because it interferes with their capacity to process and make sense of their experience. For example: "When we remember those times it is always a worry. I am always anxious, though it was worse before because we couldn't sleep. I still get infuriated by it when I feel this way because they (SL/armed forces)aren't even here anymore." Author's field research: interviewee from Unay (Santiago).

These spontaneous, unsuccessful attempts to emotionally work through the experience of the political violence are a symptom of the helplessness that confronts the traumatized. A typical testimony noted: "I was traumatized by seeing many things at age 12; even years after the shots I am still traumatized; my children are not normal; they obliterated my brothers. I used to cry a lot because my children had no water and nothing to eat." Author's field research: interviewee from Wamani (Gildas).

---

feelings of despair, suicide, fear – particularly amongst those who had been hunted down to be killed. The interviewees also said that they continue to feel traumatized and that this is responsible for outbursts of tears – sometimes lasting all night, the feeling of being physically broken (particularly amongst those who had been tortured), an inability to eat, indifference to everything around them, confusion (by those who had been abused by both sides in the conflict), feelings of guilt, an inability to concentrate, feelings of grief for those they had lost in the conflict, inability to study at school "…because the only things I could think about were those things." For the interviewees who were children at the time these feelings have not dissipated; on the contrary, the memories have not faded and they still feel traumatized.

[38] Volf, M. (2006: 22)

[39] Schreuder, B., Kleijn, W. & Rooijmans, H. (2000); Schreuder, B., et al. (2001).

By re-experiencing how suffering and extreme events feel the individual is forced to confront the fact that pain is part of their past. However, because painful memories call to life what happened during the political violence survivors are also being reminded of the experience of death and destruction and the intense fear with which these things are associated. For example, of the 44 randomly selected for interview from Otoronco everyone including children, adolescents, young adults and elderly (men and women) said that they are still afraid of SL, particularly because of fear of reprisals for having broken with SL in the early stages of the political violence.

A member of this community describes this ongoing fear: "People talk about SL coming back. If they do come, if they come back, we will have to defend ourselves. We would have to do something and things are worse now because the desire to kill any informer is much stronger than before. They say that SL is back in other places and that once they start they will start killing." Author's field research: Interviewee from Qocha (Margarita).

In this way the inner world is kept open to the presence of the past in the present and the fear from which the individual has been hiding may come to life and be relived once more.[40] In view of this survivors are reminded of the fragility and relativity of the norms and rules of behaviour which had previously governed their lives and of the realization that their own survival is no longer secure. Extreme denial and dissociation may stifle the reaction to unwelcome thoughts, dreams, nightmares, and feelings, but they cannot prevent the memory of past pain and suffering from resurfacing.[41] A victim of the violence describes how these ongoing disturbances continue to be played out: "Nightmares always come when we remember what happened because we remember everything. It was all so terrible; many of us lost our families, many of us have become estranged from each other; then we had to abandon this place as though we were criminal fugitives. If a stranger comes here we get scared because it puts us on the alert, because by ignoring his stay here we forget to think about why they are here and what their presence is for." Author's field research: interviewee from Qocha (Maximo).

To re-establish cognitive stability and emotional health survivors need to reformulate a view of reality that is able to assimilate and integrate their experiences, but this is conditional on being able to make "…a gradual shift from unpredictable danger to reliable safety, from dissociated trauma to acknowledged memory, and from stigmatized isolation to restored social connection."[42] For survivors subject to the hard struggle for satisfying basic needs the choice to confront the horrors of the past is no easy task, particularly when they are as grim and as deeply felt as those described by the following informant: "There were many dead, they burned many houses, first they killed the landowners; then they killed their animals, there was nothing to eat. They destroyed everything; there was much suffering in the village. The military came and they beat up the innocent and the guilty; they hit hard. Both

[40] Felman, S., & Laub, D., (1992: 67).

[41] Ehlers, A., Hackmann, A., Steil, R., Clohessy, S., Wenninger, K., Winter, H. (2002).

[42] Herman, J. (1992: 155).

the terrorists and the military killed many villagers." Author's field research: Interviewee from Wamani (Ismael).

In the immediate aftermath of the political violence the memories of extreme events would have been almost impossible to separate from the pain and intense fear with which these experiences are associated. For survivors who agreed to testify for the TRC this would have made any recollection of the events a considerable ordeal and likely to make inaccuracies and omissions in their testimony a real possibility. The difficulty survivors have in recalling what happened to them is illustrated by this statement: "A lot of people still don't want to talk; they keep their secrets because of what happened to those who talked during the violence; psychologically this means that they don't want to tell the people doing the surveys from the government. They are only just starting to let it out." Author's field research: interviewee from Yachaya (Flavio).

In the opinion of one informant, there is no doubt that giving testimony for the TRC was affected by having to re-experience the horrors of past pain and fear: "… When the human rights people came here for the first time, all the people (that agreed to testify) gathered together to tell them of what had happened (to them) but in many cases, they didn't want to talk about it, and that made them embarrassed about being scared." Author's field research: interviewee from Qocha (Julio). However, people also admitted to not wanting to give accurate information for fear of the consequences: "There is always latent worry amongst people, so when the truth commission asked for information no one gave reliable information. That means that the government is giving itself the right to receive any information, so just lately we gave information that was almost true, but it was only seventy percent true. There are also a lot of us that do not give information because there is always that fear which does not leave." Author's field research: interviewee from Unay (Sans).

For people from the communities studied this is further exacerbated by the fact that the present is characterised by conditions in which violence and the fear of violence are ongoing: "They say that SL is back in other places and that once they start they will start killing. Now people think nothing, our authority tell us that there is nothing, but what we hear is that it is starting in other places; we are worried because we think it will come here too, so when there is a meeting of those who were affected by the violence some people (a lot) no longer take part because they think it is better to stay quiet. We have to remember that the register of victims has the names of those who fled to the cities, not those who stayed behind and spent the time suffering; they are not listed." Author's field research: interviewee from Qocha (Margarita).

To the extent that the experiences of extreme events can only be processed if the survivor is willing and able to reconstruct and re-externalise what happened this is hardly propitious. Even when survivors are no longer fearful of resurgence in violence, they may still lack a sufficiently safe environment for them to begin the process of working through their experiences. For example, the majority (27) of 35 randomly selected interviewees in Wamani said that although they are no longer afraid in the way they used to be the fear of further violence is never far away –

especially on account of the rumours that circulate about the activities of drug traffickers and the resurgence of terrorist activity in the jungle and along the roads. The difficulty in making the shift from unpredictable danger to reliable safety is illustrated by the following: "When a stranger comes, it frightens us because it puts us on alert, because we don't know why they are staying here. We calm down once we start to ask questions about their motives, whether they are feasible or not. If it isn't, we also worry because if someone doesn't have a good reason to be here or if they try to lie to us, then we are given to believe that their presence here is not for this reason, but for other motives." Author's field research: interviewee from Otoronco (Perla).

In these circumstances the individual no longer experiences other people as a source of social support, comfort and self-realization. Instead other people become a source of anxiety and tension.[43] Over time this leads to feelings of depression and disillusionment that cause survivors to become disengaged, isolated, distrustful, hostile, fearful and selfish: "Before the violence we were closely united, I was a child then but after the military arrived people turned rebellious; the military worked people to death, both men and women. Then the military left and there was no more unity among us and we did not want anything more to do with the community." Author's field research: interviewee from Unay (Graciano).

Though subsequent developments have failed to bring closure to survivors it has brought about a situation in which they are able to remember death and destruction without remembering the feelings that accompanied these experiences. This is abetted by the lack of any counterforce to the numbing effects of depression, lack of energy and motivation, intensified feelings of guilt and worthlessness, affective liability, irritability and lethargy, loss of appetite, insomnia and lack of concentration. The following illustrates how victims are able to talk dispassionately about their experiences, not out of fear, but as a way of denying victory to the perpetrator: "I was very lucky to live, I wanted to untie my hands but they would not let me, my brothers, my dad and my sister in law all had their hands tied. They demanded that I hand over my gun, but I refused, then one of them shot me in the face and the bullet went through my ear. Then they started shooting at my family. I could not react, and then SL tried to kill me with a knife in the back saying this is how a human dog dies. After this I found that my family was dead, then someone came to search for me and then they found and helped me. I have to keep on living because I must raise my children." Author's field research: interviewee from Yachaya (Florentin).

In this respect the passage of time has made it easier for survivors to reconstruct what happened to them so long as they do not allow their memory to remember the emotional dimension of these experiences. In these circumstances survivors may come to believe that repeated reconstructions of the event have a curative effect that is able to extinguish the pain and intense fear with which these experiences are associated. This perspective is reflected in the following observation:

---

[43] "…For Freud anxiety had the quality of indefiniteness and absence or indeterminacy of an object; for Kierkegaard and Heidegger, it was the fear of something that is nothing." LaCapra, D., (2001: 57).

"Now after all of this time (since the end of the political violence) the people that were affected and all those ill-treated they just let it out: it happened to me, they did that to me, I was tortured, raped etc. They just let it out, like a child after its' been taught to sing for sweets." Author's field research: interviewee from Yachaya (Zolin). How much does this contribute to their ability to gain mastery of their experiences? Inwardly nothing much has changed. By remembering the events of the political violence without remembering how it felt survivors are still failing to assimilate and integrate the psychological wounds caused by their experiences. In this respect the reconstruction of what happened without any recall of what it felt like has created another problem.[44]

By keeping these feelings out of conscious awareness survivors are reducing their capacity to feel, with the result that their link with the memory of extreme events is weakened and they become psychically benumbed.[45] One of the consequences of this development is for people to be confined to a narrow identity that makes no concession to the complexity of their situation. Unable to undo this entrapment results in the loss of their own past experiences and a growing dissociation from local histories, traditional norms and values. This loss of the capacity to bear witness to the internal effects of psychological wounds leads not just to an enforced sense of inferiority, but to the possible loss of their identity as humans. In these circumstances feelings of impotence can make violence an almost inevitable outcome. For example, in Yachaya 42 of the 44 (95%) randomly selected interviewees said that they react violently against other people. This is consistent with the results recorded in the other communities studied as the following demonstrates:

"Anything can cause me to feel violent; it could be something somebody says because I keep remembering what happened. I don't know why, maybe it's because I saw people die and saw how they were being 'punished'; they 'punished' my father by putting him in a pit where they made him eat dog meat." Author's field research: interviewee from Otoronco (Yolanda). In this context violence is not so much a product of hate or the wish for revenge as a feeling of indignation. It highlights the fact that survivors have experienced, witnessed, or confronted an event or events that they are critically opposed to. In this way violence (or violent feelings) can be seen as the manifestation of an impulse that helps survivors prioritise their values, free up their ability to think critically and make a judgement of condemnation.[46] A witness to the killing of the community mayor describes their arrival at this emotional stage: "I react in a violent way; I don't know why, it's in my character; it goes back to when they victimized the mayor. I was alongside (him); I was at his

[44] Volf, M. (2006: 27).

[45] This was originally conceived to describe a particular type of reaction to unpleasant and painful experiences by the individual. Its purpose is to block out the feelings associated with suffering by the individual anaesthetizing themselves from the full effects of the feelings with which the suffering is associated. The numbed individual produces a feeling of detachment from other people with the result that they no longer perceive themselves as moral/thinking beings. Individualist psychic numbing is widely used to describe victims of rape and people who suffer from post trauma stress disorder (PTSD). See Lifton, R. J. (1982).

[46] Gautier, A., & Sabatini Scalmati, A., (2010: 11).

side. In front of me they killed the mayor, almost from then the psychosis has always been with me." Author's field research: interviewee from Otoronco (Icnoyotl).

Though feelings of impotence and the aggressive outcomes it produces can be viewed as a normal consequence of the political violence it is also symptomatic of: "…what has been normalized and taken for granted in the environment."[47] In order to understand the implications of this process it is important to recognise that the psychological lives of those responsible for inflicting violence on others are inconsistent with "…the idea of any norms that might exist in the landscape of internal life."[48] By failing to remember the emotional dimension of their experiences, instead of simply recalling the events with which they are associated, people unwittingly produce social conditions that allow violence to continue.

In this respect ignorance, indifference and silence collude in the development of a set of conditions that block any means by which the victim and the survivor may gain mastery of their experiences.[49] Having to endure the consequences of lived contradictions can lead to severe depression, anxiety and other symptoms of varying severity.

Faced with a situation "…in which every available choice is an insult to human dignity, every choice an impossible choice, makes people apathetic about their own powerlessness.[50] Here is the testimony of a survivor looking back on the changes it has brought to people's attitudes and behaviour: "I think that before people were more respectful, harder workers, and more reliable. Now there is no obedience, and this new generation, I don't know, they don't listen to or respect the leaders or authorities. They are lazy and just complain. They spend their lives living, they live their lives. They are always drunk and only get involved at church when one of them needs something, but when it comes to the community they don't help, because nobody helps. They are lazy. They have a misconception. They only think about easy things because during the Fujimori period, people everywhere were corrupted with little gifts. They were given government handouts, provisions and other things, and during the elections, they would use bribes. That to me is a misconception, because they do not have their own thoughts; they are easily persuaded and easily convinced." Author's field research: interviewee from Yachaya (Eusebio).

It is in these circumstances that survivors are confronted with the "…futile task of redefining decency in an atmosphere that cannot support it."[51] In the wasteland left behind by the political violence the fact that "…primary relationships with the community and the family have been cut off creates confusion, terror and a sense of persecution."[52]

Because the abuse that was performed externally has been transformed into an internal abuse the function and structure of memory "…freezes around the traumatic

[47] Watkins, M. & Shulman, H. (2008: 58).

[48] Watkins, M. & Shulman, H. (2008: 84).

[49] Watkins, M. & Shulman, H. (2008: 84).

[50] Langer, L. (1980; Langer, L., (1982: 72); Langer, L., (1993: 26).

[51] Langer, L., (1993: 26).

[52] Gautier, A., & Sabatini Scalmati, A., (2010: 35).

events and then irradiates its cone of shadow against the space or time preceding these events."[53] The testimonies from communities included in this study is eloquent on this, as the following shows: "Now, back in my village, I'm still afraid. These things are always with me. I always think that at any moment the same thing could happen all over again." Author's field research: interviewee from Wamani (Isbel).

Though any immediate danger may have receded this "...loss of the capacity to be a witness to oneself and thus to witness from the inside"[54] has disastrous consequences; not least of which is a latent tension that affects the "...particular relations of which the individual is only a part."[55] This is demonstrated by the following statements: "There is a lot of tension here in the community, especially when we think about the future." Author's field research: interviewee from Otoronco (Marisol). A survivor of the political violence reports a similar experience: "Others don't want to talk; they keep their secrets because psychologically they are afraid." Author's field research: interviewee from Qocha (Maritza).

To move beyond this situation in order that they can integrate their experience of extreme events survivors need to empathically project themselves into their own thoughts and memories of the past. In this way they can begin the process of integration so that their own painful memories can become "...infused with their present thoughts about and attitudes towards their own past."[56] However, there are constraining forces in operation that prevent survivors gaining access to the memory of their emotional experiences of extreme events.

These forces derive not from the inner lives of people, but from "...the outer environments in which their symptoms and identities evolve."[57] To integrate their experience of extreme events, survivors need to follow the social origins of their psychological wounds into the relationship between the individual and society and the particular social relations of which the individual is only a part.[58] For people in the communities studied the surrounding social and institutional context is dominated by the State.

From a national perspective it is possible to think that the state has made significant progress in addressing the suffering inflicted on thousands of families and communities across the rural highlands. However, in spite of significant efforts to strengthen democracy and human rights protection the actual lived experience in the aftermath of political violence has been repeatedly side-lined. Instead of engaging with the social experience of suffering the only authorized construction for policies and programmes tend to come from economic indicators. Faced with the problem of increasing numbers of chronic illness metrics developed to measure the burden of suffering in objective terms are used by the state to formulate health and social

[53] Sabatini Scalmati, A., (2000: 175).

[54] Felman, S. & Laub, D., (1992: 82)..

[55] Martin-Baro, I., (1994a, b, c, d: 124).

[56] Goldie, P., (2011: 193).

[57] Watkins, M. & Shulman, H. (2008: 54).

[58] Martin-Baro, I., (1994a, b, c, d: 124).

policy with respect to priorities for limited resources.[59] Though this may be important for health care reform and public health planning, economic indicators are no basis for any meaningful engagement with "…the complex, even contradictory, human side of suffering."[60] To rescue this "…slow transmutation of suffering and caring into efficiency and cost" requires an addition of narratives, ethnographies and social histories as a complement to economic indicators.[61] By ignoring these measures the state's approach to suffering is such that anything specific is left out. The notion that anything specific about suffering has nothing to add to the process misrepresents the impact of such concepts as power, culture, conflict, exploitation and hierarchy.[62]

This is an approach to suffering that is guided not by the reality of the lives and experiences of people from any specific context but by a pre-determined agenda.

Unaffected by the reality of suffering the relationship between the powerless and the state is instead guided by the historical, social and psychological explanations that comprise the mind-set of the state. This combination of indifference and lack of empathy mean that sustained suffering inspires no sympathy, no compassion and no action for change.

In its place are a series of rules and regulations based on concepts of responsibility, accountability, dignity and respect made in accordance with the legal framework of a society. It also means that objective notions of responsibility likely to foster social behaviour patterns such as reliability and trust are undermined by the consequences of de-contextualisation.[63] Indifference to matters of culture, ethnicity, political tradition, local notions of what is right and wrong and other aspects of local level morality make feelings of moral disorientation, incomprehension and incredulity on behalf of the powerless inevitable. Having encountered the full impact of the political violence at first hand the following statement illustrates the frustration this has produced amongst many people from the communities studied: "There are many things that they (the government) should help us with. If there is no support from them how can we improve? If there is no support from them how can we change our lives? The way we think has been affected by the violence and the wounds will never heal. We have so much anger towards the government and it is difficult for this feeling to leave us." Author's field research: interviewee from Wamani (Lurdes).

---

[59] Kleinman, A. & Kleinman, J., (1997a, b: 15) in Kleinman, A., Das, V., and Lock, M. (eds.) (1997a, b).

[60] Kleinman, A. & Kleinman, J., (1997a, b: 15) in Kleinman, A., Das, V., and Lock, M. (eds.) (1997a, b).

[61] Kleinman, A. & Kleinman, J., (1997a, b: 15) in Kleinman, A., Das, V., and Lock, M. (eds.) (1997a, b).

[62] "…The state's frozen objectivity means that reality has been manipulated by the state before a manipulation of the subject by reality took place." Haas, P., (1988: 78) Morality after Auschwitz, Augsburg Fortress Publishing; Kleinman, A., & Kleinman, J., (1997a, b); Kleinman, A., Das, V., & Lock, M. (eds), (1997); Staub, E., (1996a, b).

[63] For Tilly "…trust between the citizen and the state is confined to those situations in which the citizen is certain to achieve personal benefit." Tilly (1985:170).

By ignoring local information and knowledge, motivation and participation, grassroots organizations and social networks, voice and expression of discontent, moral convictions and responsiveness to local problems and access to justice the complex relationship between the powerless and the government is neutralised, leaving the way open for detachment, objectivity and the impersonal.[64] The resentment caused by this constriction in the capacities for meaningful engagement is clear from the following statement: "There is no honesty and no seriousness in what the government does; they see it as a game. The people who occupy these positions see it more as a personal convenience, which means that there is a lot of favouritism, especially for those who have the right political colours, because today there is no transparency in their work. The local authorities have their own little group and that little group does everything they want and much of what they do is driven by revenge; revenge that always exists." Author's field research: interviewee from Qocha (Severo).

By failing to acknowledge the psychological wounding caused by the political violence the institutions and organizations in the surrounding social context are blocking historical memory and the capacity for other-regarding empathy in particular. For survivors this means that the normal process of daily living has to be endured without access to any means by which they can make sense of and respond to what happened. In these circumstances basic trust is in question. For example, only 2 of the 44 interviewees (5%) randomly selected in Yachaya said that that they trust government officials or members of other institutions including NGOs. A survivor of the political violence describes the severe damage to the capacity for trust as a result of abuses perpetrated by the armed forces, the police and SL:

"During the violence we didn't know who we could report these abuses to. There was no authority because the people were too frightened by the military and SL. If complaints were made about abuses (torture, disappearances, arbitrary detentions, killings, rapes, robberies, etc.) people were either imprisoned or disappeared." Author's field research: interviewee from Otoronco (Jeremias).

This failure to engage with the original experience of the survivors can be seen as a result of the "…difficulty that mainstream Peruvian society and most of its political elite have in acknowledging their share of responsibility for the violations committed during the conflict and in accepting the history of marginalization reported by the CVR."[65] It can also be seen as a reflection of "…the low importance that the rest of Peruvian society places on the situation of indigenous people."[66]

By failing to gain access to the reality of the survivors' structures and institutions reveal the main feature of their own objective attitude to injustice and violence. This involves being unaffected by the suffering of others. The feeling of abandonment this produces has been in place for so long that it has since given way to resignation as the following statement indicates: "To tell you what the community feels about

[64] The idea that the human significance of suffering can be trivialized to a point that is morally objectionable must not be forgotten. See Frank A. W. (2001); Steiner, G. (1967).

[65] Correa, C., (2013: 1).

[66] Correa, C., (2013: 1).

the government? … Well, for example we haven't received any management or help from the mayor; the truth is we do not really know what is being done or what is being managed." Author's field research: interviewee from Otoronco (Ruben).

By blocking any emotional engagement with survivors, the institutions around them normalize the psychological wounding caused by the political violence and treat it as a part of the normal process of daily living. For many people the surrounding social and institutional context is no more than a mirror image of how they are perceived by central government. This is illustrated by the following: "With regard to central government nothing happens where there is much poverty, the government do not see anything in our community; they never have." Author's field research: interviewee from Unay (Rosalind).

Though survivors may not always consciously register the effects of this situation on their lives, the lack of any social or psychological space in which their own experiences of extreme life events could be explored encourages the belief that there is no hope for the situation to change and therefore no point in exploring what happened. This is borne out by the following statement: "In my opinion life isn't worth anything because my life isn't good. It's bad, and it is worrying. I have nothing good in my life and for someone who has a family, that is concerning," Author's field research: interviewee from Unay (Manauia).

The struggle to stand up to such a difficult environment is therefore not just about the actual situation as it presents itself; it is also about insecurity, anxiety, fear, low self-esteem, social isolation and lack of control over work and home life and lack of social integration and their impact on the internal resources of the individual. This deprives individuals and groups of human dignity and self-respect. It makes them feel that their reality has been manipulated by the government, that nobody is open to advising them and that there is no alternative but to fall back on their own resources.

In the absence of a voice, influence and independence certain motives predominate: the protection of the physical self, the preservation of the psychological self, including self-image, personal worldview and values and the attainment of some control over specific problems and outcomes.[67] For many people these feelings spill over into nervousness, fearfulness and panic, especially when faced by reminders of the political violence, such as the arrival of strangers in their community: "People here do not feel safe, we are very anxious about anyone who enters the community; we know all about the (current) attacks in nearby villages. There is a climate of insecurity, for that reason the self-defence committee was deactivated because we are afraid of being made targets for SL. But now (because of the insecurity) in the last three assemblies people have put this back on the agenda and want to reorganize the CAD." Author's field research: interviewee from Yachaya (Lino).

In these circumstances survivors are presented with "…an untenable choice: either aggressively adopt a socially stigmatized identity, or accept the closing of

[67] Staub, E., (1989); Staub, E. (1996a, b); Staub, E. (1999a, b, c, d, e, f). in Summers, C and Markussen, D. (eds.); Staub, E., (1999a, b, c, d, e, f); Staub, E. (1999a, b, c, d, e, f) in Chorbajian, L. and Shirinian, G. (eds.) (1999).

options and submit to an imposed identity that is full of dehumanizing elements."[68] Though AFAVIP has sought to take a stand against the helplessness of their situation, most survivors fail to overcome the constraining forces imposed on them by this suspension of the emotional bond to other human beings. This makes people more willing to concede to the desires of the powerful, irrespective of the perceived legitimacy of their demands.

In these ways survivors in the communities studied reinforce the position of the surrounding social and institutional context, thereby contributing to the formation and maintenance of power hierarchies.

For example, focus groups from Otoronco said that factors such as location, distance from urban areas and the lack of any government or military presence make further insurgent activity a very real threat for their community. In addition, participants said that people in the community are unwilling to regenerate the *rondas* out of fear of reprisals from SL. Focus groups in Unay said that daily life is dominated by subversive activity reportedly taking place only two days walk from their community. Participants also said that previous activities with the *rondas* make their community and all neighbouring communities a real target for further violence.[69] A woman survivor expresses such fears: "I cry so much about everything and I wonder why we have been born in this country to see all this; it has left me dead inside, worrying all the time, like I was traumatised." Author's field research: interviewee from Unay (Gaétan).

This type of situation makes feelings of intolerable anxiety, fear or shame inevitable; these evoke a negative link with knowledge that obstructs meaning "...leaving a denuded representation so as to dilute the facts and reduce the pain."[70] In this way survivors become increasingly unwilling to unify past, present and future aspects of their own psychic lives. The result of this ongoing repression of the experience of extreme life events is to weaken personal autonomy and self-confidence and devalue respect for human life; it also undermines motivation and the ability to act.[71]

The effect this has on the relationship between people and their surrounding social and institutional context is illustrated by the following statement: "My countrymen don't know much about their rights, a lot of my fellow villagers don't know their rights, and so they are fooled in every way.

They don't know their rights because they aren't informed or trained, because for this, one has to be trained, one has to analyse, to study, or at least know it. Sometimes everyone tells us that we have rights and when they ask us about it, they don't know how to answer, because they are very humble people." Author's field research: Interviewee from Qocha (Maximo).

---

[68] Martin-Baro, I., (1994a, b, c, d: 132, e, f).

[69] During the political violence some subversives had been killed by the *ronda* and others disappeared.

[70] Gautier, A., & Sabatini Scalmati, A., (2010: 117).

[71] Lira, E., (2001).

Before the violence the sense of responsibility people had for each other meant that people were aware of the duties attaching to any social role they were responsible for as well as well as for ensuring that other people were fulfilling their roles. This happened because the rules and conventions that people used to meet their basic psychological needs were generally respected. The help they would have received was of a kind that enabled them to overcome their stressful experiences and move toward a stronger integration and involvement in the life of the family and community. However, the moral and emotional framework that protects people from the psychological effects of difficult life conditions is conditional on a relatively contained social environment with established rules and a degree of social stability. An informant noted how political violence brought irrevocable damage to this arrangement: "Before the violence all our needs were organised through the community leaders and the *organizaciones de base* (grass roots organizations), but all that finished during the violence because they didn't do anything to help." Author's field research: interviewee from Qocha (Pastor).

The impact of the political violence on this moral and emotional framework is such that any emotional connection with "...other people's feelings (which is the affective basis for empathy)" has been incontestably damaged.[72]

The effect this has had on the rules and conventions that used to help survivors meet their basic psychological needs is illustrated by the following: "The main people (leaders) here have a particular type of conformity because they have no vision for the future; they don't plan their activities for the period whilst they are in positions of authority or for any period in the future. In the same way they don't plan any short, medium or long-term projects. It is so bad that they are more concerned about their own interests than those of the community." Author's field research: interviewee from Wamani (Ismael).

Under such conditions it is difficult for people to re-establish what used to give meaning to life. This frustrates the basic needs for safety, control predictability and self-respect, thereby making adaptation of and reduction in the old values of solidarity inevitable.[73] In this respect psychological resistance to the problem of suffering has brought greater independence from other individuals and groups but it has also encouraged fear, envy, violence, hatred and other symptoms of social isolation.[74] Instead of a place of safety and support the legacy of political violence has brought loneliness, instability and danger. The consequences this has had for community life are illustrated by the following: "Before the people were united but now they live their own life. Now there is no pity, just selfishness, no support for orphans or widows. Now there is no such solidarity; when I was young there was mutual support, not now." Author's field research: interviewee from Qocha (Necahual).

The idea that acts of kindness and selflessness are seen as unusual and potentially suspicious are a major step towards the idea that traditional norms and values are not carved in stone.

[72] Krznaric, R., (2014: 15).

[73] Staub, E., (1989: 45).

[74] Pawelczynska, A., (1979: 126).

That they are no longer an effective means of building solidarity makes traditional norms and values appear increasingly vulnerable to revision, rejection and ultimately cancellation altogether. That the supposedly tightly woven fabric of society can easily unravel is attested to by an informant: "Here *ayni* and *minka* are almost no longer practiced, either in communal work or in meetings, because people are no longer interested; here everyone works to get ahead in their own way and this means working individually." Author's field research: interviewee from Qocha (Isabel).

From being a safe place, the rural highland community has become associated more with fragmentation and danger. For example, only 3 of the 35 randomly selected for interview from Qocha said that they no longer feel nervous, tense or worried. Of the remaining 32 interviewees some said that they lived in a more or less constant state of nervousness, tension and worry on account of concern for their family (7), others on account of having been tortured (2), despair for the future (16), fear that the violence will resume sometime soon (2), the fear of being killed (2), the military (3). In the case of Unay the memory of horrific experiences is kept alive by external difficulties that only make people want to withdraw into themselves still further, or leave their community altogether: "Here people are stressed all of the time because in the small hours of the night unknown groups come walking through the community which makes women and men think that it must be SL fleeing the area." Author's field research: interviewee from Unay (Tlacotl).

By bringing into question the ways in which people used to make sense of their environment the political violence has created a new way of thinking in which the individual has come to feel that there is nothing left to lose, nothing left to provide support (emotional, material or informational) and no status to maintain. This shattering of basic assumptions about the self and the perception of the community as a meaningful place is described in the following: "Before the political violence started, the community was quiet. The only thing people cared about was having their family, their land and the community. People had a good time and sang at the *fiestas*. Before the terrorism appeared, there were police and control and respect. That all went after they (SL) destroyed the community leaders and the magistrate." Author's field research: interviewee from Wamani (Jerome).

A survivor summed up the aftermath of the violence as follows: "No authority is even bothered about what happened to us, and no one is sorry." Author's field research: interviewee from Wamani (Martirio).

In a context of hunger, deprivation, ill treatment, injustice and poor health this makes survivors insensitive to the suffering of others and removes the act of meaningful human interaction from the difficulty of decision-making. In this respect the most powerful legacy of the political violence has been to reproduce in survivors' minds the feeling that they are on their own and that this will always be so from now on. This is demonstrated by the following: "Here you get tired of people. They are really egotistical, opportunistic, so for this reason we are going to leave and live elsewhere because the people from here do not share anything; they are not sociable, I don't know why people are so selfish; perhaps it's in the breed." Author's field research: interviewee from Unay (Momoztli).

By shifting the emphasis onto the individual the political violence has created a schism between personal and social identity.[75] Instead of living via their social group survivors are more autonomous and independent, more internally driven, and less inclined to follow traditional leaders, duties and obligations when told to do so.[76] This has impact on young people and their relationship with the community: "Now people are less disciplined, young people no longer respect the old, now young people say that these community activities are pathetic, we also say that; earlier it was the only thing that people cared about." Author's field research: interviewee from Unay (Rafael).

Such distancing from the group mindedness of social norms represents a major step towards the idea that the deepest and most profound guide to the demands of everyday life has lost its authority. To have no moral framework to fall back on, no emotional support system; to have nothing left to lose, no status to maintain and to be without pride or dignity is to live in a world that is devoid of meaning and outside of what we, who do not have to endure such conditions, understand as ordinary life. In this environment of low trust, anxiety, high vigilance and low safety nets the lack of state recognition for their plight make people believe that nothing can be done to improve their situation.

From this perspective it would seem that the surrounding social and institutional context has little to offer those survivors of the political violence seeking to confront and somehow find an appropriate outlet for the abuse that has come to acquire such a hold over their lives. In the absence of state assistance, the prospect of ever being able to work through their experiences of the political violence is, for the majority of people, pure fantasy.

This has generated indignation: "Up 'till now, no authority, local, provincial or regional, is sorry or cares; the national government is even worse. I appeal to the current leader to make policies which will change things, and for him to also realize the reality of the situation and to fix his electoral manifesto, which people are unhappy about as he only uses it to receive votes. It was entirely through deceit and broken promises, as he is not really concerned about the situation of this country. It is urgent that the government respects us. It is all just lies. They do not respect our rights and there are continuous rises in cost. Currently, all production is for self-supply only. People live in total chaos. Public and basic services, roads and other such things are only for those with money. In reality, we need them to hear us." Author's field research: interviewee from Yachaya (Vivian).

From this perspective the deeply internalized perceptions of their helplessness make it difficult to confront what has been normalised and taken for granted. Instead of speaking out about the ways in which the psychological wounding caused by the violence is treated as a part of the normal process of daily living people seek to

---

[75] Lykes, M. B. (2000); Martin-Baro, I., (1989).

[76] For Bracken P. J. & Petty C. "Modern warfare is concerned not only to destroy life, but also ways of life. It targets social and cultural institutions and deliberately aims to undermine the means whereby people endure and recover from the suffering of war." In: Bracken, P. J., & Petty, C. (eds.) (1998:3).

distance themselves from the troubling realities around them. In a context of hunger, deprivation, ill treatment, injustice and poor health this leads unconsciously to the pretence that immersion in the present and the resumption of routine and regular activity are enough to re-connect people with the ways in which they used to make sense of the world.

Being forced to submit to an imposed identity that is full of dehumanizing elements makes it particularly difficult for people to reach out toward and relate to the experiences of others through emotion. This undermines the emotional bond between people thereby making any meaningful human interaction impossible.

This is demonstrated by the following statement: "Participation (in the life of the community) is little because there is no interest; people are conformists with what they have; they do not want to progress. Anything new doesn't work because people are not interested; they are very conformist." Author's field research: interviewee from Qocha (Severo). These conditions threaten the exercise of the faculty of empathy that in turn impairs moral judgement. In this way the perception and the experience of other people becomes distorted.

These survival strategies are not just a source of psychological comfort, but a means of avoiding the harshness of their situation and of evading self-knowledge; they also help to sustain people in the belief that the old values, systems, rules and customs still have meaning. In this way people feel less alone, less vulnerable and better placed to retain their identity without any of its burdensome responsibilities. So long as people lack a sense of control and this continues indefinitely these survival strategies are almost bound to feel like being the only realistic choices.[77] It would therefore be incorrect to assume that people support what disconnection, scapegoating, passivity, selfishness, fatalism and lack of empathic connection stand for; they make use of them, not out of respect for established rules, fixed beliefs and practices, but because the individual is in a state of denial about information that is as painful as it is unwanted. In these circumstances human intelligence becomes severed from feeling, intuition and imagination.[78] By striving to separate themselves from their own experiences of extreme events survivors are allowing the psychological wounding caused by the political violence to decompose their identities.

5.1 Conclusions

I have focused on what happens when the presence of terrifying experiences in human beings gets left untold. By restoring the context in which people overwhelmed by brute force live with what has indelibly marked them the chapter seeks to bring much needed attention to the internalization of abuse and its consequences.

---

[77] See Fiske, S. T., (1993); Boehm and Flack, (2010: 46) in Guinote, A. & Vescio, T. K., (2010); Fiske, S. T. & Neuberg, S. L., (1990); Saakvitne, K. W., Gamble, S., Pearlman, L., & Lev, B. (2000); Staub, (1989, 2003).

[78] Watkins, M. & Shulman, H. (2008: 69).

In this way the thoughts and memories of the victim and how their past merges with their present thoughts about and attitudes toward their past has been brought into focus. This merging of the internal and external worlds was found to suffuse everyday reality to such an extent that it alters the way in which survivors live their lives.

For people in the rural Andean communities studied this was borne out by feelings of helplessness, fear, numbness, mistrust, anxiety, sleeplessness and nightmares, all of them characteristic of a traumatized mind. In addition, the chapter shows how being able to emotionally work through their experiences was severely compromised by the overwhelming struggle to satisfy the demands of the immediate present and the fact that their present is characterised by conditions in which violence and the fear of violence are ongoing. Unable to confront and somehow find an appropriate outlet for their experiences means that survivors have been compelled to adapt to a new reality characterized by isolation, depression, anxiety and selfish and erratic behaviour.

Chapter 6
Overcoming Past Trauma

Chapter 5 explored the merging of the internal and external worlds of survivors of the political violence commingle with everyday reality to such an extent that it transforms lives. For survivors in the communities studied the struggle to satisfy the demands of the immediate present and the fact that their present is characterised by conditions in which violence and the fear of violence are ongoing impels them to adapt to a new reality fashioned out of an intolerable internal homelessness. This chapter focuses on how survivors adapt to living under conditions that prevent them from confronting and finding an appropriate outlet for their experiences.

Instead of acknowledging the obligation they have to themselves and their own past experiences trauma encourages survivors to believe that immersion in the present and the resumption of routine and regular activity are enough to re-connect them with the ways in which they used to make sense of the world. By minimizing their own psychological discomfort and responsibility past painful experiences have become sufficiently detached as to be treated as a part of the normal process of daily living. In this way the memory of extreme events is split off and silenced.[1] For the survivors this has been critical to their own survival.[2] However, this disavowal of the past does not also mean that they remain locked into an on-going and exclusive identification with the present. Though this process enables survivors to adapt to and carry out the tasks needed for daily survival it also produces a susceptibility to anxiety, rage and depression, a sense of helplessness, an inability to concentrate, fear and a retreat into dependency. These are powerful symptoms.

---

[1] For Carnes, P.J., trauma splitting is defined as the aspect of betrayal bonds that ignores "traumatic realities by splitting off the experiences and not integrating them into personality or daily life." Carnes, P.J., (1997: 14–17); see also Kristeva, J. (1982); (1984); LaCapra, D. (2001:39ff); Blustein, J. (2003); LaCapra, D. (2004); Lepore, S.J. Revenson, T.A., (2006); Staub, E. (2003); Blustein, J. (2008).

[2] Psychic splitting also provides people with a means by which they can protect their children from knowing about what they lived through. See Erdinast-Vulcan, D. (2012: 314) in Lothe, J. Suleiman, S. R. & Phelan, J. (2012).

T. J. Bowyer, *Beyond Suffering and Reparation*,
https://doi.org/10.1007/978-3-319-98983-9_6

They not only mask the full impact of what survivors still have to live with as unprocessed memories; they also diminish capacity to feel. A survivor of the violence describes these feelings: "There is no confidence between people in the community because they cannot afford to drop their guard." Author's field research: interviewee from Otoronco (Jeremias).

By closing off their capacity for empathy with their own past survivors reduce exposure to experience of their own suffering. Over time this undermines motivation and encourages blind obedience. This process produces a state of 'psychic numbing' that blocks out all feelings associated with memories of extreme life events. By anaesthetizing themselves from the full effects of their own experiences of extreme life events people are able "…to minimize psychological discomfort and responsibility about actions and thoughts that would otherwise be prohibited."[3] However, this attempt to skirt around painful memories "…allows no room for the validating formalization of one's knowledge or, at best, refers it to an extremely restricted social circle."[4] Unless this process is "…supplemented by practices of working through and integration,"[5] its capacity for preventing the experience of extreme life events from continuing to interfere with survivors lives will not diminish.

For people in the communities studied no such opportunities for exploring and expressing the experience of extreme events exist. By living in an environment of injustice, violence and repression people become "…resigned and submissive through the everyday demonstration of how impossible and useless it is to strive to change their situation."[6] For example, 33 villagers were randomly selected for interview in Unay and everyone of them said that they did not trust government officials or members of NGOs.

The explanations they gave were as follows: (1) the government promised to help them and it never has; (2) the rampant inflation that accompanied the escalation in violence during the first government of President Garcia,[7] and now the cost of living is rising again and this looks likely to continue; (3) the first government of Alan Garcia was the worst of times for the killings and this looks set to return; (4) NGOs are not to be trusted, because although some have done some good things, many are devious and never fulfilled their abundant promises.[8]

Increasingly alienated by the dissolution of boundaries between their own internal and external reality leaves survivors mistrustful and suspicious of malevolent intent that can prove especially resistant to change as the following illustrates: "Sometimes they lie to you; they tell you that they come from such and such an office and that they are going to do such and such work to help us when it isn't true;

[3] Watkins, M. & Shulman, H. (2008: 85).

[4] Martin-Baro, I., (1989).

[5] Schwab, G., (2010: 20).

[6] Martin-Baro, I., (1994a, b, c, d: 211).

[7] The first government of Alan Garcia was between 1985–1990.

[8] In Wamani 36 of the 60 (60%) randomly selected interviewees said that they have no interest participating in the lectures or the workshops provided by NGOs and other public institutions and organizations.

they always steal from you in one way or another." Author's field research: interviewee from Qocha (Rosa).

From a psychological perspective this is responsible for "...depressive feelings of inferiority, worthlessness and hopelessness about the larger context of daily life, lack of a sense of agency, of the impossibility of affecting a future or even of being able to hope for a future different from the present, the abandonment of the past and too often the erupting of violence born of futility."[9] This process is aided by the growing influence of the dominant culture and the spread of consumerism, material goods and alternative life styles. Its' capacity to pressure survivors to get on with life and confront the new encourages survivors to treat the past as "...a chronically debilitating experience rather than an opportunity for growth, integration, *communitas* or transformation."[10]

These conditions are not conducive to working through the pain and harshness of extreme experiences. Instead they have made the search for relief in the immediate present inevitable; they have also caused survivors to become increasingly vulnerable to outside influences.

This is demonstrated by the following: "These days the community has an atmosphere of envy because some people are going about with the aim of having a better economy than others. Seeing these things makes some villagers envious of how these people work and the effort they took to take advantage of this opportunity." Author's field research: interviewee from Wamani (Miguel). Increasingly alienated from the surrounding social and institutional context by the dissolution of the boundaries between internal and external reality leaves survivors with an abstract relation to reality as the following suggests: "I see that people are changing their lifestyle, in their food, in their way of living, everything." Author's field research: interviewee from Otoronco (Ramon).

By blocking off any opportunity to work through and integrate the subjective or internal side of emotional experience the long term psychological and community consequences of extreme experiences are constantly being revived in the constricted relationship people have with each other and with the surrounding social and institutional environment. The idea of being able to disengage from the passive and submissive behaviour of this overwhelming cocktail of emotional poison is risible to the extent that its enduring legacy is responsible for shaping the beliefs people have about the nature of the world and their lives.

The despair this produces in those traumatized is demonstrated by the following: "I suffer from constant nightmares, and sometimes see different ghosts. The foreign helicopters flying over remind me of the days of conflict. My scars from the torture cannot be erased. I think that in the future my rights could still be trampled on again; I have lost confidence in everything because now we are going through harder times than ever and we do not have the slightest bit of peace." Author's field research: interviewee from Unay (Santos).

[9] Wakins, M. & Shulman, H. (2008: 112).

[10] Watkins, M. & Shulman, H. (2008: 138).

For Martin-Baro the lack of emotional support means that people feel stuck "… in the here and now without a before or after."[11] This being so, what people in the communities studied are confronted with is a condition that is uprooting them from any deep and living connections with their environment. It is aggravated by the rupture in their access to shared values, common humanity and shared responsibility. That this is contributing to the undermining of people's relationship with place, conditions of birth, forms of employment and social environment is beyond question, but however strong the lure of the dominant culture and its alternative ways of living might be the hunger it promises to satisfy won't compensate for the loss of their connections with the past and a sense of their own intrinsic place in the world.

In the words of one community activist: "I've been seeing this new situation lately. I believe that this exclusion should not exist because it stems from the government. If they steal, they cover it up, but here, if a poor man steals a chicken, he is brought to justice. I remember those years that passed us by. I feel great remorse; nothing they do will ever bring back the people who died. Most of the population here are unhappy; it's not like the people that suffered the most are still alive. They only use money to appease us and calm all those who were mistreated." Author's field research: interviewee from Qocha (Julio).

Belief that nothing can be done and that it is all hopeless is often a trigger for people to abandon individual uncertainty for the sake of collective identity. However, this is a nihilistic feeling triggered not so much by ethical ideals of decency or good as by the powerful sway of mass society and state authority. Instead of helping to make people morally grounded and responsible, the decision to submerge themselves into the group is taken, not because the individual is attracted to what it stands for, but because any other alternative is too painful to bear.[12]

This is contrary to the idea that groups can be a powerful source of validation and support during the early stages of recovery for survivors of prolonged, repeated abuse.[13] In the words of one survivor: "The biggest tensions in the community come from conformity. People have no interest in looking for ways to overcome the problems in the community. They are always saying that the best thing to do is leave. They claim that nobody is going to get anything and that the best thing is to leave before SL gets any stronger." Author's field research: interviewee from Yachaya (Victor).

The emotional condition of people ranges from states of intense confusion to death-like feelings, and defensive ambiguity (through which they can avoid inner conflict and criticism) and diminished subjectivity.[14] To avoid humiliation people (and in particular, survivors) need to hold on to a modicum of self-respect, but the

---

[11] Martin-Baro, I., (1986).

[12] See Fiske, S.T., (1993); Boehm and Flack, (2010: 46) in Guinote, A. & Vescio, T.K., (2010); Fiske, S.T. & Neuberg, S.L., (1990); Saakvitne, K. W., Gamble, S., Pearlman, L., & Lev, B. (2000); Staub, (1989, 2003).

[13] For the use of groups as a resource of validation and support in the first stage of recovery, see Herman, J. (1992: 218ff).

[14] Gautier, A., & Sabatini Scalmati, A., (2010: 4).

idea of keeping feelings of indignation, shame and guilt alive can seem fanciful and meaningless in a context of daily survival. In this respect unconscious adaptability, collusion and complicity with the surrounding social and institutional environment are a symptom of people "...who cannot atone for what cannot be undone."[15]

A survivor of the violence describes the way in which apathy, despair and indifference have conspired to undermine the sense of connection between the individual and the community: "Another thing that affects the community is that people don't want to hold office. They don't want to make arrangements for the community in case they get stopped and searched any time by SL, the local authorities or any other occupying authorities. For example, the community board won't get involved in anything outside the community; they only enforce internal agreements of the community assembly. The community leaders don't seek to strengthen the organization or help to keep the peace. They don't make security decisions because they don't want to upset SL because during the violent times the authorities were completely fucked and after that the authorities and the villagers prefer to do nothing." Author's field research: interviewee from Wamani (Herberto).

In practice this abandonment of individual uncertainty for the sake of collective identity leaves the individual's internal world unaffected. This is tantamount to an admission of failure to find any rational solution to the effects of their extreme experiences. It means that the decision to submerge themselves into the group happens not because the individual believes in what the group stands for, but because it alleviates their feelings of severe emotional stress borne in isolation.[16]

Though people (and survivors) may be aware of how worthless this makes their decision, they do not necessarily respond with a moral feeling to the consequences of this decision. In this context feelings of apathy and indifference are as much responsible for the failure to adopt the right attitude to the emotional dimension of their experiences of extreme life events as wilful compliance, selfishness or manipulation.

For people in a state of ambiguity critical thinking and anything that passes as an alarm mechanism is suspended, with the result that they become easily swayed.[17] In the words of one former community leader: "People don't want to support the community authorities if they are asked to do something. Support for the community leaders is in name only and means nothing practical; things like that have no substance; people don't care anymore." Author's field research: interviewee from Wamani (Ordell).

By destroying their own emotional capacities to feel survivors are able to persuade themselves that what is happening has nothing to do with them.[18] This

[15] Herman, J., (1992: 193).

[16] For Baumeister and Leary "...much of what human beings do is done in the service of belongingness. Empirical findings conclusively show that the need to belong shapes emotion and cognition." Baumeister, R. F. & Leary, M. R. (1995: 521). See also Baumeister, R. F., Twenge, J.M., & Nuss, C. K. (2002).

[17] Gautier, A., & Sabatini Scalmati, A., (2010: 5).

[18] Haas, P.J., (1988).

reinforces the outsider's impression that people are simply passive victims or the servile instruments of local and national government policy. However, this abandonment of individual uncertainty for the sake of collective identity is primarily a pragmatic response to the absolute powerlessness of their situation. It underscores the fundamental distinction people (and survivors) make between strategic conformity to necessity and an absolute conformity to necessity.[19] In this way the abandonment of individual uncertainty for the sake of collective identity is made morally acceptable and in so doing transforms the meaning of participation and social capital.[20]

However, although this escape into the group enables survivors to disburden themselves' of responsibility it does not alter the enduring responsibility they have to themselves and others, irrespective of how submerged in the group they may become. This means that no matter how the individual feels about the situation they find themselves in they still bear some responsibility for it.[21] Is this the point at which what remains of traditional norms and values dissolves into assimilated poverty? To address this question, we need to return to the individual's internal world and consider how experience of extreme events prevents them from being able to respond emotionally and cognitively to the present.

The destruction of the normal ways in which survivors think, act and relate to others undermines their access to effective forms of social support. This is responsible for unprecedented levels of isolation and loneliness that ultimately destroy human connectedness and any relationship with the outside world. In this context any opportunity to work through their emotional experience of extreme life events and obtain some form of integration is more or less meaningless. This can cause emotional ruptures in experience so profound as to produce changes in the psyche. These include loss of self-confidence, depression, problems with physical health, and the immune system.[22]

A survivor of the political violence reveals how the effects of what happened continue to resonate in her own life: "With all of the problems I have had to face and remembering all that happened during those years, I am always afraid of strangers. I never stop worrying and this has caused me to suffer from some health complications." Author's field research: interviewee from Otoronco (Jacinta).

The psychological effects of violence live on as recurrent dreams, intrusive recollections and images of the terrible past. Having been forced to confront malevolence, meaninglessness and terror survivors now find themselves "…consigned to something from which they cannot in any way distance themselves."[23] Because the psychological effects of extreme events are easily triggered by factors that remind

---

[19] Des Pres, T. (1976); Pawelczynska, A., (1979).

[20] By social capital I am referring to "…features of social organization, such as trust, norms and networks that can improve the efficiency of society by facilitating coordinated actions." (Putnam, 1993: 167).

[21] Staub, E. (1989:38ff).

[22] See Bugental, D. B., (2010: 209ff) in Guinote, A. and Vescio, T. (2010).

[23] Agamben, G. (1999: 105).

survivors of what happened they are unable to separate themselves from the fact that these events are part of their historical past and of their present and as such are unforgettable.

Those who have lived through such debased psychological experiences often live in a state of constant dread as the following statement illustrates: "At night, I have nightmares and am permanently scared, having suffered a lot of torture. Due to all these factors, I am very concerned about everything that is currently going on." Author's field research: interviewee from Otoronco (Sanchez).

Because it is not possible to rebel against this situation survivors are compelled to recognize that these are not forms of suffering that are healed but only ones that are endured. In these circumstances the belief that some important social norm has been violated makes humiliation and feelings of abjection inevitable.[24] This is responsible for adjustments in their attitudes and behaviour that are inconsistent with traditional patterns, routines and emotional support.

The cognitive implications of these adjustments have outward consequences that undermine civic mindedness, diminish social cohesion, encourage non-conventional behaviour, destroy solidarity and lead to the suppression of pain and suffering. A survivor describes the difficulties this presents: "People do not forget, but those that try not to hold past atrocities against people who did bad things end up thinking the same way they did during the terrible past and that is a disaster for everyone that gets involved." Author's field research: interviewee from Qocha (Julio).

Though this loosening of moral constraints frees survivors from obedience more than ever before, it also undermines their ability to resist effectively, to cooperate, and to participate in helping others. This has structural implications that are reflected in the survivor's perceptions of GROs, NGOs, community assemblies, local authorities, central government, etc.[25]

The survivors' attitudes towards the conduct and impact of NGOs and their activities are especially noteworthy as the following demonstrates: "I distrust the NGOs because I don't believe what they tell us. They (NGOs) come here to trick the people and not to serve. They have taken us for a ride and in the end, we have received nothing. Here they have betrayed us and the people know it." Author's field research: interviewee from Qocha (Ramiro).

However, the sense that resurgence in violence is a growing threat signifies a further constriction in the survivor's willingness to be actively engaged in the protection of their community.

---

[24] The interpretation of abjection most appropriate to this study is the one developed by Julia Kristeva who described abjection as "...that which is rejected by/disturbs social reason - the communal consensus that underpins a social order." Kristeva, J. (1984: 65).

[25] In some cases, this destruction of the normal ways in which people think, act and relate to others is the result of a particular war strategy that often has very specific aims. For example, the use of rape as a political act designed to break down existing socio-cultural structures by unsettling the community structure, feminizing men, changing the ethnic makeup of a society, creating a state of fear and silence, and demonstrating total control over a community. See for example: Hague, E. (1997) in R. Lentin (ed.) (1997); Hayner, P. B. (2002); Yuval-Davis, N. (1997); Boesten, J. (2007a, b) in Pankhurst, D. (ed.) (2007); Brinkerhoff, D. (2007a, b); Kleinman, A. & Kleinman, J. (1991a, b); Boesten, J. (2007a, b).

In every one of the communities studied the issue of security is producing confusion and anxiety; the following is typical: "The community leaders want to start the CAD again but the people stay quiet and others say that they have no time; that they have to work on their farm; that if they are engaged in work for CAD it will upset the family because there will not be enough food and clothing." Author's field research: interviewee from Yachaya (Marcelo).

To the extent that the destruction of the normal ways in which people think, act and relate to others causes them to believe that nothing can be done and that further misery and suffering is inevitable – a compelling indictment of the absolute powerlessness of their position. Having to live in such a debilitating environment leads to "…depressive feelings of inferiority, worthlessness and hopelessness about the larger context of daily life, lack of a sense of agency, of the impossibility of affecting a future or even of being able to hope for a future different from the present, the abandonment of the past and too often the erupting of violence born of futility."[26]

For example, in Yachaya 24 of the 44 (55%) randomly selected interviewees said that they often feel violent towards themselves. This social 'normal abnormality' especially affects children because they have no alternative but to "…construct their identities and develop their lives within the network of these dehumanizing relations."[27] The severity of this situation is reflected in an interview with a health professional responsible for Yachaya: "A lot of teenagers, experience psychological problems that are a legacy of the conflict, of whom there are about 20 cases with psychological trauma. Other adolescents who did not experience political violence exhibit suicidal tendencies of which 3 cases were nearly fatal." Author's field research: interviewee from health centre responsible for Yachaya.

This lack of recognition and respect for what the response to the experience of extreme events does is a breach of normative expectations. From a moral perspective this has happened because the capacity for other-regarding empathy has been effectively annihilated by the deliberate destruction of their basic beliefs, including those mechanisms used to counter misuse of traditional knowledge and traditional cultural expressions.

By eliminating those members of the community that best embodied its relationship with the government SL bequeathed to the surviving population a situation in which all moral/value based assertions lack authority/credibility. From having built their lives on assumptions that made them feel safe and secure the political violence has forced survivors to come face to face with their own vulnerability.

Though some people are clear-sighted enough to see what is happening they feel powerless to do anything about it: "People nowadays just receive and take; they are used to handouts and don't fulfil their duties to the community. They are so far from understanding their commitments because they have an idea that everything is free, that everything falls from the sky like manna and it's not like this; there are things you have to work at." Author's field research: interviewee from Otoronco (Jeremias).

---

[26] Watkins, M. & Shulman, H. (2008: 112).

[27] Martin-Baro, I., (1994a, b, c, d: 124).

Through the violation of their rights and dignity by means of physical or psychological abuse the deepest and most profound guide to the lives of survivors has been all but destroyed. Instead of being treated in a way that fosters self-worth the failure to respect particular norms and values has led to a state of helplessness that undermines self-determination, weakens self-confidence and devalues identity. The isolation of the survivor thus persists long after the political violence has ended, as the following demonstrates: "Some of us have become almost useless because during the violence we were forced to do things and we have to try and forget those things but we can't." Author's field research: interviewee from Yachaya (Nohemi).

In the aftermath of the violence these are conditions in which "…misery has penetrated into internal time consciousness, disrupting the relationship between past, present and future. By this skewing of time, it destroys identity, one's relationship with oneself. It locks survivors into an eternal present."[28] Though this enables survivors to free themselves from obedience to ineffective norms and values, it also undermines their sense of propriety and self-respect and with it a capacity for self-determination. This makes anomie, selfishness and other forms of social fragmentation commonplace. The emotional bond with other human beings is suspended and acts of kindness and selflessness are perceived as unusual and potentially suspicious.

This destroys the survivor's capacity for empathy to the extent that they are as likely to cause hurt to others or treat them as mere objects.

By failing to connect with other people as human beings with their own thoughts and feelings, the individual is failing to acknowledge their subjectivity.[29] This not only prevents them from being able to respond to the thoughts and feelings of other people with an appropriate emotion, it also alienates them from others. Being unable to empathize therefore undermines the individual's capacity to understand others position. For survivors in the communities studied this makes them feel devalued because there is no one to reassure them that their thoughts and feelings about what happened have been heard, acknowledged and respected.[30] These feelings may be awkward and ambiguous, but practically everyone gives recognition to this personality change in the same way as the following suggests: "In general people are conformists with what they have; they do not want to progress, we used to bring professionals here because of the contacts I have but people are not interested; the people are conformists." Author's field research: interviewee from Unay (Plinio).

To challenge these deeply internalized perceptions of their own helplessness survivors have to confront what has been normalised and taken for granted. However, this is an extremely painful process. Learning to create cultural alternatives to what has been learnt over a lifetime does not simply happen. How then can survivors move from a position of detachment about their own past to one that enables them to reclaim it? To answer this, we need to recognize that submissive behaviour is not

[28] Amery, J. (1980: 62ff).

[29] Buber, M., (1958).

[30] Baron-Cohen, S., (2011: 13).

an essential characteristic of human conduct, but "…the fruit of an historical and sociological situation."[31]

From the suffering born out of living in a context of hunger, deprivation, ill treatment, injustice and poor health survivors feel powerless to change their situation. This inhibits them from struggling against their situation and encourages survivors to internalise the experiences, achievements and values of the state and other institutions and organizations. This increases the feeling of inferiority and a lack of self-confidence.

The following testimony supports this: "Even now none of the authorities are sorry or cares and the national government is even worse. I appeal to the current leader to make policies which will change things and for him to realize the reality of our situation. It is urgent that the government does something about this. Everything they tell us is just lies. They do not respect our rights. People live in total chaos. Everything is entirely done through deceit and broken promises. None of them are really concerned about our situation." Author's field research: interviewee from Qocha (Nacho).

If the only certainty is lack of empathy and compassion how can survivors avoid the drift towards even greater desensitization and indifference? For survivors whose deeply internalized perceptions of their own helplessness cause them to live in ways in which they believe they have no control over their situation this "…does not signify an absence of response, but rather a response which lacks a critical quality."[32] In these circumstances the memory of past injustice, suffering and misery becomes subject to the fatalism that so often overwhelms survivors.[33] For example, one interviewee said: "…I don't know what else to do. I don't have the courage to leave my village and anyway it doesn't matter. I will stay here and if I die I die, what else is there?" Authors field research: interviewee from Unay (Lucita).

For Martin-Baro (1994a, b, c, d) this "….is an attitude caused and continually reinforced by the oppressive functioning of overall social structures."[34] Though this outlook can be changed through suitable social support and dialogue no such environment has emerged in Peru, in spite of the work being carried out by AFAVIP. Through their increasingly narrow worldview survivors lose the connections between the context in which they live and any capacity to transform it. In these circumstances survivors have an enormous capacity for a moral blindness that manifests itself in states of denial, dissociation, forgetfulness and identification with ideologies of the dominant culture.[35]

To bring the influence of the past into full view and make it as self-evident to others as it is to themselves the sufferer must reassess their own strict separation of the past from the present.[36] However, the lack of suitable social support and dialogue

[31] Freire, P., (1980: 48).

[32] Freire, P., (1972).

[33] For further information about fatalism, see Martin-Baro, I., (1994a, b, c, d: 200ff).

[34] Martin-Baro, I., (1994a, b, c, d: 210–211).

[35] Watkins, M. & Shulman, H. (2008: 131).

[36] Kleinman, A. & Kleinman, J., (1991a, b).

makes any opportunity to enhance their own sense of responsibility for their situation very difficult. From the perspective of survivors this is consistent with the normal functioning of the existing social system because it reflects their position within particular social structures. For example, one informant said that their situation is explained by the fact that "…we are poor and ignorant, so it is easy for the government to forget us." Authors field research: interviewee from Otoronco (Joviana).

This is consistent with the opinions of survivors from the other communities studied as one of them explains: "The political authorities are very important in the life of the people, because without these authorities there is nothing to help people after what happened. The trouble is we are not perceived to have the same importance as more influential people." Author's field research: interviewee from Qocha (Mario).

Though remembering what happened may help to re-establish the subjectivity that the political violence denied them, the circumstances in which they find themselves are such that survivors are obliged to repress their own anger – if they value their own survival.[37] These constraining forces comprise the social structures, discourses and ideologies that cause survivors to live in conditions of 'marginalized dependency' and 'oppressive misery' "…that is forcing upon them an inhuman existence and snatching away their ability to define their own lives."[38]

For survivors the failure to properly acknowledge suffering and how it should be dealt with makes any natural interval between past and present meaningless.[39] The non-recognition and misrecognition of suffering is not only humiliating, it deprives people of material security, self-respect and self-worth. In the words of one survivor: "Its' exactly like they (government officials) are ashamed to talk about what happened; if we don't have a dialogue it's as if we know nothing." Author's field research: interviewee from Unay (Santiago).

However, the idea that survivors can separate themselves from memories of trauma, is unthinkable. In this respect the capacity to forget is not so much in question as the ability to wilfully abandon the memory of what happened. These events retain a powerful emotional charge that has the capacity to "…become more alive and powerful, not as model but as spectre, as a past that is establishing itself as a present, or as a sword of judgement hung over the present."[40]

For those unable to free themselves from this bondage to the past the lack of any means by which they can make sense of the world and begin to work through their experiences of extreme events is enough to ensure that the past will continue to interfere with their lives.

---

[37] McCullough, M. & Worthington, E. L., (2001: 107–8).

[38] Martin-Baro, I., (1994a, b, c, d: 26–7).

[39] See Pedersen et al. (2010) for research examining the intersection of cultural norms, past and current events, and expressions of distress in the Quechua population of Northern Ayacucho. See also Pedersen, D., Tremblay, J., Errazuris, C., & Gamarra, J. (2008); Pedersen, D., Kienzler, H., & Gamarra, J. (2010); Llaki and Ñakary.

[40] Maier, C.S., (1997: 15).

This is responsible for the erosion of trust, the escalation of uncertainty and an increasing disillusionment with the future of shared values and norms of behaviour.[41] It also increases the risk of exploitation and conflict and makes humiliation and inhumane treatment by society endemic. Inside this powerful unwelcome experience, the immediate question of self-preservation is likely to be so overwhelming that suffering will feel like the only reality as the following demonstrates: "I feel bad about both the military and the terrorists because both sides abused us: my children hid in the caves. I could not eat; I was like crazy, desperate. I could not study because I was always thinking of how my mother had died. I was desperate to see so many deaths; I felt bad, I just cried day and night, I had no desire to eat; there is so much sadness here. I thought I was going to die because my father was killed with a bullet. I have lived with my mother and my grandparents ever since. I suffer so much; I have nothing. At any time, I thought they would come to kill me and the rest of my people. I used to go crazy about the things I've seen and I've spent the rest of my life living with it." Author's field research: interviewee from Wamani (Rollande).

To the extent that the psychological effects of extreme events are easily triggered by factors that remind survivors of what happened they are unable to separate themselves from the events that are part of their past and of their present. In the aftermath of the violence the cumulative effect of this is not just overwhelming misery and suffering but "…a compulsion to be free from the suffering of their experiences."[42] Through this need to relieve themselves of the distress and discomfort of their situation survivors have the means by which they can begin to search for an interpretation and understanding of what they are going through.

In order to develop a critical consciousness an understanding of the larger frames of culture and history is required in which "…the interdependent relationship between the intra psychic, interpersonal, community; economic and environmental contributions to the structure of experience are embedded."[43]

To make the link between the sufferings of symptoms with these outer environments requires survivors to confront what they take for granted. In order to transform the experience of extreme events from something indigestible and unprocessed into "…an engagement that cannot but be perpetually catching up with its own inadequacy"[44] survivors need to restore the historical context to their memory of what happened. In this way survivors are able to bring to awareness "…the remembrance of those who have suffered and died as victims of human efforts to dominate over nature and/or human beings."[45] Only through the recovery of the historical past is it possible for people to begin to understand what has caused the current situation

[41] McCann, I. L., & Pearlman, L. A. (1990a); (1990b); Pearlman, L. A., & Saakvitne, K. W. (1995).

[42] Leder, D. (1990).

[43] Watkins, M. & Shulman, H. (2008: 10).

[44] Avelar, I., (1999: 3).

[45] Morrill, B.T., (2000: 28).

to come about.[46] Failure to unify past, present and future aspects of their lives undermine efforts to overcome existential fatalism and, in doing so, deny survivors control of their own existence.

For Gutierrez "…memory is the present of the past…that calls to life and rejects every form of unjust death."[47] This idea that memory gives back life to those who are dead is consistent with the idea that it is resistant to the time of historiography and "…to the ideological tendency to adopt fixed ideas of the past, interpretable only according to a cultural logic advocating the acceptance of death, allowing the other who has died to become nothing but the past."[48] In this way memory reverses what has happened and puts back into question the past to which it refers.[49] In this way memory becomes "…vigilant memory… memory that sets itself apart from the continuity of survival and history to serve as an ethical resistance inscribed within our knowledge in all its utilitarian or commemorative forms."[50]

From this position an opportunity for the vanquishing of suffering presents itself because it has the capacity to "… (1) render a critique of the evolutionary world view and (2) to stimulate human imagination for social-political action."[51]

The importance of this form of critical consciousness motivates efforts to remember past suffering and awaken survivors from apathy and indifference. This takes place "…not so much by remembering traumatic events and their accompanying emotions as by interpreting memories and inscribing them into a larger pattern of meaning."[52] For many people this often means that remembering what happened is not so much about the re-unification of past, present and future aspects of their psychic lives as a re-injuring: "I still feel nervous. It's because of what happened in those years. I don't go back. I only remember everything that happened from the age of eighteen or nineteen years after it was all over." Author's field research: interviewee from Qocha (Pomposa).

The notion that remembering wrongdoing and suffering is harmful and something to be avoided is a powerful emotion, not simply because 'dangerous memories' revive feelings of pain and suffering, but because they make people vulnerable and open to exploitation. This is because these types of memories "…illuminate for a few moments and with a harsh and steady light the questionable nature of things we have apparently come to terms with."[53]

---

[46] In this way people remain true to themselves and this helps them to retain something fundamental about their own identity. For Elie Wiesel, "…salvation, like redemption, can be found only in memory." In Wiesel, E. (1990: 201) This theme was subsequently commented on by Miroslav Volf who said that "…faith in the saving power of memory – faith that it will heal the individuals involved and help rid the world of violence is his (Wiesel's) central obsession." Volf, M., (2006: 19).

[47] Gutierrez, G., (2004: 258ff) in Gutierrez, G. (2004) *Textos Esenciales: acordarse de los pobres*, ed. Andres Gallego Lima*: Fondo Editorial del Congreso del Peru*).

[48] Spargo, R. Clifton (2006: 46).

[49] Levinas, E., (1999: 56).

[50] Spargo, R. Clifton (2006: 46).

[51] Metz, J.B., (1980: 117).

[52] Volf, M., (2006: 28).

[53] Metz, J.B. (1980: 109).

In this way the revival of memories about what happened is something to be feared because of its association with questions of truth and justice that relate to the events being remembered, as the following demonstrates: “People were brought here blindfolded, both with and without children; then after three days or four days they began to disappear and all that’s buried in the river and when I returned to the village all the people could do was talk about was how well the dogs are eating and later on I found that the dogs had eaten the corpses because the guerrillas had destroyed the military here. Then I went back for my son and we fled and hid in the highlands.” Author’s field research: interviewee from Otoronco (Carlos).

For survivors struggling hard to satisfy everyday basic needs remembering is less about the redemption of the past and more about something from which they cannot escape, even if they wanted to, as the following demonstrates: “The nightmare is when I’m sleeping and into my mind comes those times of violence that we passed through; sometimes those things occupy every aspect of my sleep and I feel very desperate.” Author’s field research: interviewee from Qocha (Jose).

How survivors manage the memory of past injustice and misery depends on the way in which they choose to carry on with their life after their experience of extreme events: they may prefer to ignore the past altogether; they may deceive themselves about its significance; they may deceive themselves about the extent of their blameworthiness; or, they may be crippled with feelings of loss, shame or guilt.[54]

Because survivors often prefer not to be reminded of their past they tend to continue to repress the memory of what happened whenever possible. This makes it easier for the political violence and memory to intersect in nightmares, fear, anxiety, insecurity, and tension, humiliation, and so forth. In this way the memory of what happened remains outside and incapable of being integrated into anything that came before and outside anything that has happened to survivors since the events took place. Should we be so surprised when these ‘dangerous memories’ consist of such episodes?

The following experiences recounted by one survivor are typical: “I remember when the army was here and that helicopters were passing by overhead. The Shining Path took my brother away, he was 15 years old and I have never seen my brother again. I remember that during those years people were dropping like flies (a lot of people were being killed), the corpses smelled horrible and the dogs would eat them; there was no time to bury the corpses. I was totally traumatised and we were afraid to go back. We slept with our shoes on in case we had to escape in a hurry. I am afraid that the violence will come back because with this government it was war… we lived on the run going from hill to hill; we fled because the Shining Path could have arrived at any moment. The Shining Path surprised people while they were sleeping and would kill them. They killed my neighbour and took our animals. Because of all this I left my village.” Author’s field research: interviewee from Unay (Julian).

---

[54] Blustein, J., (2003:: 57ff).

Thus, terrible events and the misery of daily survival causes suffering to remain an unappeasable experience; it does not diminish with time.[55] The idea that time should be left to heal the wounds of the past is dispossessed of any value.

Is it really possible for the future to redeem the past when the present is experienced in the way described by the following survivor: "Before now there was rubble everywhere. It was so bad that everything was burnt black; many of our houses didn't even have a roof. Now we are all afraid because it would be easy for the terrorists to get into our houses if they came back; if I hear a dog bark I think it must mean that the terrorists have returned; I am very afraid of them." Author's field research: interviewee from Yachaya (Perla).

These events constitute a catastrophic emotional rupture in how survivors perceive themselves, their community and their relationship with the outside world.[56] By losing their connections with the past and a sense of their own integral place in the world survivors are living their lives in ways that are incompatible with their own culture. Because this is aggravated by the lack of participation in community life they are increasingly cut off from all relationships that give meaning to life, as well as those needed to sustain life.

This is inconsistent with social norms that make for "…a lack of deep and living connections with their environment."[57] The result is for the social norms of Quechua culture to have increasingly given way to individualistic behaviour and other symptoms of uprootedness. For example, in Otoronco 37 of the 44 (84%) randomly selected interviewees said that they prefer to do things alone, in spite of the threat of sanctions from the community authorities should they fail to carry out work for the community.

A survivor describes the difficulties this presents in the period since the conflict ended: "Before solidarity meant that we gave support to people, support for orphans and widows. None of that exists now; everything is about isolated self-interest, every man for himself. Before you were with people to get the water because there was a single wash stand, a single well; now everyone has their own water, everyone has their own light and no one turns to their neighbour and the neighbour to you and so we are like a city. Here there is no compassion, the people are just selfish, and no one listens to you. There is no such unity that used to exist when I was little." Author's field research: interviewee from Wamani (Rainerio).

To the extent that survivors endure severe emotional stress in ways that are incompatible with the social norms of Quechua culture, the memory of what happened and the wrongs inflicted on them are still in process. Though this increasingly individualistic behaviour provides opportunities for survivors to enter into a deeper relationship with themselves and others, it also deprives them of any deep and living

[55] For Mathew Ashley "…no progress can be made as long as one sees in memory only the cybernetic recall of facts from the past." Mathew Ashley, J., (2014: 131) in Bingemer, M.C. & Casarella, P., (eds.) (2014).

[56] Broucek, F. (1991: 5); see also Regel, S. & Joseph, S. (2010: 18–19).

[57] Weil, S., (2002: 41ff).

connections with their environment.[58] A survivor of the political violence describes the difficulties this presents since the conflict ended: "All people think about is how to get ahead, but we once thought that it was not just about bringing up our family but also for the community and for that we would be coordinating, but now it is not like that." Author's field research: interviewee from Otoronco (Flavio).

This means that the benefits of individualistic behaviour ("…being able to listen more deeply, speak directly from the heart, encounter feeling fully, bear suffering in the self and other and at the same time, experience the joyful and mysterious presence of other unknown souls")[59] have to be weighed against the loss of their previous identification with collective social narratives.[60]

For people living with hunger, deprivation, ill treatment, injustice and poor health the opportunities for realizing the advantages of individualistic behaviour must sometimes appear slim as the following testimony indicates: "Now there is no pity, just selfishness, no support for orphans or widows (from the violence). Now there is no such solidarity; when I was young there was mutual support." Author's field research: interviewee from Yachaya (Marco).

This is also an environment in which the resources by which people used to protect themselves from misery and loss have all but vanished. Is it therefore possible for survivors to "…faithfully submit to the tutelage of their symptoms?"[61] To address this question we need to recognise that the meaning survivors give to their memories (and the symptoms arising from those memories) changes over time. In this respect survivors may assume greater responsibility for their past as a result of the ways in which their own changing situation alters their perception of the past and their relationship with it.

From this perspective remembering what happened can be understood not simply as a psychological phenomenon, but as the subject of a moral imperative.[62] For Blustein this "…makes sense if for no other reason than that moral responsibilities endure over time and have implications for future conduct and that in order to fulfil them [people] have to remember them."[63] Instead of breeding indifference and apathy this enables survivors to look back at painful events and the emotional reactions with which they are associated in ways that can help them move forwards. To hold that the changes in the way survivors look at their past enables them to transform their own psychological wounding into personal growth experiences makes for a particularly powerful claim.[64]

---

[58] Watkins, M. & Shulman, H. (2008: 149).

[59] Watkins, M. & Shulman, H. (2008: 149).

[60] For the individual to benefit from collective social narratives respect for collective obligations such as those suggested by Simone Weil are needed: order, liberty, obedience, responsibility, equality, hierarchism, punishment, freedom of opinion, security, risk, private property, collective property, truth, liberty, obedience, honour. See Weil, S., (2002: 41ff).

[61] Watkins, M. & Shulman, H. (2008: 61).

[62] Blustein, J., (2008: 30).

[63] Blustein, J., (2008: 31).

[64] Calhoun, L.G., & Tedeschi, R., (2009: 29) (eds).

In the communities studied the capacity to respond emotionally and cognitively to the psychological damage inflicted is increasingly challenged by the breaking down of social norms and values and the increasing exposure to the dominant culture. Though the survivors' memory of what happened continues the loss and destruction of important relationships within their own community makes the revival of cultural traditions, history, values and a sense of solidarity with others increasingly hard to conceive. A survivor of the violence describes the difficulties this presents since the conflict ended: "There is a lack of participation of the members of the community in the decisions of community development. The leadership should always be present in these processes of community development but many have been affected by the attitude of the people and by the authorities who have no respect and importance for the needs that the population or the families are going through." Author's field research: interviewee from Qocha (Maximo).

To better understand "…the way in which the individual faces up to their responsibilities, what courage they manifest in suffering, what dignity they display in doom and disaster"[65] we need to look at how successful they are in defending themselves physically and psychologically. It is important to recognize that survivors taking responsibility for the psychological damage inflicted on them is not something done in isolation from other responsibilities (or from other people).[66] For survivors that have witnessed the disintegration of trust, respect, self-esteem, security, and supportive relationships, an appreciation of the current situation and of the individual's own place in the wider context including spiritual needs this is a formidable challenge.

In the communities studied the idea of taking responsibility for the past by deliberately seeking to integrate it into the present is likely to seem both impracticable and unrewarding to survivors, authorities, NGOs etc. A survivor of the political violence describes the resignation so many continue to feel since: "Well as I'm getting old, I'm not afraid anymore. I'll only live another five years, give or take. The people here are humble so they just get on with life. What happened happened." Author's field research: interviewee from Yachaya (Eufemia).

In these circumstances it is pertinent to ask if the failure to unify past, present and future of their psychic lives is really so important? If the past does not directly interfere with the present does the lack of any genuine control over their existence really matter when the present survivor's outlook is already so overwhelmingly fatalistic? These questions have implications for how we should assess the survivor's emotional response to trauma.

The temptation to deny responsibility for the psychological damage that was inflicted on them may give the impression of being particularly difficult to resist in a context of daily survival. Because survivors feel powerless to change their situation they are more likely to think of themselves in ways that damage their capacity to act on their most important motives. Feelings of impotence and helplessness would therefore seem to destroy their motivation to act in relation to a past injustice. These

[65] Frankl, V., (1955).

[66] Blustein, J., (2008: 69).

are factors that cannot be ignored, but at the same time they are not enough to deflect attention away from "…the belief that a moral wrong or injury has been done or that an important norm or expectation has been violated."[67]

A survivor describes how these feelings have impacted on their own life since the conflict ended: "I would watch from here people being thrown out of helicopters and hitting the ground like a sack. They would cover them with little handkerchiefs. The soldiers didn't want us to look, but I would anyway. They didn't want us seeing them shoot everywhere, but I would hide here and watch them. Seeing this made me cry, as I thought this must have been how my parents were killed…. I used to cry all the time." Author's field research: interviewee from Unay (Salud),

To explore the way these feelings of impotence and helplessness have been understood and how they are transforming the way in which individuals and groups are adjusting to their new environment is not a precise science. It is an evolutionary process that has the capacity to inform critical thinking in ways that nothing else can. Who can confront the experiences of political violence and not be challenged to evaluate their own preconceived ideas and paradigms? New situations and information compel the individual survivor to recognise that if they are to survive they need to be tougher and more unscrupulous than everyone else. In this respect trust, compassion and solidarity are suicidal.

The following statement by a survivor reflects the alienation and inner deadness that feelings of impotence and helplessness can produce: "There are so many mass graves all over the place that you can't even count them all. In one place there are 8 graves all belonging to the same family. Around here people would be brought from all over, and then killed here. They would bring men, women and children, all blindfolded. Wherever did they bring all the people from? A helicopter would bring people here every day." Author's field research: interviewee from Otoronco (Ilhuitl).

By failing to acknowledge the feelings that people have about what happened to them and how these experiences have destroyed their world the social structures, discourses and ideologies that act upon people have blocked the way to forgiveness and reconciliation. This impersonal disregard for the moral relevance of the psychological damage inflicted on survivors imposes an inhuman existence upon survivors and deprives them of any ability to define their own lives. A survivor describes the difficulties this presents: "They haven't opened some of the graves as they say there aren't any witnesses. They've only opened two. And how will we carry all those [remains] from the mass graves in the highlands? My friend's mother and her neighbour's parents are buried here. There are also graves from where the mudslides happened. Now, back in my village, I'm still afraid, because these things are always with me. I always think that at any moment the same thing could happen all over again." Author's field research: interviewee from Qocha (Valentin).

In this way the wider social and historical environment is responsible for a set of conditions that make anger "…pivotal to self-affirmation and liberation" and "…the healthy response of a self to violation and a crucial avenue to self-acceptance and

[67] Brudholm, T., (2008: 101).

acceptance of others."[68] Because the anger survivors feel is deeply personal and linked to their trauma, it helps to keep the past alive and in doing so helps to sustain their commitment to particular moral standards as the basis for normal human behaviour. In the following testimony the sense of alienation and inner deadness commingle with the loneliness and isolation that the political violence has left survivors with: "I was told that my husband had escaped when he was about to be killed, but they got my brother-in law and killed him. All the people who were "disappeared" have all been done away with completely. When I heard all this, I went back to my village crying but I never did find my husband; they must have killed him." Author's field research: interviewee from Yachaya (Mora).

For survivors compelled to live under conditions of an indifferent present this can strengthen the values they hold and give renewed impetus to the motivation to act. Though this cannot undo what has happened survivors may also feel that if nothing is ever done the emotional rupture to their lives and their way of life will simply be allowed to continue.[69] In this respect the motivation to do something can only benefit from their growing independence from cultural norms and its influence on people's increasingly individualistic behaviour. Even so, this view is not shared by those who continue to regret the loss of the old ways and in particular of community unity, as the following statement illustrates: "What is lacking is unity; each person is separated from everyone else; everyone lives and works separately." Author's field research: interviewee from Unay (Plinio).

By making identities stronger and more independent disillusionment with cultural norms not only makes people more autonomous; it also has the capacity to make them more internally driven. From this perspective survivors are better placed to keep the memory of past injustices alive because it is easier to depart from the familiar and explore alternative orientations.[70]

Because existing social structures, discourses and ideologies have never given any indication that the moral concerns of survivors will ever be taken seriously it is unlikely that others will ever feel reconciled with them. In such circumstances any attitude other than resentment would be inappropriate. By showing little remorse or regret for what happened existing social structures, discourses and ideologies have created an environment in which outside indifference and objectivity about past injustices can only be challenged through resentment.[71]

---

[68] Brock, R. N., (1988: 19).

[69] Brudholm, T., (2008: 169).

[70] Watkins, M. & Shulman, H., (2008: 158).

[71] Much of the contemporary interest in the subject of resentment began with the work of Jean Amery (1980). Some of the key contributions since then include Zygmunt Bauman (1989) who described resentment as "…a discharge, a by-product, of social settings that set interests in conflict and those who hold those interests at loggerheads." Some important recent contributions to the subject include work by Jeffrie Murphy (2003) and Jefffrey Blustein (2008) and most recently from Thomas Brudholm (2008) who suggests that resentment gives insights into the moral implications of what happened.

Though this is contrary to the fashionable idea "…that negative attitudes and emotions are detrimental to being truly human,"[72] their continuing outrage and refusal to forgive can be seen as a moral protest against what happened and a justifiable reaction to the disrespect shown to them thereafter. Its capacity for exposing the need for amnesia on behalf of existing social structures, discourses and ideologies also means that resentment is an invaluable resource for survivors continuing to live under the threat of resurgence in political violence. In this respect resentment can be seen as "…the reflex expression of an honourable emotional response to inexpiable wrongs and legitimate moral expectations that have not been properly dealt with."[73] From this perspective resentment has "…a constructive and positive role to play in the maintenance of social harmony and human relationships."[74]

However, this does not detract from the fact that its capacity to reverse the overwhelming influence of isolation, friction, tension, hatred, disunity and disharmony is conditional on the survivor's willingness to keep the past alive. In many situations this does not happen. The explanation for this is likely to involve social, cultural and economic factors and their interaction with attitudes and responses at the individual level.[75]

For people in the communities studied the breaking down of social norms and values and the increasing exposure to the dominant culture may be responsible for conditions that give rise to a lack of self-understanding. By living in ways that are increasingly incompatible with their own culture people are moving ineluctably towards a situation in which they are much less sure of themselves. This can be demonstrated by the following: "Some of us have become almost useless because (during the violence) we were forced to do night patrols (vigils) and we have had to try and forget those things but we can't." Author's field research: interviewee from Yachaya (Fabricio).

Inevitably, the impact of the violence has brought about significant alterations in human relations from outside the family and the community as well. This is particularly striking because this is exacerbated by the hard struggle for satisfying everyday needs and the fact that their present is characterised by violence and the fear of violence. In their relationship with local officials and other representatives from the surrounding social and institutional environment it has introduced "…misunderstandings in the form of equivocation, paradox, and confusion, which may provoke unknowing compromise."[76] Though unavoidable in the aftermath of the violence this can have devastating results.

A survivor describes the difficulties this has produced in their relationship with representatives responsible for the management and administration of the government reparations scheme (PIR): "Most people are not informed about what the PIR actually is, and this includes the persons who were worst affected by the

[72] Brudholm, T., (2008: 49).
[73] Brudholm, T., (2008: 49).
[74] Brudholm, T., (2008: 17).
[75] Blustein, J. (2008: 83ff)..
[76] Gautier, A., & Sabatini Scalmati, A., (2010: 6).

violence. They are not well informed because of their own negligence; they fail to attend the meetings that we community leaders have been trained for and this is why I am thinking about leaving office." Author's field research: interviewee from Qocha (Porfino).

In the aftermath of the violence it is inevitable that the distressing effects of shame, anxiety, and loss of meaning and a distorted sense of self-identity will give rise to feelings of immense personal insecurity. Having their shared contextual environment of safety destroyed drives people "...towards conformism, incapacity to criticise, suggestibility and easy manipulation."[77]

As one survivor explained: "In the community there are many people who cannot face the politicians because they feel unable; they feel ignorant. Its' the same with the community authorities; they are afraid to act, to perform any action, which is why we have problems with people from here who retreat to avoid problems or making problems." Author's field research: interviewee from Otoronco (Ramon).

In this climate of uncertainty, the evasion of moral responsibilities has made reality sufficiently ambiguous for people to take only a superficial interest in the past and their relationship with it. Speaking of the troubled relation of memory to the violence Honoré (an interviewee from Unay), said that survivors are so focused on the future that they do not have the time to acknowledge their own past. These changing conditions and the corresponding psychological changes they give rise to indicate a failure to appreciate the consequences it has for their understanding of themselves, their abilities, interests and concerns. From this perspective any lack of self-understanding is because the failure to assume ownership of their own past experience of extreme events has deprived people of links between their own past and present lives and given rise to a situation in which they are unable "...to make sense of who [they are] on the basis of important truths about what happened to [them] in the past."[78]

Failure to take responsibility for their own past means that any temptation to ignore or deny the past is unlikely to prevent survivors from being reminded of what happened and of the injustices with which the past is associated.[79] For Murphy "... the individual who let's go of his resentment for psychological, spiritual or material reasons linked with his own daily survival 'let's go' of useful anger and has less psychic energy to put forward toward obtaining justice. Overcoming resentment may therefore compromise values of genuine importance."[80]

This raises an important question: To what extent is resentment able to help transform the psychic fragmentation and apathy that force survivors "...to learn submission and expect nothing from life"[81] into critical consciousness?

Because survivors consider the societal response to what happened as inadequate the memory of their experiences is likely to continue to fester. An informant explains

[77] Gautier, A., & Sabatini Scalmati, A., (2010: 6).

[78] Blustein, J. (2008: 87).

[79] Ehlers, A., Hackmann, A., Steil, R., Clohessy, S., Wenninger, K., Winter, H. (2002).

[80] Murphy, J., (2003: 115).

[81] Martin-Baro, I., (1994a, b, c, d: 26–7).

that their frustration with central government is the result of its lack of interest in rural poverty: "…they are not interested, even where there is much poverty; the government do not see anything for them in our community." Author's field research: informant from Wamani (Marco).

So resentment and the refusal to forgive what happened can be seen "…as the reflex expression of a moral protest and ambition that are as permissible and admirable as the willingness to forgive or forgiveness proper."[82] This is not just about their resentment of the response to what happened; it is also about the violation of their traditional, norms, values and expectations, as is demonstrated by the following: "It is difficult to convince people to remain active in the community because they disregard the ways we used to do things. They do not want to obey and comply because they say they have no time, no time because they are more worried about their farm and their animals." Author's field research: interviewee from Unay (Santos).

Though social structures, discourses and ideologies have moved on the resentment survivors feel about what happened and what has since been done to honour their suffering has not. By pushing the memory of what happened to one side social structures, discourses and ideologies are neutralizing the moral impact of their existence and impeding the development of a democratic political culture. In this context survivors have no answer to the question 'why?' This frustrates the basic need for safety, control predictability and self-respect, thereby making adaptation of and reduction in the old values of solidarity unavoidable.[83]

To regain their self-esteem, their self-pride and the life that was lost to them people need to transform the psychological damage inflicted on them into personal growth experiences. Though positive psychological change is not inevitable what happened and what has since been done to honour their suffering has transformed some survivors' understanding of the world and their prior worldview.

By changing the way in which people perceive the world around them they develop a new consciousness for determining how they respond to their situation. In these circumstances the significance of what happened can cause survivors to adopt a bad faith by trying to ignore what happened and what has since been done to honour their suffering. In a context of daily survival this is likely to happen not because survivors are entirely aware of switching off or blocking out the memory of the psychological damage inflicted on them, but because they choose to set up a barrier which prevents the memory of what happened from reaching conscious knowledge.[84]

Though this type of passivity and complicity is normally associated with the bystander and their failure to respond to some past injustice, the changes in the way survivors perceive the world around them can also cause them to respond to the psychological damage they suffered by being indifferent and dysfunctional about

---

82 Brudholm, T., (2008: 171).

83 Staub, E., (1989: 45).

84 Cohen, S., (2001: xii ff).

their own past. This draws our attention to the fact that "...a definitive part of human experience is the way in which we react to outside circumstances."[85]

A survivor describes the difficulties this presents since the conflict ended: "The people here are conformists and very depressed because the community has been forgotten (by the state authorities); the only development programmes take place in the urban parts of the district, not out here in the villages; also there is no work for anyone, no help for the school or the health post." Author's field research: interviewee from Qocha (Mario).

For an individual to transform the psychological damage inflicted on them into personal growth experiences they need to "...reconfigure their thoughts, beliefs, and behaviours to adjust to ongoing and changing demands."[86]

For survivors in the communities studied this means that the forging of new links between depressive feelings of inferiority, worthlessness and helplessness with the social structures, discourses and ideologies responsible for states of "marginalized dependency" and "oppressive misery" is undertaken by individuals acting alone.[87] In many cases this makes survivors reluctant to separate themselves from fixed understandings of themselves and make the connection between their private lives and the public events associated with what happened.[88] This can take place even when the failure to assume full responsibility for themselves' has consequences that undermine their own ability to meet current and future needs. Typical is the following statement: "The poverty in this community is because the population is conformist and individualist[89]; they only look out for their family and not for the whole community." Author's field research: interviewee from Otoronco (Sanchez).

The psychic fragmentation and apathy that forces survivors "...to learn submission and expect nothing from life"[90] also has the capacity to transform the psychic pain of humiliation[91] into a radical search for meaning and orientation.

Because this is positively associated with "...the reconstruction of meaning, the renewal of faith, trust, hope, and connection, the redefinition of self, self in relation

---

[85] Barnett, V. J., (1999: 9).

[86] Lepore, S. J., & Revenson, T.A., (2006: 27) in Calhoun, L.G. & Tedeschi, R.G., (2009).

[87] Martin-Baro, I., (1994a, b, c, d: 26–7).

[88] In spite of its close association with the political violence and its aftermath, individualism has also been associated with conflicts among families in the administration of land belonging to the community. See Gonzalez, O.M., (2011: 103ff); Galvez, M., Ansión, J. & Degregori, C.I. (1981).

[89] In spite of the long history of individualism within the indigenous peasant population its current use in the communities studied is not overtly related to its earlier usage, which referred to the figure of the *gamonal*. The history of the *gamonal* is discussed in Gonzalez, O.M., (2011: 103ff). Until the Agrarian Reform of 1969 the *gamonal* was perceived as a feudal lord and regarded as an "... economic and political power in the highlands during the colonial period." Though this brought its original role to an end the image of the *gamonal* as the embodiment of exploitation remained.

[90] Martin-Baro, I., (1994a, b, c, d: 26–7).

[91] For these purposes the act of humiliation "...involves putting down, holding down and rendering the other helpless to resist the debasement. The feeling of being humiliated emerges when one is unable to resist the debasement and one deems it to be illegitimate as well as unwanted." See Lindner, Evelin G. (2001).

to others, and sense of community"[92] it offers survivors a means by which they can assume ownership of their own past experience of extreme events by forging new links between their own past and present lives.

Thus, the search for meaning and orientation "...may be viewed as natural human strength that represents the very life force of adversity that can compensate for the coexisting posttraumatic distress,"[93] even if it's overall effectiveness is ultimately contingent on the interplay of a diverse range of personal and environmental resources. These include personal resources that facilitate adaptability and assertiveness such as self-esteem, self-efficacy and social support as well as environments that promote: (i) physical and mental health, (ii) normative development; and (iii) social cohesion and the development of social capital.[94]

From previous studies relating to the aftermath of trauma we know that people suffer much less psychosocial distress in circumstances where high levels of personal resources are available.[95] However, from the evidence presented earlier in this study (and presented later) these resources are so manifestly deficient in the communities studied as to make coping difficult and vulnerability to stress, breakdown and disease inevitable.[96] As one survivor put it: "People in the community don't communicate with each other like they used to, even though there has been a lot of training. It's because they are selfish, because they aren't humanitarian." Author's field research: interviewee from Otoronco (Ninon).

In this respect the ability to assume ownership of their own past experience of extreme events by forging new links between the survivor's own past and present lives can seem like nothing more than a fantasy. To moderate the effects of extreme experiences such as the loss of identity and feelings of being worthless requires survivors to shift their perception out of the local dimension where their feeling of belonging is traditionally located. Entering this new perception of the world is inclined to leave people adrift in a meaningless oblivion from which there is no apparent escape since this shift in perception goes hand in hand with a lack of confidence that it will ever be effective.

In addition, the lack of social spaces that "...support the development of critical consciousness, the strengthening of dialogue and the nurturing of imaginative practices of representing history and conceiving the future"[97] mean that survivors lack the opportunity to articulate their concerns and build solidarities. This is reflected in the low level of social commitment, a low level of emotional involvement and a

[92] Lev-Wiesel, R. & Amir, M., (2006: 257) in Calhoun, L.G., & Tedeschi, R.G., (2009).

[93] Lev-Wiesel, R. & Amir, M., (2006: 259).

[94] Lepore, S. J., & Revenson, T.A., (2006: 32); Ben-Sira, Z., (1991); Folkman, S. & Lazarus, R.S., (1984).

[95] See for example Amir, M. & Lev-Wiesel, R., (2001); Lev-Wiesel, R. & Amir, M., (2000).

[96] See for example: Folkman, S. & Lazarus, R.S., (1984); Brewin, C.R., Andrews, B. & Valentine, J.D. (2000); Ozer, E.J., Best, S.R., Lipsey, T.L., & Weiss, D.S. (2008); Ullman, S.E., Filipas, H.H., Townsend, S.M., & Starzynski, L.L. (2007); Ullman, S.E., & Filipas, H.H.(2001); Yamawaki, N., Darby, R., & Queiroz, A. (2007).

[97] Watkins, M. & Shulman, H. (2008: 210).

growing independence from cultural norms and increasingly individualistic behaviour. The result of this breakdown in the natural order and the increasing "…liquefaction of social frameworks and institutions"[98] means that the range of opportunities conducive to personal growth experiences are restricted and short-lived.

6.1 Conclusions

To make people more alert to the aftermath of violence, this chapter has brought the experiences with which it is associated into full view. Only in this way can we hope to better understand the convoluted ways in which survivors adapt themselves to living under conditions that prevent them from being able to confront and somehow find an appropriate outlet for their experiences. It is important to begin by identifying some of the common emotions and behaviours associated with survivors affected by political violence and living in a context where their priority is daily survival.

This helps to ground the determining influence of such concepts as power, culture, conflict, exploitation and hierarchy, and the meanings survivors give them. The starting point needs to be the needs, duties and obligations that provide survivors with expectations about the world and about their identity as human beings. The bedrock upon which this moral and emotional framework rests involves respect for the essential needs of others. These comprise physical needs and non-physical needs that involve the moral aspects of life. Both are indispensable, so that being deprived of these needs can make survivors blind to the situation in front of them.

Provided the moral obligations that arise out of respect for the essential needs of others are not violated the normal mechanisms by which the demands of everyday life can be addressed are likely to be upheld. This lubricates the relationship between the individual and the moral and emotional framework, and protects survivors from the psychological effects of difficult life conditions. Though the actual activities, which obligations require from survivors, depend on the circumstances the deficiencies of any social order can be determined by the range of conflicts between obligations that it involves.

This being so, what survivors in the Andean communities studied are confronted with is a condition that is uprooting them from any deep and living connections with their environment. It is aggravated by the rupture in the survivor's access to shared values, common humanity and shared responsibility. Only through the recovery of the historical past will it be possible for survivors to begin to understand what has caused the current situation to come about. If survivors fail to work through their experiences of extreme events the past will continue to interfere with their lives, undermine efforts to overcome existential fatalism and, in doing so, deny them control of their own existence.[99]

---

[98] Bauman, Z., (2004: 51).

[99] For Finkelkraut, "…those who refuse to forget are besieged by a cultural suspicion that demands to know how the past may prove useful to the future." Finkelkraut, A., (1980).

Chapter 7
Disillusionment After Change

Having explored the experience of political violence and how survivors from the communities studied have sought to process what happened to them, this chapter looks at how disillusionment informs the perception of individuals and groups across the social, political and economic spectrum and how this is subsequently confronted and managed by community members.

For survivors struggling to satisfy their basic needs the idea of being able to overcome existential fatalism in the aftermath of political violence is not normal. It is the overwhelming urgency of the situation that shapes local reality and defines the meaning of normal behaviour, not the rupture in people's access to shared values, common humanity and shared responsibility. Nevertheless, this is a highly aversive state which is likely to make people want to change a situation that denies them control of their own existence.

To assess the impact of this devalued identity more closely the reader is reminded of the need for an understanding of what was done to ordinary people and ".... the principle of brute force that lay behind it."[1] In giving voice to individual and communal responses this chapter shows that avoidance rather than confrontation is the most common strategy. By abandoning and then trying to recover the relationships that give meaning to life, as well as those needed to sustain wellbeing survivors no longer share what they have and what they know. They may not help others as they would have done in the past. However, they are still able to do so, on condition that the behavioural strategies they adopt in their relationship with other people are meaningful and of practical significance.

This and the following chapter explores how the Andean experience is very relevant to many other situations around the world, drawing out some of the wider lessons from the research cases.[2]

[1] Sebald, W.G. (2004: 151); Wessells, M.G. & Monteiro, C. (2004a, b); Baglishya, D. (2000); Martin-Baro, I. (1989); (1994a, b, c, d); Staub, E., (2003).

[2] de Lemus, S., Spears, R. & Moya, M. (2008); Tiedens, L.Z., & Fragale, A.R. (2003).

T. J. Bowyer, *Beyond Suffering and Reparation*,
https://doi.org/10.1007/978-3-319-98983-9_7

7.1 Legacies of the Past

Failure in human connectedness is a reminder of how people are capable of causing extreme suffering to another without inflicting actual bodily harm. By turning people into objects, the capacity to prevent one person from hurting another has been suspended.

To overcome the psychic pain generated by this type of suffering people are likely to resort to a range of psychological defences including: avoidance behaviour, emotional numbness, psychic paralysis, passivity, reduced awareness, scapegoats, shame, withdrawal (e.g., selfishness, fatalism), counter behaviour (e.g., resentment, aggression, prejudice), and altered state of consciousness.[3] Though the range of choice from these or other defence responses varies they usually reflect the individual's own personal and cultural attitudes and values. For survivors from the communities studied the psychological responses to the legacy of the past extend across a broad spectrum.

Of particular importance is the loss of charity and the compassion they had been accustomed to extend and to expect from others.[4] This loss of social structures, cultural values, self and group identities is at the centre of the individual's deepest and most profound assumptions. Its impact is such that it brings about a radical transformation in the relationship people have with such basic psychological needs as security, safety, trust, esteem, positive identity, feelings of effectiveness and control, positive connections to other people, a comprehension of reality and of one's own place in the world, and transcendence (or spiritual needs).[5]

An informant said that their situation is explained by the fact that "…there is no confidence in the community because the bad times have caused a lot of mistrust; people don't support the leaders of organizations like they used to." Author's field research: interviewee from Otoronco (Gustavo).

This is consistent with the opinions of informants from other communities studied as one survivor of the violence explains: "Before (the violence) the people were united and now they have a bit of money and people move away and live their own life. Each one practically lives his own life, today everything is about money. Now there is no pity, just selfishness, no support for orphans or widows. Now there is no such solidarity; when I was young there was mutual support, not now. Author's field research: interviewee from Yachaya (Claudia).

In this respect the experience of violence is not the absolute limit of all possible suffering. New situations and information compel people to recognise that if they are to continue to survive they need to suppress and forget the impact of direct

---

[3] Frommberger, Ulrich (2014); Regel, S. & Joseph, S. (2010: 7).

[4] Theidon, K., (2013: 314).

[5] For a discussion of cultural bereavement, see Eisenbruch, M., (2007) in Pouligny, B., Chesterman, S., and Schnabel, A. (eds.) (2007: 71–96); See also McCann, I.L. & Pearlman, L.A. (1990a); Pearlman, L.A.& Saakvitne, K.W. (1995); Saakvitne. K.W. et al., (2000); Staub, E., (1989, 2003).

exposure to violence.[6] The following shows that, however horrific experiences have been, the current situation make avoidance behaviour more or less essential to their own survival: "During the conflict both terrorists and the army killed people in the community. This has left the community with much fear. Everything was neglected for such a long time: land, animals… So many people were killed from the community. Now people migrate to get away." Author's field research: interviewee from Wamani (Nelli).

In more predictable circumstances a stressful event is likely to increase an individual's affiliation and integration into their own socio-cultural system.

Before the violence local beliefs, values and practices that used to help people meet their basic psychological needs were often respected. This is reflected in the following testimony: "First we lived all together but when the terrorists came that was the end of that arrangement." Author's field research: interviewee from Qocha (Frida).

For survivors the violence has so impaired the system that any emotional connection with "other people's feelings (which is the affective basis for empathy)" has been irrefutably damaged.[7] This deadens the ability to share in the suffering of others and heightens the most terrible aspect of suffering, which is "…not so much the pain itself but the loneliness therein."[8] For example, a survivor felt their situation is explained by the fact that: "…the people who live among us are damaged; there is envy, there is abuse, there is indolence; there is a lack of culture." Author's field research: interviewee from Wamani (Herminio).

This means having to deal with deep distortions in people's sense of responsibility that lead to wrongdoing and toleration of wrongdoing. In addition, it means having to deal with the feeling that people no longer support each other in their judgements about what is wrong and in matters of responsibility.[9] By failing to rebuild trust powerful expectations about a sense of wrong, standards and responsibilities are utterly compromised and replaced by feelings of fear, anxiety and intimidation. Increased violence in the form of robberies, attacks on soldiers, drug trafficking, and extrajudicial killings ensure that these feelings remain at the forefront of people's lives. This is clear from the following: "The issue of security in the community is creating confusion among people here, because they have heard that there is evidence of the presence of Shining Path in communities in other parts of the country, which make them think that terrorism can return to this community." Author's field research: interviewee from Qocha (Maximo).

This undermines civic agency because it makes people reluctant to take action if it risks confrontation with organizations and institutions and other powerful actors. From this failure to provide any adequate moral and political response to their situation people have made the reconstruction of their own standards of trust difficult if not impossible.

---

[6] Carlson, N. (2012).

[7] Krznaric, R., (2014: 15).

[8] Bingemer, M.C. & Casarella, P., (eds.) (2014: 8).

[9] Walker, M.U., (2006: 74–5).

How to replace their own moral comfort with the charity and the compassion they had been accustomed to extend and to expect from others? How to uphold human dignity in spite of being subject to the effects of irremediable, shocking and incommunicable suffering? In the absence of a public forum where survivors can speak their truth and their suffering can be formally acknowledged the prospects for rebuilding trust and other past assumptions are not good. For survivors to lead others to greater truth about their experiences of the violence their experiences "…must be received, affirmed and proclaimed by the community that is nourished by their testimonies and in which witnesses will endure."[10]

From a national perspective it is perhaps still possible to think that significant progress has been made in addressing the suffering inflicted on thousands of families and communities across the rural highlands. The implementation of collective reparations for a significant number of communities, the policy of providing documentation for massive numbers of people and adding them to the Civil Registry testify not just to the state's commitment to address human rights violations but to the factors and conditions that led to those wrongs as well.

Though much work still needs to be done there is a sense in which people in government circles have come to believe that the past can now be left to fend for itself. However, for survivors who have to live with the suffering inflicted by the violence it is a different matter.

If the state is to make sense of the reality of sustained daily suffering and what the legacy of violence does to people it needs to recognise that these disruptive experiences are part of the historical past and of the present and as such are deep-seated and indelible.

By paying no attention to the actual lived experience of human suffering the system has deprived the sufferer of any access to the traditional norms and values from which all meaning used to emanate. Unless the state and people affected by the violence can come to some mutual agreement about the injustice of this disregard for the past there will be no change in the reality of daily suffering.

To reframe the concept of policies and programmes so that large scale forces relate to the aftermath of the political violence the state needs to recognise the relevance of the past for understanding contemporary suffering. In this way the moral impact of human existence can be brought into the mainstream of political life. Even so, recognition for the actual lived experience of human suffering continues to be repeatedly side-lined through policies that emphasize social unity, nation building and an overall outlook which insists that no future is possible unless the past is left behind. Not only does this encourage impersonal attitudes and reification, it also makes it easier to refer to survivors *en masse*. In addition,"…[e]quity, justice, participation and freedom were peripheral and were raised only as afterthoughts in the national and international development policies."[11]

By failing to gain access to the reality of other people the state is able to exclude issues of moral/practical import from entering their field of perception. In practice

---

[10] Bingemer, M.C. & Casarella, P., (eds.) (2014: 30).

[11] TRC Final Report, Sengupta *supra* note 12, at Vol. IX, Part 4, Ch. 2.2, at 849.

this means that individual needs, interests and priorities can be ignored so that survivors of political violence can be thought of in stereotypical as opposed to individuating ways.

Vetlesen noted: "...for the state the exchangeability of one person for another result from the liquidation of their uniqueness as individuals and prepares for the indifference between people that made the holocaust possible."[12] For survivors of violence this means that feelings of anxiety, shame, desperation, fear, confusion, withdrawal and self-loathing are of no relevance to their relationship with the state.

By making interpersonal compassion subordinate to the demands of a task oriented and performance-oriented culture the state has effectively purged the subjective content from the lived experience of other human beings. This is clear from the following: "We villagers do not trust the state; it didn't protect us during the political violence and since returning to the village no one has helped us. The community is very bitter because there is no state support: my people are saying that only in the elections do we see the state and then it disappears along with all the promises they made; they forget us." Author's field research: interviewee from Wamani (Victoria).

In addition, focus groups from the communities studied said that state-funded social programmes designed to 'mitigate' the effects of the violence and the impact of extreme poverty did not take effect until more than 15 years after the abuses had taken place. These conditions make it difficult for survivors to share their traumatic experiences with others. A survivor commented on the reparations: "I'm unhappy with the collective reparations because it is not like the people who were worst affected are alive; they only want to appease us, neutralizing our memories of all the mistreatment with money." Author's field research: interviewee from Wamani (Rosa).

Because the sharing of traumatic experiences is a precondition for the restitution of a meaningful world this means that survivors cannot even begin to rebuild the most minimal form of emotional connectedness with other individuals and groups. The following informant voices a widely held view: "We should have the same value those in power have and there should be no discrimination. Whatever claims poor people make are not heard by those in charge. Having peace in Peru is like banging your head against a brick wall." Author's field research: interviewee from Qocha (Julio).

This leaves survivors alienated and burdened with an unprocessed past, ultimately diminishing the individual's tolerance and ability to cope with their traumatic experiences; it also encourages them to distance themselves from others. This is demonstrated by the following: "People laugh at us because they don't know how to love their fellow men. My father's house was big. They burnt it down using bombs and setting it alight. Three days later, I sent for my husband to come and see. They had taken all of my things. Those people are so bad. I'm suffering and they didn't feel sorry for me at all. This is why I no longer trust people; I only trust God." Author's field research: interviewee from Qocha (Frida).

[12] Vetlesen, A. J., (1994:112).

By making past human suffering subordinate to justice and reconciliation the *Plan Integral de Reparaciones* (Comprehensive Reparations Program) (PIR) and its reparations programmes have brought about a set of conditions that generate unrealistic expectations about the future social inclusion of the historically marginalised. If suppression of the painful memories had been respected as no more than a temporary expedient it might have created conditions suitable enough for survivors to begin to make sense of their situation. Instead the opportunity to work through trauma and obtain some form of integration is blocked by a system that encourages the prolonged suppression of painful memories out of political expediency.

This disregard for the past is borne out of a system of detachment: it blocks any new meaning about people; it prevents silenced people from asking questions, it separates and isolates and it keeps survivors locked into a stage of development that never goes beyond those past events, as the following demonstrates: "Others don't want to talk; they keep their secrets [about what happened to them] because psychologically they are afraid." Author's field research: interviewee from Qocha (Mario).

This failure to reassure survivors that the importance of what happened is properly acknowledged and that the appropriate responsibilities are assumed strips them of their own moral sense. It makes meaningful dialogue and a shared moral understanding unfeasible. Having been stripped of their moral sense all distinctions between one individual and another disappear, thereby eliminating anything that lends distinctiveness to the individual or group. The negation of the on-going suffering of the victims of the violence, the lack of any recognition of what has gone before underscores the vital role of compassion in what it means to be human.

To reduce the meaning of human suffering to reparations projects that focus on the primary, economic and social needs of the survivors is to misrepresent the process and the consequences of human suffering. Over time this has a deadening effect on the survivor's intellectual, mental and emotional life. This has the capacity to break the resistance of the survivor and the group and lead to a level of disconnectedness that is unprecedented. By failing to align itself with the actual lived experience of human suffering the state has reduced everyone to sameness thereby ignoring factors such as culture, ethnicity, and political tradition, local norms and values and other aspects of community level morality.

This is clear from the following: "Does the government think it can make the pain and suffering of those years easier to bear just by giving communities collective reparations and even make us believe that we will be given individual reparations? But this is business for the government because it benefits the people who have economic power." Author's field research: interviewee from Wamani (Ordell).

For survivors this application of the universal to the detriment of the particular effectively blocks any emotional connection with 'other people's feelings' (which is the affective basis for empathy). The following shows how the community has been impacted: "I remember those years that passed us by. So, what can the government do to soothe that pain, that fury, the courage that the people from the village have because of what they went through? Well, these days, the government is simply giving some of us collective reparations, including making us think that they will give us individual compensation. But nothing they do will ever bring back the people who died." Author's field research: interviewee from Qocha (Julio).

The effects of this situation make survivors less willing to think critically about themselves and more inclined to follow authority regardless of where it leads. By letting go of their own subjectivity survivors give up any demand for their right as human beings to be recognised and affirmed as individuals. This constitutes a major revision of what passes for acceptable behaviour. It has redefined the meaning of satisfactory relationships between individuals and group, as the following testimony demonstrates: "The government doesn't care about us. I think about how many people must have been killed and about the abuse that we were subjected to. They shouldn't lie to us; they should just say that there won't be any reparations if there indeed won't be." Author's field research: interviewee from Qocha (Aurora).

By absolving people from responsibility for their own actions this type of relationship effectively separates the powerless from their own capacity for private and individual judgement, logic and a sense of justice. Insofar as it has the power to "… join people who have separate or conflicting interests, who do not feel good about each other, who are unequal, or who simply do not understand one another"[13] it looks like something, which it is not.

Forged out of the frustration of basic psychological and material needs this is an unequal relationship that makes no allowance for any subjective felt-experience. Instead it is cynical, manipulative and pessimistic; there is no space for compassion and (for local people) it is motivated entirely by survival. This is clear from the following: "There is a lot of resentment amongst villagers about collective reparations because nothing has arrived and because no one thinks that anyone will ever be awarded individual reparations. The only things to have come out of collective reparations are money for the construction of a communal meeting house and an irrigation system in the neighbouring community." Author's field research: interviewee from Unay (Jesus).

Not being in touch with the emotional states and goals of others means that government policies and programmes have brought this unequal relationship into contention with the idea of effective cooperation.[14] By abrogating their own individuality and personal responsibility people invalidate their own basic beliefs and precepts, thereby encouraging the belief that everything is determined and that everything can be explained. This is a process that does not pass unnoticed, as the following statement demonstrates: "There is no chance that one of us from the community who is in conflict with the mayor is able to take a step forward and say 'I'm willing to negotiate' The imposition of the power of the mayor is always worth more than any other opinion." Author's field research: interviewee from Qocha (Severo).

Through non-recognition of the reality of the survivor, the state shows its moral insensitivity, reaffirming how government policies and programmes fail to bear witness to the reality of the social context. For many survivors the lack of official accommodation to the expectations of the powerless is enough to justify the feeling

[13] Sennet, R., (2012: 6).

[14] De Waal, F., (2010).

that the past cannot be 'dealt with', and needs to be kept open and unfinished. This is clear from the following statement: "There are people who still need to be recognized and the damage repaired. For example, we have several mass graves here which the truth commission has been unable to establish the facts about and we ask that these facts are clarified for the good of the country and their relatives from this community." Author's field research: Interviewee from Qocha (Marcelino).

The lack of remorse and unwillingness to rectify past mistakes of the state make resentment almost inevitable as the following testimony demonstrates: "We have lost our families (mother, others lost their parents, siblings, others were disabled, traumatized) so far we have not been given justice; we cannot sue the state or the people responsible for the murders they committed. Why? Because we have no money, we are country people." Author's field research: interviewee from Otoronco (Ruben).

For the survivors the failure to properly acknowledge human suffering and how it should be dealt with makes non-recognition and misrecognition of human suffering humiliating; it also deprives survivors of material security, self-respect and self-worth, as the following testimony indicates: "I'm unhappy with the reparations programmes; they only want to appease us, neutralize our memories of all the mistreatment with money." Author's field research: interviewee from Qocha (Jorge).

It is therefore important to look at what has not been acknowledged and not incorporated into the relationship between the government and the survivors. In this way it is possible to highlight the discrepancies between legitimate moral expectations and the conduct of the state to which the resentment felt by survivors is directed. For survivors the long-awaited response to these and other atrocities has not been forthcoming.

By failing to give up on insisting what is right, survivors are able to retain a belief in resentment as a means by which they can challenge government indifference, objectivity and other assorted moral disengagement mechanisms such as the diffusion and displacement of responsibility. In this respect resentment has "…a constructive and positive role to play in the maintenance of social harmony and human relationships."[15] This is clear from the following statement: "Having peace in Peru is like banging your head against a wall. I remember those years that passed us by. I feel great remorse; these types of abuse should never happen again. So, what can the government do to soothe that pain, that fury, the courage that the people from the village have due to what they experienced? After all this time we are still waiting." Author's field research: interviewee from Qocha (Plinio).

For powerless survivors the experience of the violence (and the subsequent behaviour of the government makes a reassessment of their life and what is deemed important highly probable. The experience of physical and psychological persecution has so reduced the lives of the survivor to the barest essentials that it makes an interrogation of the worth of their previous life and the norms and values that governed them more or less inevitable. In their efforts to try and better understand what happened to them survivors often undergo a transformative process in which their

[15] Brudholm, T., (2008: 47).

suffering finds a meaning. This can be nothing short of a realization that suffering has a future role that is both positive and affirmative.

Though the experiences they were forced to endure were unwanted the personal insights gained from what happened have the potential to rescue people from past illusions about their way of life, including what can be trusted and what should be feared.[16] The realization that their own survival and their own socio-cultural system are no longer secure is able to trigger an instinctual emotional response to features of the environment associated with some aspect of the experiences from the past. This situation is described by one: "I've been seeing this new situation lately. When I look at the situation, I believe that this exclusion should not exist because it stems from the government. It is the government that has provoked all this violence." Author's field research: interviewee from Wamani (Ordell).

7.2 Disillusion with Reparations and Their Consequences

The range of problems associated with government reparations are grouped together under four different headings: political, economic, social and security. These four types of government reparations problems overlap with each other and are not mutually exclusive. Both political and social-state reparations problems are mentioned most frequently across all five communities. The frequency of reparations problems is variable and reflects the contextually specific nature of the issues involved. For example, the most important reparations problems in Qocha have focused around people's belief that individual reparations to survivors will never happen whereas in Yachaya the most commonly experienced problems associated with reparations are a result of people having failed to use the monies available to them wisely.

Disillusionment threatens the ability to think, feel and behave in a manner that allows individuals and households to perform effectively. People who perceive the social setting as a place of fragmentation and danger tend to feel less secure and less engaged.

A survivor of the violence describes this loss of the primordial senses of self and basic belonging for the life of their community since the conflict ended: "We are a population with many fears and terrors, but we cannot be sure what direction things are going because there is no official information; it is all just rumours." Author's field research: interviewee from Unay (Porfirio).

In a context of unpredictable change, disillusionment can leave people with feelings of helplessness that so diminish the self-concept, that there is nothing and no one with whom they can identify. This encourages survivors to detach themselves from their immediate environment so that the practical attitudes they have towards the security available to them do not come to be seen, let alone experienced as arbitrary or outlandish. This is clear from the following: "We do not trust the government;

[16] Frankl, V., (1985 105–7); Janoff-Bulman, R., (1992: 132ff).

it didn't protect us during the political violence and since we started to come back here no one has helped us. This community is very bitter because there is no state support: my people are saying that only in the elections do we see the state and then it disappears along with all the promises they made; they forget us." Author's field research: interviewee from Qocha (Pomposa).

For individuals and groups in the communities studied disillusionment encourages stress that serves to emphasize and make more severe the suffering in their lives. To improve their life conditions, survivors need to align themselves with social and political groups that can help to remove factors that threaten the self-concept and identity. However, the social and political groups available do not help to protect the individual self-concept and identity so much as underscore how removed people are from meaningful interaction and issues of moral and practical importance.

This constitutes a profound threat to survivors' assumptions about the world and their comprehension of reality. In particular it profoundly threatens their respect for and valuing of social and political groups (including their own) because the individual self-concept and identity has been harmed, as the following demonstrates: "…in the community everything is dangerous, no one is really safe; those who are most affected are the women and children." Author's field research: interviewee from Qocha (Godofredo).

Financially, an informant explained that the results can be extreme: "…I haven't enough money to meet my needs, because the money that I have doesn't cover the cost of eating." Author's field research: interviewee from Qocha (Tiburcio). The following comment is telling about the breakdown of community security patrols: "… people here aren't interested in reviving the *rondas* because we don't have the time." Author's field research: interviewee from Otoronco (Rufo).

Other symptoms of disillusionment are directed towards the community and its leadership as the following account makes clear: "There are no active leaders within the community; only those who make decisions affecting the internal affairs of the community. Nothing is done to promote the future of the community; instead leadership is just decisions about when crop planting should start. The village leaders are farmers and the positions they occupy are of secondary importance." Author's field research: interviewee from Otoronco (Juanito).

Another survivor of the political violence describes the implications of a weak and ineffectual leadership for ongoing security problems affecting the community:

"Many authorities are afraid to leave the community because the area is threatened by dangers from highway robberies, rape, attacks on soldiers, extra-judicial killings and backpackers on the high passes and on the route to the jungle. Insecurity is everywhere, not just far off, but in areas close to the community. The military and the police are mostly in the capital district". Author's field research: interviewee from Yachaya (Raquel).

A survivor of the violence describes the lack of respect and attention from government officials and the implications this has for their community: "The district mayor is authoritarian and makes decisions without consulting any of us" (Author's field research: interviewee from Qocha (Maximinio).

In spite of the loss of traditions and values resentment about past injustices remains a meaningful response to the situation. This is because resentment has the capacity to motivate people to challenge the status quo, including such social and political processes as state indifference and objectivity. To uncover the extent to which this allows the individual survivor to keep the past open and unfinished this chapter (and the following) looks at the relationship between the terrible past and the indifferent present from the perspective of the survivor. The socio-psychological consequences of these experiences bring survivors ever closer to a psychological state in which social rules collapse and individual survivors find themselves at the mercy of their own impulses.

Because the lack of meaningfulness and purposefulness this produces is beyond the control of the individual and incapable of change particular types of attitude emerge: social withdrawal, hostility, isolation, and an inability to trust.

In the aftermath of the political violence this is responsible for a sense of agitation and confusion and the feeling of being haunted by a past that intrudes into every aspect of the individual survivor. Though these unhealthy attitudes encourage disillusionment and apathy the idea that it has caused survivors to become passive and devoid of social and political activity is not borne out by this study. Resentment arises from the inability to express psychological reactions to the political violence through lack of opportunity, oppression and indifference.

The more the state and NGOs fail to engage effectively with collective responsibility and the acknowledgement of shame and guilt, the more likely it is for the feelings of injustice experienced by local survivors to become submerged into the psyche and the cultural unconscious. This perception by social and political groups reaches across the realms of the social, political and economic spectrum to include the individual survivor's emotional responses to the resurgence of violence, the military, government reparations, other state programmes, NGOs, local officials and the community as a trusting social environment.

7.3 Disillusionment with NGOs

For people affected by violence and struggling to survive the consequences of what happened and the conditions under which they live are with them all the time. To help survivors rebuild a positive sense of self NGOs need to take an emotional interest in the human impact of the situation. In practice this does not happen. Instead, the emotional consequences of suffering and all the various and convoluted processes with which the violation of normative expectations is associated tend not to feature in NGO agendas or their projects.

This is clear from the following statement: "There are some very important facts about the involvement of civil society in NGO projects: the first contacts they make with us never pick up from us different ideas, proposals and visions. They don't consult the community or the authorities. NGO projects are not about what are the most urgent community priorities." Author's field research: interviewee from Unay (Rafael).

By preventing survivors from making sense of their situation NGO interventions encourage further psychological and physical withdrawal from the social arena. Though NGO activities have become increasingly commonplace in recent years, of all those active in the study region the number working to promote reconciliation, mutual respect and mutual tolerance is negligible. Their impact on the life of the community is described by one survivor: "Here NGOs are actually cashing in, and the work that they leave us with is not worth much. Some of them don't take their work very seriously. Instead of improving things NGOs are destroying the best of what we had." Author's field research: interviewee from Qocha (Marcelino).

In spite of the high level of interest in peace building, focus groups from all five communities included in this study only identified two NGOs (from an average of 0–5 NGOs per community) specifically involved in projects intended to foster increased security, mutual regard, truth and justice. This included one national NGO working with 120 widows from the conflict in Unay and one national NGO working on women's rights, rape, discrimination and exclusion of women in Wamani. Focus groups from all five research communities said that they had no knowledge of any type of NGO activity involving peace and conflict impact assessment with local GROs.[17]

This means that any NGO contribution to reconciliation and trust is left to NGOs working on social issues, such as health, education, nutrition, agriculture, etc. Precisely how significant these NGOs and their projects are to overcoming the terrible legacies of the past is difficult to assess.

The fact that the link between NGO activities and the promotion of increased security, mutual regard, truth and justice is so tenuous makes their contribution to reconciliation; mutual respect and mutual tolerance insubstantial, if not meaningless. However, the overwhelmingly negative impressions of NGOs have less to do with their failure to contribute to the various components of reconciliation than lack of prior experience. Consider the survivors in the immediate aftermath of the political violence looking for any means by which they can overcome the worst aspects of their experiences and move on.

In such cases survivors are likely to be more receptive to assistance from various hitherto, unknown sources (including NGOs)] than would ever have been possible prior to the violence. For survivors struggling to cope with psychological upheaval and anxiety their awareness of the mismatch between their own expectations and reality only began to emerge as the negative impressions of NGOs and their activities started to accumulate.

In spite of the intense difficulties in the aftermath of the political violence, it should be emphasised that local scepticism and mistrust of NGOs are also a product of the recent history of political violence. Prior to the violence the isolated, inward-looking nature of rural highland community life meant that contact with anyone

[17] More specifically this refers to the activities AFAVIP which are discussed in more detail in relation to its contribution to a safe environment below.

outside their own immediate environment was limited. For many local people this means that the military, SL and other terrorist activists would have been their first major encounter with strangers.

That their experiences of these 'strangers' was responsible for so much suffering and abuse are reason enough for them to remain fearful and mistrustful ever since.

How these feelings are likely to work to the disadvantage of NGOs is described by a survivor of the political violence as follows: "Sometimes we think the NGO mandate comes perhaps from terrorism; we just wonder why we are being approached. Mistrust of others has never left us because when unknown people come here we think it could be SL coming back." Author's field research: interviewee from Qocha (Severo).

Though this has helped to make the post-conflict situation intensely threatening it has brought a level of detachment and objectivity to people's perceptions of NGOs and their offers of help that might not otherwise have been there. People's experiences of NGOs have arisen within the context of an uncertain and unpredictable environment and this has helped to protect them from the feeling that any pre-existing assumptions about NGOs have been violated. This has helped to make criticism and evaluation of NGOs easier because people have never felt the need to rebuild any past assumptions about their benefits and advantages. To the extent that people have learned from painful experience they recognise that NGO activities and projects do not always correspond with local expectations, as the following indicates: "The NGOs are always providing training, but we are tired of it because we work on the land and already know a bit about the practical work. NGO training should be more practical according to their specialities." Author's field research: interviewee from Qocha (Isolda).

In the aftermath of political violence, the need for financial assistance, material resources and vital services has increased survivor awareness of the need for informational support to help them better understand the declared intentions of single NGOs.

A survivor of the violence describes the anxiety people have about the real objectives of NGO activities and the degree to which NGOs are willing and able to accommodate the needs, interests and priorities of the community itself: "I mistrust the NGOs. They have policies that are just to benefit their NGO. Here, in my community they are actually cashing in, and the work that they leave here is just a small investment. With some they don't take their work very seriously. Instead of improving this, the NGO is destroying what we ourselves had, in their use of materials, and their minimization of costs to create more savings for them." Author's field research: interviewee from Yachaya (Zelin).

Negative assumptions about NGOs are widespread. Nowhere is this impression more immediate, powerful or convincing than in the opinion people have of NGO projects and activities: the emphasis on unnecessary (and useless) training to the exclusion of everything else. This is clear from the following: "We are tired of NGO lectures, trainings, and interviews. They are just a waste of our time and only of benefit to the NGOs themselves. Yes, I distrust NGOs, but you cannot generalize. I can only say that I distrust the ones I know." Author's field research: interviewee from Qocha (Luna).

Lack of trust also manifested itself in the nature of people's attitude to NGOs working on social issues such as health, education, nutrition, agriculture, etc. A mother with two children stated that: "…the NGO work on community health and hygiene hasn't changed a thing; we are just the same now as when they first arrived," Author's field research: interviewee from Unay (Gracias).

While another woman in the same community said that two major projects started up by NGOs (one for an orchard and one for maize production) had both failed: "I have no confidence in NGOs because they do not work with a conscience; they do not work for the good of society. This is because the things they are responsible for have not been properly addressed; they have not solved the problems. They come here thinking they are going to do things and they fail to fulfil their objectives." Author's field research: interviewee from Unay (Fulgencio).

Many focus groups cited accusations of broken promises and corruption against NGOs. An informant said that they did not trust NGOs even when they show enthusiasm because this is used to mislead people about what they actually end up doing: "…some of the projects they carry out are not what they told us would happen." Author's field research: interviewee from Otoronco (Alvaro). Another said that it was impossible to trust them because they do not always tell the truth: "…they tell you that they come from such and such an office and that they are going to do such and such work when it isn't true." Author's field research: interviewee from Wamani (Jerome). A further informant said that this also led to NGOs using the worst materials for construction projects to minimize costs and create more savings for themselves (paraphrased) Author's field research: interviewee from Unay (Santiago).

Underlying this feeling of distrust is the suspicion that NGOs are also financially dishonest: "They are always focused on profits; even congressmen have called for an audit of them. I have knowledge that NGOs has funding but that they have not used 100% of the funding for the community or the projects for which it was intended; many NGOs just leave people with promises." Author's field research: interviewee from Yachaya (Zolin).

The overall failure to acknowledge the potential of NGOs to promote reconciliation, mutual respect and mutual tolerance in the research communities suggests that community members do not identify NGOs with solutions to problems associated with security, mutual regard, truth and justice. Instead, they tend to think about NGOs either having a fundamentally different agenda to those NGOs they present to the community or simply identify solutions to their own economic, social and political problems without the assistance of NGOs: "We have given up with NGOs. That's why lately we decided to work on production projects because this way we will at least generate some income for the village." Author's field research: interviewee from Qocha (Tiburcio).

Another interviewee acknowledged that any change in the relationship between the community and NGOs would be difficult to achieve, if only because this is contrary to the handout mentality that people have become accustomed to: "…in order to be successful we need productive projects because we want to learn and produce for ourselves so that we can improve our lives, but still some of my fellow villagers remain closed off as a result of the endless habit of obeying to the end." Author's field research: interviewee from Yachaya (Tenyoa).

7.4 Fear of the Future: The Prelude to Resentment

In the past, before political violence in the Peruvian Andes, it was perhaps easier to control and modify behaviour through a set of beliefs that affirmed acceptable behaviour and confronted deviancy. Such beliefs worked because the way of life was relatively enclosed and relatively free of external influences. Isolation made interactions and relationships between local people easier to recreate over time, reducing tendencies for suspicion and mistrust, since penalties for transgression of social norms were generally respected and enforced.[18]

However, with the societal disruption resulting from violence, relational rules and expectations about other people's conduct and obligations were broken and came to be regularly violated. Disobeying social norms became commonplace, which made it stressful talking and communicating with other people. Individuals were no longer confident of the truthfulness of others, creating social tensions and internal stress. Instead, distraction and misdirection became part of obtaining reliable information, and if a stranger was involved, these feelings of stress and distrust would be particularly powerful, given that local people had grown accustomed to thinking of strangers as untruthful and potentially dangerous, divisive and violent.

Repeatedly in the testimony of survivors the feeling of fear and mistrust towards strangers is emphasized as this survivor describes: "With people who come here from outside we are quiet; we show distance and distrust and link it to the uncles (SL) who came here before the political violence started and who gave us speeches about how they work for poor people. In the community we are aware of all the facts about the community. If people see any attack in the community most stay away and keep their eyes closed. They no longer want to have their lives threatened. After having lived experiences in cities it's much easier to flee if there is any more trouble. Before when we fled the community, we had to trek for a week, day after day, going carefully up in the hills." Author's field research: interviewee from Yachaya (Emilio).

In the aftermath of the violence people are faced with the tremendous anxiety of having to live in a world that they perceive as dangerous and threatening, and one in which their own survival cannot be guaranteed.[19] There are several kinds of fears that dominate the relationship survivors have with the external world. The main fears include: fear of resurgent political violence, fear of strangers and a fear specifically of military and the police.

---

[18] See for example La Serna, M., (2012: 19ff).

[19] Janoff-Bulman, R., (1992: 65).

7.5 Fear of Resurgent Political Violence

In the aftermath of the violence, survivors often exhibit extreme fear in response to reminders of what happened to them and their families. To avoid these anxiety-provoking situations survivors learn to develop avoidance and escape strategies. For rural highland communities' rumours about resurgence of political violence mean that these mechanisms are well established. This is clear from the following: "I think that maybe the Shining Path or the army will return. If the army comes back they will want to 'punish' us to spite us, telling us that we are terrorists. The terrorists will start to kill us again, telling us that we are '*yana humas*'[20] Author's field research: interviewee from Otoronco (Ofelia).

Feeling helpless to resist these ongoing threats to survival and self-preservation makes the reconstruction of a viable, nonthreatening environment seem remote and unrealistic. The sense of impending menace increases the survivor's vulnerability to further psychological disintegration and is exacerbated by the fact that highland communities are no longer closed entities. Instead the static, inward looking socio-cultural system of the past has evolved into something much more transient and subject to external influence. This is explained not just by the resurgence in political violence or the activities of various kinds of drugs and alcohol-related lawlessness and anti-social behaviour.

Those who survived the political violence have no illusions about the implications of this for the life of their community: "I am afraid when workers from public institutions come here and for that reason we do not talk with them. For that reason, we do not talk, we talk when they talk, as we do with the NGO workers. For example, in other places people ask where you are from; but here we are so afraid of them that we talk only if we are spoken to. "Author's field research: interviewee from Yachaya (Luisa).

In the aftermath of political violence, survivors resort to economic migration that can help the individual to split off trauma-related experiences from their daily life, dispensing with the legacy of the past, at least temporarily. However, the search for better employment opportunities is both threatening and unpredictable. In most cases the work is short-term, poorly paid and conditional on long periods away from the community and their families. This increases the sense of impermanence and makes survivors more vulnerable to further stress particularly if it is associated with the intense impact of victimization. This is nowhere more apparent than in the threat posed by the increasing number of strangers regularly encountered by local people in and around their community.

[20] Quechua = "fighting with the army".

7.6 Fear of Strangers

For many, encounters with the military, with SL and other strangers was strictly limited prior to the political conflict. The first major encounter with strangers was often a violent experience, and resulted in suffering and abuse. This can explain why local survivors remain fearful and mistrustful even of strangers who claim they want to help them, as the following demonstrates: “In a small community like ours you never know who is coming or going. If there are strangers walking about we may suspect them of being a cattle rustler and if so we cannot do anything because here there is no police station we can use to confirm it.” Author’s field research: interviewee from Yachaya (Rebecca).

Having to confront strangers in an environment where there is little by way of a legitimate authority structure is an important aspect of psychosocial stress as it is experienced in the Andes and elsewhere in post-conflict settings. Ever since strangers first began to appear amongst them rural highland people have learnt to be on their guard.

From their experiences during the violence through to the present strangers are synonymous with acts of subterfuge and deception. This is clear from the following: “Before the military arrived we were afraid; we were afraid of strangers, we did not know why people suddenly arrived asking us for something. For example, strange people arrived in civilian clothes; we did not know who they were. These were *Senderistas* who said that they had come because ‘we love poor people’ and that ‘we are poor like you and that everything will be fine, and that all your needs will be attended to.’ Then they forced us to give them our names so that they had a record of all of us. When there were problems between us we were punished; we were lead into the public square and there we were whipped to make everyone talk. When they were here there was a lot of theft, then there was abuse of women, rape and being thrown in the public square to be whipped.” Author’s field research: interviewee from Otoronco (Gustavo).

Because the intention to deliberately mislead people is inextricably linked with the political violence duplicity has become as much a challenge to the individual’s basic assumptions as the memory of the events that threatened their survival. The survivor of the political violence is usually extremely nervous and apprehensive of anything likely to trigger associations with the past as the following testimony demonstrates: “I think that maybe the army will return. If the army comes back they will call us terrorists. If the terrorists come back they will start to kill us again by saying that we are – ‘*yana humas*’- (fighting with the army).” Author’s field research: Interviewee from Unay (Porfirio).

Before the arrival of SL individuals mostly thought of other people as truthful and reliable; it was possible to maintain this belief because the socio-cultural system under which they lived did not tolerate individuality.

Instead life was governed by a set of beliefs based on solidarity and cooperation.[21] One survivor said that "…before the political violence the community always lived in the same way and nothing changed but now nothing is the same." Author's field research: interviewee from Wamani (Julia). Another looked back to a time that seemed increasingly remote: "…the community was quiet (before the political violence); people took their products to the local town by walking through the hills for two days where they would get hold of a truck for the transport of essential products such as salt, sugar, bread, and fruit." Author's field research: interviewee from Otoronco (Ramon).

Nevertheless, the memory of being forced to confront brutality, malevolence and helplessness is an incentive for people to recognize that they still have responsibilities that require them to find the right answers to their situation. To prevent any potentially negative impact it is likely that survivors will want to maximize control and minimize their own helplessness. The type of precautionary behaviour most commonly adopted by people from their community since the conflict ended is described in the following statement: "When I see some unknown person I have to know who that person is, so I go over and since he is unknown I ask him whatever. When it comes to some unknown person we ask where they are from or what they do. The thing to do is to identify them; it's easy now as they don't find it so easy to deceive us. But during the political violence we used to see strangers so we hid because they would be carrying weapons and grenades." Author's field research: interviewee from Yachaya (Percy).

However, these behavioural strategies are of limited value. In recent years the dominant *mestizo* culture has brought the outside world into the rural highland community to devastating effect. Improvements in transportation, education, health and commercial opportunities (as well as lawlessness) have utterly transformed people's respect for their own language and culture.

Its impact on their respect for the core value: "Let's live with just one heart"[22] has so violated social norms that it has cut people off from each other. To the extent that people can have some – even marginal – impact on their environment, they perceive that there are motives to defend their assumptions about the world and their comprehension of reality as effective.

This has structural implications that can prevent civic mindedness from being further undermined, can improve social cohesion and can encourage the suppression of pain and suffering. This can be seen from the fact that living in stressful economic and social circumstances helps survivors understand that there is nothing about their situation that should be exempt from thorough interrogation. The problem this presents people with is that there is no counterforce to the insights obtained from this self-interrogation into their situation. This has the effect of making survivors feel that their situation is uncontrollable and unavoidable. To advance understanding of the disillusionment this produces we therefore need to extend our range

[21] Individuals from other cultures have also borne witness to the importance of solidarity and cooperation for human survival. For example: Wiesel, E., (194:55) Davidson, S., (1984: 555–572).

[22] In Quechua: *Jucshungulla cawashun.*

of analysis from the fear of strangers to other ongoing threats to survival and self-preservation.

7.7 Fear and Mistrust of Military and Police

Nearly 80% of randomly selected interviewees from the communities studied said that they are still afraid of the military and police.[23] Participants reasoned that any return by the military and police to the area would result in further abuses of the type they had experienced during the violence. For example, the majority (29) of 35 randomly-selected interviewees in Otoronco said that they are still afraid of the military and police. For some interviewees (9) any return by the military and the police would trigger great fear because they do not want to be tortured, raped or beaten up again as they had been during the violence.[24]

Close to the end of a focus group discussion on the role of the military and the police one survivor of the violence described her feelings: "The police were the same as the terrorists as they too were responsible for people's disappearance. The police took my brothers away and I have never seen them since and this is why I hate them." Author's field research: interviewee from Qocha (Celestina).

This misconduct of the police and the military is an abiding and longstanding cause of fear and mistrust in relation to the legacy of the past and varies inversely with feelings of security. Though the events have been recorded the far-reaching psychological implications of what was done to people by the police and the armed forces have not been properly acknowledged. Instead the particular brutality they experienced and the stress it has been responsible for are endured in an environment of official silence and indifference.

This minimalist approach makes it possible to objectify the survivors[25] and "… render their suffering abstract and difficult to identify with."[26] For the survivors this violation of moral norms is tantamount to a transformation from human beings into things. By failing to obtain adequate social recognition for the physical and psychological injury done to them the memory of what was done serves to reinforce the belief that the past is unappeasable. Though survivors struggle against their humiliation as best they can, for example through mass protests, they are held not just by

[23] Between 35 and 40 randomly selected interviewees from each of the five research communities were asked for their opinion about the military and the police.

[24] The respondents who said that they no longer fear the military or the police was either because they had served in the army as regular soldiers or because they had worked with them in the rural patrols. Some also said that their fear of the military had diminished since the conflict because they know that human rights organizations exist to protect people from further military abuses.

[25] For example, "...Quechuas say the *mestizo* only looks on the external circumstances and insults them for not speaking Spanish, for not wearing shoes, and for being dirty. In the social stratification of Peru, the peasant farmers are often considered only slightly more civilized than the "jungle savages" (*chunchu*)." Smith, Terry P. (2006).

[26] Dean, C.J., (2010: 114).

the horrors inflicted on them but by the lack of recognition of their betrayed innocence.

It is not by chance that rebellion against official silence is fed by the subversive power of remembering as the following makes clear: "Having found out about the ongoing rebel attacks on the local population the police and military installed a police post in the community. From then on, there was a lot of violence and the people then knew that their lives were in danger. The police arrived and began to accuse the entire population of being *terrucos*.[27] They set out looking for the authorities and the other locals who they had accused of being *terrucos*. In their rush to escape the locals were shot, and in many cases, they were taken into custody as suspects at the police post to be interrogated and tortured. The police then returned to the homes of these people to sexually abuse any of their family members. During the day they stole everything they could find, as they believed that everyone from the community was a *terruco* or part of the *senderistas* and so they were not well regarded." Author's field research: interviewee from Qocha (Tulio).

Having eliminated the far-reaching psychological implications of human suffering from official business survivors have no alternative but to accept that their protests about the conduct of the police and the armed forces will not be acknowledged and that the injustices visited on them will not be recognised. In this respect history remains an 'open wound' that not only keeps traumatic memories alive but is being continually aggravated by official (and unofficial) calls to forget the past and move on.

A survivor of the violence describes how memories of inhuman treatment remain "insurmountable obstacles to peaceful social coexistence and to political reconciliation"[28] "…two or three days after my husband and the others were imprisoned their clothing was piled up at the army barracks gate and people said that the prisoners were being away taken by helicopter.

There are so many mass graves all over the place that you can't even count them all. There are also graves where there were mudslides. I don't know why the military brought them here. I guess they thought that they would never be found in those gullies, and that everyone was too afraid to denounce them. Seeing all of this completely traumatized us, and we haven't been the same since. How would you feel if your neighbour were taken away, killed and made to disappear? It's terrifying, and that's why I'm scared even today." Author's field research: interviewee from Qocha (Frida).

Though this feeling of dehumanization makes people passive and depressed it does not dispel their feeling of having been wronged. Instead the memory of these experiences lives on inside of them because they are unable to forget. A survivor of the violence describes their own "…forgotten site of memories and feelings, dreams, gaps in understanding symptoms and discomforts, shame and reconciliation"[29] by way of the following: "One night, while my son was studying, some soldiers seized

[27] Peruvian slang for *terrorist*.

[28] Lira, E., (2001).

[29] Watkins, M. & Shulman, H., (2008: 152).

him and several others. He escaped and the soldiers followed him. They entered the house and brought him out with a sack over his head, and then made him 'disappear'. Then I went to the police station to ask after my son, but on the way there, I ran into some soldiers. One of the soldiers grabbed me and said 'here's a leader', and took me to the barracks. From there they started to beat me. I don't remember anything more. I woke up at about 4pm, and I realized that I was stark-naked. My back hurt and I was crying. The women asked me why I was crying. Then they saw my back and said that I had been stabbed with a knife. The soldiers told me, 'Motherfucker, are you a terrorist? Yes or no? Are you going to talk or not, damn it? Are you a leader or not? Tell us the truth and we'll set you free right now.' Then they told me that if that they saw me walking down the street the following day, they would kill me." Author's field research: interviewee from Qocha (Maximo).

Irrespective of the powerlessness of their situation the sense of injustice is likely to persist for as long as people are unable to work through their experiences. In this respect a kind of anti-history develops in the memory of people as the following makes clear: "I am the first complainant against the military. I presented my complaint before the attorney general in Lima before filing this as an abuse of human rights they told me that I had every right to present my complaint about the abuses. A week later my complaint was published in the newspaper and it said that my community had become a clandestine cemetery. After a few days they kidnapped me in my house from where I was detained. They made me disappear for twenty-five days. They refused to provide my family with information but this did not stop my family looking for me everywhere. Finally, they got me out of a dark cell; there was a visit from the International Red Cross to see the health status of prisoners, nothing more. So, I told people about what had happened. I felt very sad, because here they have killed illiterate, innocent people; people who had nothing to do with the insurgency." Author's field research: interviewee from Otoronco (Feliciano).

The events in these accounts draw attention to the variety and complexity of what was done to people by the police and the armed forces. Though they record events and report the facts of a historical occurrence accounts do **not** testify to the long-term stress they are responsible for. In this way the memory of suffering continues to confound the national consensus that it is time to move on and leave the past behind as the following demonstrates: "Sometimes when the army comes I always think that they will immediately start to abuse us again." Author's field research: interviewee from Otoronco (Juna).

Being outside the boundaries of normal reality the events these accounts describe are associated with feelings that have "…no beginning, no ending, no before, no during and no after."[30]

Instead they involve acts of injustice which people were powerless to prevent and for which there has been no official acknowledgement, as the following demonstrates: "…during the dangerous time we fled to the hills, our animals wandered off, we lost everything, and we were left with nothing. It was very sad, I was not well, and I saw the terrorists killing people. They killed people by rounding them up and

[30] Felman, S. & Laub, D. (1992: 69).

after killing them they would bury them in a pit. This is what the terrorists and the army did to us. I felt sad for my village because my village was completely destroyed. We all had to leave during the violence." Author's field research: interviewee from Otoronco (Imaculada).

Through a combination of detachment and objectivity the state has been able to successfully deflect attention away from its own responsibilities for any legitimate moral expectations, as the following makes clear: "There are very few police and military personnel in the entire area; there is also a lack of police vehicles; they are also badly paid, which is why many of them are corrupt and commit crimes." Author's field research: interviewee from Wamani (Ofelia).'

By neutralising the moral impact of what was done to innocent people the uniqueness of the individual has been dishonoured and the human being displaced from its role as the centre of moral concern. This affects the perception survivors have of themselves to the extent that it undermines their competence (biological, social, psychological and economic) and the decision-making process. In these circumstances memories of the violence seep through into people's consciousness to provide new and devastating insights into the present: "Now whenever we see the military we are still scared. My father was repeatedly hit by them during the violence. They didn't let us leave the house and they shot my brother in the night when he came back from the city. Death is safer. They also shot people who went out during the night." Author's field research: interviewee from Qocha (Frida).

The quality of 'otherness' about the events inflicted on people makes the prospect of there ever being any *rapprochement* between the parameters of normal reality and the events that they were subjected to hard to conceive. This can be demonstrated by the following interviewee comments: "…the military did whatever they wanted. They stole the livestock, the animals, and the wheat. People had to abandon their farms and suffered so intensely that we no longer thought about living. Then the military took 10 people, claiming that they were "terrorists" and took them to a place up in the mountains. There they killed 6 of them and 4 disappeared. No one knows anything about their whereabouts to this day." Author's field research: interviewee from Yachaya (Nopaltzin).

Having been forced so far beyond the bounds of normal reality the memory of events retains a powerful presence in survivors lives because they refuse to align themselves with the rest of their reality. In this respect the events in these accounts must be understood in relation to the cultural space that they occupy. First and foremost, this is because memory "…is not just individual, nor is it just a binding activity for groups; it is their cultural inheritance, whether actively or passively maintained."[31]

[31] Olick, J.K., (2007: 6).

7.8 Conclusions

The idea that the "…response to the past, primarily of crimes and atrocities, has priority over the attempt to shape the future,"[32] ignores the ongoing challenges of living in conditions of extreme poverty and the emergence of new forms of violence.[33] In these circumstances the legacy of the past has fused with new forms of psycho-social stress that are a continuing problem in all the research communities.

As this study has shown, this means the legacy of the past remains unresolved, an open wound. Instead of healing, the violent past influences and shapes local people's perception of social and political groups across the social, political and economic spectrum.

Viewing the process of healing, forgetting and forgiveness as somehow natural assumes that the past can be overcome. Yet for most survivors healing has little practical or moral meaning. Neither do government reparations ensure that social relationships are morally repaired. More importantly, having failed to take on its collective responsibility for post-conflict communities' well-being, the government's attitude has brought about a set of conditions that can even actively deter people from working through the past towards healing and recovery.

By failing to engage effectively with the psychological reactions to the political violence government (and NGO) policies and programmes are in contention with the idea of effective cooperation. In this way lack of opportunity, oppression and indifference prevents people from making sense of their situation and thereby encourages further psychological and physical withdrawal from the social arena. To help survivors rebuild a positive sense of self government and NGO policies and programmes need to take an emotional interest in the human impact of the situation. But this does not happen.

This situation is not unique to the Andes, and has become a feature of post-conflict traumatisation in other rural communities that have witnessed large scale destruction through political violence.[34] A certain amount of psychic splitting is therefore necessary for survival, since otherwise the unprocessed historical past would deflect the attention of local people away from the urgencies of new and pressing issues.[35]

However, the burden of an unprocessed past is not just about the failure to properly acknowledge people's suffering from among key individuals, organizations, institutions, and local authorities.

---

[32] Heyd, D., (2004: 191).

[33] Miller, K. E. & Rasmussen, A., (2010: 7–16).

[34] See for example Martin-Baro, I., (1994: 124); Anckermann, S; Dominguez, M., Soto, N., Kjaerulf, F., Berliner, P. and Mikkelsen, E. (2005); Bagilishya, D. (2000); Staub, E., Pearlman, L.A., Gubin, A. Hagenigimana, A. (2005); Wessels, M. and Monteiro, C. (2005) in Christies, D. & Wagner, D. (eds.) (2005).

[35] Dissociation is a defensive strategy that is used to ward off the overwhelming impact of massive trauma. "...it is an extreme form of psychic splitting that helps to sustain people under catastrophic circumstances." Schwab, G. (2010: 20); Kilborne, B., (1999).

It is also about the psychic pain that emanates from this failure in human connectedness and moral repair. In this respect it is the sheer awfulness of living with the burden of a past that has not been fully adjusted to. Whilst survivors continue to live with wounds that are not healed, and perhaps not even acknowledged, and often in conditions of extreme poverty, where new forms of violence emerge, there is neither closure, nor what can be termed mastery of the subject.[36]

[36] See for example, Olick, J., (2007: 31); Lifton, R.J. (1986: 417).

Chapter 8
On the Margins of the Visible: Daily Survival in the Rural Andes

The purpose of this chapter is to look at the lives of people unable to re-establish cognitive stability and overcome existential fatalism from perspectives not already discussed.

In Chap. 6 failure to properly acknowledge the suffering of survivors from among key individuals, organizations, institutions, and local authorities was found to exacerbate the psychic pain they experience from having to live with the burden of a past that has not been fully adjusted to. Because of this failure in human connectedness and moral repair the overwhelming urgency of survivors struggling to satisfy everyday basic needs was also found to be affected.

The disillusionment and feelings of hopelessness this is responsible for is what now shapes local reality and defines the meaning of normal behaviour, not the rupture in people's access to shared values, common humanity and shared responsibility. Nevertheless, to live with psychic wounds that are not healed, and not even acknowledged, and in conditions of extreme poverty is a highly aversive state and one which is likely to make survivors want to change a situation that denies them control of their own existence. This chapter looks at how the failure to properly acknowledge suffering among key individuals, organizations, institutions, and local authorities has the potential to change people in highly positive ways.

8.1 Beyond Disillusion and Fear?

To counter the disillusionment created by this situation the state has sought to promote reconciliation and improve its own legitimacy through a range of policies and programmes. In addition to collective reparations and compensation the Comprehensive Reparations Plan (PIR) includes initiatives that are intended to

T. J. Bowyer, *Beyond Suffering and Reparation*,
https://doi.org/10.1007/978-3-319-98983-9_8

provide repair when individual assessments of harms suffered by each survivor is not possible.[1]

To effectively counter the effects of objectification, however, requires an explanation of suffering that extends beyond the all-too easy list of adverse effects of violence and poverty.[2] In this respect, recognition is vital to individual survivor and group survivor self-confidence, self-respect and self-esteem.[3]

In the aftermath of violence, the talk of reparations and the business of getting on with living have sent out a message that is at odds with survivor experiences. For people not linked to survivors in some meaningful way government reparations can give the impression that the actual experience of suffering and what it does to human beings has been obliterated. If suppression of the painful memories had been respected, as no more than a temporary expedient this might have been possible. But this has not happened. Instead the opportunity to work through trauma and obtain some form of integration has been blocked by a system that encourages the prolonged suppression of painful memories out of political expediency. This disregard for the past: "…keeps silenced people from asking questions, it keeps the judged from judging, it separates and isolates, it keeps people locked into a stage of development that never goes beyond those past events."[4]

The notion that output oriented legitimacy and service delivery are the most important means of promoting opportunities for reconciliation and justice has overlooked the human dimension of the situation. By failing to regard survivors in rural highland communities as individuals who have been unjustly treated the state has turned them into an abstract category. Through reparations there is a risk that the government will seek a one-size-fits-all solution, de-contextualizing experiences of physical and psychological injury as if all victims experienced damage in the same way.

For survivors this failure to identify with the particular individual is tantamount to exploitation and the violation of the one thing that ought never to be abused: the pain and death of others. This has turned government reparations into a trigger for the memory of past events to return and disturb the surface of apparent calm. However, memory is also able to provide the material through which the systematic detachment and objectification of survivors' work can be questioned and even

[1] In addition to the programmes to help victims obtain their civil documentation implemented by the *Registro Nacional de Identificación y Estado Civil*, or (RENIEC) (National Registry for Identification and Civil Status) efforts to improve civil registration (especially in rural areas) have also been implemented. See Correa (2013:21).

[2] "...Western diagnostic classifications are problematic when applied to diverse non-Western survivor populations. The view of trauma as an individual-centred event bound to soma or psyche is in line with the tradition in this century for both Western biomedicine and psycho analysis to regard the singular human being as the basic unit of study." Summerfield (1997: 150).

[3] See in particular, Taylor (1992); Honneth (1995). For more recent contributions see Schmidt am Busch, H-C. & Zurn (2010) (Eds.).

[4] Galeano (1993).

challenged outright. In this way every rebellion against the dehumanization of suffering "…is fed by the subversive power of remembered suffering."[5]

Because the Truth and Reconciliation Commission (TRC) was intended to restore dignity to those who had suffered damage and hurt, and to help them become full citizens, makes its capacity to counteract the destruction of memory and the screening out of human suffering particularly important. The TRC sought to contribute to the vision of a new kind of future, rather than restore the insecurities of the past, moving: "…beyond the precarious conditions of their prior life."[6]

In the TRC document *Hacia una politica nacional de reparaciones* (Towards a national reparations policy) the TRC explains that "… with its application, (the PIR) will contribute to improving the quality of life of the population and open possibilities of cultural, social and economic integration for those who many times not only suffered poverty and exclusion but also suffered directly the consequence of recourse to violence."[7] For survivors in the communities studied, this effort to ensure "recognition and reaffirmation" of specifically Civil and Political Rights (CPR) violations on behalf of the PIR, is judged as a strictly limited success story.

The long delays before reconstruction efforts began were responsible for widespread bitterness, particularly amongst survivors. And not allowing regional government to participate in implementation of the PIR only aggravated the problem. People despair of ever gaining official recognition for their suffering. One expression of the hopelessness this gives rise to is expressed as follows: "Here no one knows anything about individual reparations; no one knows anything about mental health, none of the health workers (HWs) know anything about what the conflict does to people's lives. Here no one knows much about the recommendations of the TRC; the community has heard about individual reparations from the radio, but they don't know how to file their claims. Anyway, it's difficult, because this is a Quechua speaking community." Author's field research: interviewee from Wamani (Rosa).

This lack of knowledge about government reparations reinforces the considerable breach between citizens and the state, but for some people this is a situation that is exacerbated by the attitude of survivors.

In the words of one survivor: "Even the people are not well informed about what the PIR actually is, and this because of their own negligence; they fail to attend the meetings that we community leaders have been trained for." Author's field research: interviewee from Qocha (Maximo).

Though measures of 'recognition and reaffirmation' cannot rub-out what was done or reinstate what has been destroyed the feeling that government reparations fail to capture the outrage of what happened is widespread. The survivor needs to mourn for the harm that was done to them and to find their own way to come to terms with what cannot be undone. This demands from the survivor a willingness to come to terms with the impossibility of getting even. This is supremely difficult in any circumstances, but for the lack of any meaningful acknowledgement from the

[5] Metz (1980:110).

[6] TRC Final Report, *supra* note 12, at Vol. IX, Part 4, Ch. 2.2: 146.

[7] as cited in Laplante (2007).

state makes it a source of immense frustration and anger for survivors: "There are many aspects that the state should improve. If there is no support from them how can we improve our communities? How can we change our lives after being affected by the violence? We will never be healed from what happened. The anger we have is inside us and we do not forget." Author's field research: interviewee from Unay (Orlando).

By failing to restore survivor dignity, government reparations have created a situation in which the feeling of abandonment amongst survivors is bound to continue. Having created a situation in which people remain "…unable to trust, unable to forgive and unable to reconcile,"[8] government reparations have created a fertile environment for the unfettered expansion of cynicism, apathy and disillusionment. On-the-one-hand, this can underpin future violence; on the other- hand, resentment *may* help to transform post-traumatic despair into some form of post-traumatic growth.[9]

Nevertheless, a climate of optimism and positive thinking cannot be created in a climate of overwhelming apathy and despair as the following statement illustrates: "I remember those years with great remorse and those types of abuse should not happen again because if they do the people will not let themselves get hit in the same way. So now the government makes attempts to ease that pain, that anger that came from the courage of the people who were affected and this amounts to simply giving us collective reparations and even encouraging us to believe that we will be given individual relief, but this is business for them and we see this because they are the same people who have economic power. These collective reparations do not bring back those that died because these things are irreparable, and that is why most people here are unhappy with what is happening." Author's field research: interviewee from Qocha (Severo).

From this position of complete helplessness, it is inevitable for survivors to feel that nothing will ever bring relief let alone restore their own sense of power. In contrast to the safe social environments that facilitate resilience people from the communities studied are less optimistic about making the shift from unpredictable danger to reliable safety: "No 'real' reparations mean that no one can return to life like it used to be. No 'real' state help makes it hard for us to re-build our lives. It has had an impact on us that is not easy for the outsider to understand." Author's field research: interviewee from Qocha (Frida).

By refusing to endorse the pseudo-empathy of government reparations survivors are in a position to demonstrate that what was actually done to them is not the only issue of importance.

Focus groups in Wamani describe collective reparations as nothing short of a mechanism for the manipulation of people at election time. This mechanism, and this feeling, of suffering being misused, is not confined to the Andean context of this

[8] Govier (2002: 146).

[9] Calhoun and Tedeschi (2009: 29) (eds).

study, or just to Peru, but has been frequently reported by other researchers in, for example: Cambodia, Rwanda and the Balkans.[10]

Participants in focus groups from the communities studied reported that whilst various promises were made to them under the reparations scheme, nothing concrete had happened. Although construction of a mill was proposed, for example, once built people said it was more symbolic than useful. It became the symbol and reminder of sufferings the community had undergone. Focus groups from Qocha said that money for construction of a communal assembly hall had been given to them. But because the amount provided fell far short of the total cost, the building had been left unfinished. Several years ago, the community leadership submitted a request to the local authorities asking for financial support to construct a small museum to remember the victims but no response was ever forthcoming.

Interviews with people directly affected by the political violence from all communities studied said that the monies received for their particular community had been too modest to bring much tangible benefit. In addition, the money had very often not been wisely spent. Instead of investing in qualitative improvements the funds tended to simply be spent on construction projects. Nobody had ever informed community members how much money they were entitled to under the reparations scheme and this caused them to lose interest.

Focus groups also said that no reparations had ever been made available for the loss of education, the destruction caused to the local economy, to infrastructure and housing. Even access to justice was not provided under the TRC.

It emerged that there was a great deal of confusion about what and who the collective reparations scheme was actually intended for. The difficulty this presents people with is demonstrated by the following statement: "I don't know what the collective reparations for the community involve because I don't go to the meetings for those who were affected, as I'm not classed as an affected person. They say the meetings are for those who were affected, but we were all affected. The military robbed my house and when I told them this they weren't willing to put me down as an affected person, they told me it was only for those who lost their family." Author's field research: interviewee from Otoronco (Herminio).

It is clear that despite its emphasis on repairing damage caused by CPR violations, the lack of adequate funds, information and advice means that collective reparations have brought little benefit to survivors (and the region in general). However, it is important to remember that the experience of trauma is so far outside the boundaries of normal reality that no response will ever undo or cancel out what was done to people. Let us be clear about one thing: no compensation, no opportunity to work through what happened can ever be commensurate with the pain and suffering

[10] For commentary on reparations see for example Bevernage (2012: 61); Colvin (2006: 176–215) in South Africa. In De Greiff (2008); Hayner (2002: 133ff). For commentary on the interpretation of suffering see Agger et al. (1999); Agger (2001) in Christies; Wagner (eds.) (2005; Anckermann et al. (2005); Beneduce (2007: 41–70) in Pouligny et al. (Eds.) (2007).

that people were subject to; there can be no mastery of the subject and no closure.[11] The falsification or disregard of the past is therefore as much a breeding ground for the return of memories about what was done as the survivor's own feelings of impotence and despair.

The lack of information and misinformation about individual reparations from the government is a source of great resentment and frustration. One survivor, faced with a future of unremitting uncertainty and pain described the difficulties this presents: "The community does not know if the state will ever provide support for individual reparations even though many people were made orphans by the violence and they have no type of support from anyone." Author's field research: interviewee from Wamani (Ordell).

In 2008 the National Register of Victims (RUV) began a programme in Otoronco to initiate individual reparations. The responsibility for this work lies with the district authorities, together with support from the *Comision de Alto Nivel.* However, lengthy delays in the collection of information and the processing of claims have generated considerable tension amongst the families of the survivors. Focus groups said that many people are ignorant of the fact that they are legally entitled to individual reparations as specified by the RUV. Inevitably, these feelings interfere with the development of a safe social environment needed to facilitate coping and post-traumatic growth: "The people in this community don't know much about their rights; they let themselves be deceived in every way. They don't know their rights because they are not informed, they are not trained, because for this you have to be trained, to analyze, to study at least to know. Then when you hear people say that they have rights but they don't know how to answer questions, then these people are very humble." Author's field research: interviewee from Otoronco (Flavio).

In recent years ongoing delays and lack of further information about entitlements have led many survivors to lose hope that individual reparations will ever be made to them. The following account offers a more specific explanation for people's scepticism about the government's willingness to provide individual reparations: "I reckon that individual reparations will probably not happen because when it comes out there will be another government that will not have the same concerns about who the reparations are for and that the compensation will be given to the relatives of the *terrucos,* because they were the only ones that stayed behind when everyone else was running away. I know because during that time I was a member of the local authorities and that if I hadn't escaped I would have been killed as well." Author's field research: interviewee from Qocha (Tiburcio).

[11] The scale of the destruction can be demonstrated by the following average figures based on some of the official results for each community studied: deaths 8, disabled 5, tortured 7, widows 8, orphans 6, displaced 60, undocumented 35, communal property destroyed 82, family property destroyed 151, organizations affected 6. Following visits from the TRC investigators local people subsequently passed the names and details of an additional 150 (approx.) missing, tortured, killed, displaced. None of this takes into consideration the unmarked mass graves found in the communities studied, but only discovered after the TRC investigators had completed their own inquiries. The most recent unmarked mass graves were found whilst the fieldwork for this study was being carried out; it was expected that other unmarked mass graves would be discovered in due course.

In such circumstances helplessness, powerlessness and lack of all mastery make the individual incapable of any resolutely forward-looking progression. The more the government refuses to share in the passionate and impossible wish, that what was done was never done, the more people will lose any expectation of help and concern for their pain and suffering. One survivor reflects on the unrelenting hopelessness this has produced in their life: "Here in Qocha we victims of political violence are still waiting for the state to recognize and compensate the victims of violence; there is still the hope that we will achieve justice. No individual is receiving reparations for what happened to them and their family." Author's field research: interviewee from Qocha (Tezcacoat).

Frustrated by their own sense of helplessness, some survivors attempt to bypass their outrage altogether through expressions of cynicism and contempt for those seeking reparation, in spite of everything: "Of course there are those who are seeking individual redress; yes their families were affected, if they killed your mum, your dad or you have been raped because most were *terrucos* mind, because they were going to die if not more besides; to me all the authorities have been killing therefore they have been as bad as the *terrucos*." Author's field research: interviewee from Otoronco (Paulino).

The fact that the survivor needs assistance of others in rebuilding a positive sense of self is a problem, which to a high degree determines the individual's capacity for trying not to think about the past. In this respect the loss of any expectation of help and concern for their pain and suffering undermine any exercise of the faculty of empathy. This failure to take an emotional interest in the human import of the situation in which victims and survivors find themselves deepen the survivor's feelings of injustice and destroys the idea of a natural interval between past and present.

To help survivors rebuild a positive sense of self the state needs to take an emotional interest in the human import of the situation. In this respect the subjective felt-experience of the survivor is invaluable for an "…understanding of experience and its aftermath, including the role of memory and its lapses in coming to terms with or denying and repressing the past".[12]

To ground the determining influence of culture, context and institutions (and the subjective nature that the individual brings to their situation) the common feelings, emotions and behaviours associated with people affected by violence and living in a context of daily survival need to be brought into full view.[13] However, government programmes pay little attention to the emotional consequences of suffering and all the various and convoluted processes with which the violation of normative expectations is associated. Instead state funded social programmes such as PRONAA,

[12] LaCapra (2001: 86–7); Dussaillant and Gonzalez (2015: 233–251) Lifetime Suffering and Capabilities in Chile in Anderson (ed) *World Suffering & the Quality of Life*, Springer.

[13] See Suarez (2013); Charbonneau and Parent (eds) (2012); Justino (2009); Srinisvasa Murthy and Lakshminayaranah (2006); Brinkerhoff (2005); Moser (1996); Moser (1998); Dussaillant and Gonzalez (2015: 233–251) Lifetime Suffering and Capabilities in Chile in Anderson, R.E. (ed) *World Suffering & the Quality of Life*, Springer; Harvey (2015: 269–281) The Cultural Geography of Community Suffering in Anderson, R.E. (ed) *World Suffering & the Quality of Life*, Springer.

PRONAMA, PRONAMACH, *Vaso de leche*[14] and JUNTOS[15] are governed by the values of a unified national culture and not specific individuals and groups.

Such a reductive minimalist approach to state sponsored development programmes forces people into a position of passivity thereby making their suffering abstract and difficult to identify with. This dehumanizing of the powerless means that the cognitive (recognition) element of empathy is only partially intact and that the affective element (the emotional response to someone else's feelings) is kept firmly out of action.[16]

So long as participation and inclusion of the powerless are determined according to a system with minimal interest in the reality of what it is like to live in conditions of low trust, extreme anxiety, high vigilance and low safety nets, government programmes are only likely to exacerbate suffering and not relieve it. For people in the communities studied government sponsored social programmes have brought increasing dependency and a stultifying attitude that destroys hope and the prospect of a better future.

Instead of an integrated set of rural development policies, programmes and projects there is a lack of contextually specific development efforts which make it difficult for people to exercise voice and for state institutions to actively listen and respond. This is responsible for making survivors feel that no one is interested in allowing them to make sense of their situation and that nothing can be done and that further suffering is inevitable.

Focus groups from all five communities studied said that government programmes tend not to involve the community authorities or its' members because it was assumed that everyone would want the programme, irrespective of what it was for. Participants said that the failure to consult with the community encourages a handout mentality and deepens conformity. State programmes also promote tensions, such as disputes about the date/location of their implementation and the failure to identify who the beneficiaries are.[17] The difficulties this produces is illustrated

[14] The Glass of Milk board meets every 3 months as well. The leaders of this organization only receive and distribute food to beneficiaries; they have no training or experience in management, administration that could improve the organization or its activities. Communal dining is another organization that exists thanks to the vertical inputs they receive from PRONAA, a state organization that makes a donation of beans, rice, oil, morón, wheat, peas, tuna, every 3 months and distributed to ½ kilo, about a certain amount for communal services. This organization also meets every 3 months.

[15] JUNTOS is a state program created to eradicate extreme poverty through the promotion of primary education, reduction in child mortality and improvements in maternal health. To benefit the individual must meet certain requirements: identity, nutrition, health and education after which they are entitled to collect the incentive money 100 soles a month from government agencies in cooperation with the *Banco de la Nacion*. Monitoring and control of the participating households is undertaken every 3 months. If the household fails to meet its commitments payment is suspended for 3 months. The selection of beneficiaries is made through the ministry of economy using the INEI survey on extreme poverty once the individual's first and last names have been verified by RENIEC.

[16] Baron-Cohen, S. (2011: 85).

[17] Focus groups said that state programmes never gave enough consideration to the interests, needs and priorities of the elderly, widows and single mothers.

by the following statement: "I criticize the JUNTOS organization as its bad, because it's a small group that receives support from the State, and it should be in general. I'm critical because it should be more for single mothers, the disabled and the elderly. The JUNTOS programme should be for everyone because nobody here is a millionaire. We all work in the field and we all eat with difficulty. It is for this reason that I say this so that there is no envy; it should be for everyone." Author's field research: interviewee from Yachaya (Luisa).

By failing to introduce and implement an appropriate policy regime the state awareness of economic suffering is restricted to the use of economic indicators to measure the burden of suffering in objective terms.

In the context of recovery from the political violence this seriously undermines state legitimacy, authority and effectiveness. For the survivor the lack of an integrated set of rural development policies, programmes and projects evoke past experiences of injustice, indifference and ill-treatment. In this way government programmes are not perceived as a right, but simply as support for poor people. Focus groups from the five communities studied said that government programmes encourage conformity because they do not encourage people to think or find other ways of generating income. For some participants this attitude is particularly dangerous since a government programme may be suspended or cancelled at any time. Participants said that there are no government programmes available to help them promote or invest in income generation in agriculture or livestock production, and no incentive to recover traditional craft work (blanket weaving, making their own clothing, and so forth).

For the survivor struggling to come to terms with the meaning of the trauma in their own life this is hardly conducive to helping people come to a better understanding of the issues involved: "There are many rights that need to be reinstated in this community. Many villagers are still psychologically ravaged by the violence and evil from that time. People need help to remedy such harm. That kind of investment could give people encouragement and help them to change their lifestyle." Author's field research: interviewee from Qocha (Guillermo).

Hidden behind discussions about the need for a more integrated set of rural development policies, programmes and projects an entirely new explanation for the root causes of human suffering has begun to emerge.

This involves acknowledging the adverse effect of geography and how people's perception of the effects of geographical isolation is changing over time.[18] Though regional physical barriers have long been recognised as an obstacle to effective communication, market access and provision of public sector services, its only real significance, until recently, has been from its association with the new growth theory which highlights the productive advantages of access.[19] This means that in spite of its 'rugged complexity' the geographical difficulties associated with rural highland communities are largely unrecognized.[20] Being unable to make the gradual

[18] Webb, R. (2013).

[19] Romer, P. (1986); Krugman (1991: 483–499).

[20] Webb (2013).

shift from humiliated isolation to restored social connection increases the negative effects of intrusive thoughts and other memories which make demands on people as the following statement indicates: "Their projects are meant to generate employment but we don't think they do. What we need are projects that help us to improve our capabilities (such as how to set up micro businesses)." Author's field research: interviewee from Qocha (Jose).

8.2 Resentment Towards Local Authorities

To understand what constitutes legitimacy from the perspective of local people it is important to consider the extent to which local authorities actually respond to their concerns and demands. This study began by asking local people about the extent to which local authorities actively listen and respond to their concerns. No one from any of the focus groups in Unay said that they had any confidence in the local authorities because "…they never fulfil their promises." Participants said that a transnational mining company had been given authorization by the local authorities to begin mining activities on community land but with no prior consultation with the community.

The feeling that this had done irreparable damage to their relationship with the local authorities was palpable.

Every focus group held in Otoronco said that that none of the local authorities had any respect for local people. Participants said that the extent to which local authorities explain and justify their decisions and the consequences lack the voluntary consent of local people is all too apparent. The fact that local authorities fail to actively listen and respond to people means that the checks and balances normally used to ensure that local officials are made responsible for their actions are not in place. This raises questions about the legitimacy of local leaders and officials, and the extent to which local people are prepared to tolerate this form of local governance, given the lack of shared ideas and values between local leaders and the local population. It was felt in most focus groups that women and marginalised people in particular were not listened to.

More generally it was felt that the local authorities needed more respect for transparency in their activities, including in infrastructural projects that were intended to improve the local environment and to build trust between the government and the community. Being unable to disclose in confidence to significant others only serves to reinforce the negative effects of intrusive thoughts and other symptoms of stigmatised isolation as the following makes clear: "The authorities and officials of the Ayacucho region are only present at the opening of the work done or the laying of the first stone; this makes people unhappy that the authorities do not come to the community to see what kind of needs the community has." Author's field research: interviewee from Otoronco (Carlos).

The distrust this produces is widespread: "…we don't trust them; they didn't protect us during the political violence and they haven't helped us since." Author's field research: interviewee form Unay (Alicia). Every focus group held in Qocha were adamant that the lack of local authority investment was responsible for widespread disillusionment and increasing levels of delinquent behaviour. Participants also said that the local authorities exploit their traditional cultural identity and customs for political gain, especially in the run up to elections. Nearly all focus groups held in Yachaya said that local community representatives tend to be excluded from contact with local authorities, in spite of the new commitment to decentralization and greater social inclusion. Participants also said that the local authorities fail to help them with the development programmes promised by the regional government.

In this way people are less able to stretch and improve their coping skills, which mean that they are less well placed to present a positive face and make the necessary shift from unpredictable danger to relative safety. For example: "I think that local authorities are well established organically but that they are socially corrupt and mafia like; there can be no trust of them because if one presents a document on behalf of a community it is not attended to right there, but if a document is presented by a powerful organization then everything gets facilitated fast but if you are a peasant farmer then they let your papers sleep for two years or more. If it is approved as a project they will say come back in half a year here and when you return they say that there isn't enough money to cover the budget and that its' got to be made lower and so on. I think the authorities are manipulative; I think that when you are paid you shut up, I think that true justice does not exist in Peru." Author's field research: interviewee from Yachaya (Marcos).

All focus groups in Wamani said that the local authorities fail to respond to requests submitted by the community for training in attitudinal change and capacity building. In spite of the effort people put into the preparation of their project proposals beforehand local authority support is rarely if ever forthcoming. This reinforces the belief that priority for local authority support is always given to projects located in the district capital. One interviewee noted tellingly, that this is because "…there is corruption in the bureaucracy which means that they (local authorities) don't do anything about our complaints and requests for help…so we have to complain to them all of the time if we are ever going to get them to comply." Author's field research: interviewee from Wamani (Sabino).

The strength of feeling behind this observation becomes clear in the following statement from a community representative: "This is the sixth time I've been elected - all because I am the one who is willing to take on the local authorities. In my position I have denounced them to the *[Peruvian] Home Office, the Oficina Nacional de Procesos Electorales (Peru's National Office of Electoral Processes),* the Civil Governor of Ayacucho, and the General Command of Ayacucho, because there are bad people here." Author's field research: interviewee from Wamani (Ignacio).

Every focus group held in Wamani said that the government refuses to recognise their objection to the fact that most local officials (municipal workers) do not live in the District. Participants said that this only confirms their belief that local authorities deliberately neglect rural highland communities and indigenous people in particular because the government does not regard them as a priority.

This opinion is unanimous across all communities studied and shows that there are demands for better local authority officials and representatives in future.

The case of one survivor of the political violence reveals how the experience of complete helplessness can sometimes lead people to look to bring about change in highly positive ways: "Ill-willing authorities are happy to sacrifice the people. They are betraying the humility of the peasants. What we need are good civil servants who want the village to progress and who are willing help us to move forward, because most of us are illiterate." Author's field research: interviewee from Qocha (Pepita).

Most focus groups held in all five communities studied reserve some of their most hostile criticism for their Mayor. Participants in Otoronco said that the mayor takes decisions without consulting the community. One informant said: "…we do not know anything about what he is doing. I do not really know what they (local authorities) are managing. Just tell us this, when are things going to be better?" Author's field research: interviewee form Otoronco (Saturnin). It was generally accepted amongst all focus groups held in all five communities studied that the reason why their local mayor lacked credibility was because he spent most of his time in Lima. This also reinforces the belief that local authorities fail to listen and respond to legitimate concerns and demands. It is responsible for much tension and confusion and serves to reinforce the authoritarian nature of the relationship between people and local authorities and with the mayor in particular.

These top-down relationships promote a cycle of mutual antipathy and mistrust; the lack of commitment promotes negative relationship acts that reinforce mistrust and increase people's reluctance to become dependent on the relationship, as the following demonstrates: "Here in our community, people are afraid to speak out against the mayor, because we are told 'who speaks ill of me will have to have money'." Author's field research: interviewee from Qocha (Julio).

This inability to hear expressed concerns and the lack of any willingness to explain and justify government decisions and their consequences are symptomatic of a wider preoccupation relating to accountability.

In Qocha one focus group specifically organised to discuss the community and its finances said that the public presentation of quarterly accounts by local authorities was so general and lacking in detail that people did not bother to attend.[21] Participants said that because the Mayor was unfamiliar with accountancy procedures no explanation about how the money was spent and on what was ever given. When he asked about the finances, Jorge said that he was just "…given smooth words" and accused of attempted slander.

The same informant said that when other people saw this "…they did not talk because they were scared; that's why people don't ask local officials questions, and just [remain] cheerful."

[21] This study found that people consider community participation for the presentation of the quarterly accounts to be lower than for any other public activity.

Many focus groups in Qocha said that local authorities are not accountable because they do not take their responsibilities seriously.

Drawing on his experience as a former community leader an interviewee said that "…there is a lot of favouritism (amongst local officials), especially amongst those who have the right political colours, because today there is no transparency in their work. The local authorities have their own little group and that little group does everything they want and much of what they do is driven by revenge; revenge that always exists." Author's field research: interviewee from Qocha (Plinio).

Though this has generated much bitterness amongst people their objections to the way in which they are being treated has failed to bring about change. Participants said that this has led to a serious deterioration in relations with the local authorities. Another member of the community offered this comment on local authorities and their attitude to accountability: "The local government does present its accounts but it does this in such a way that people do not understand. Sometimes (most of the time in fact) people go along with what they have heard (conformists) but what the authorities present in terms of accountability is never done in any detail. I would like them to inform us exactly what they have been spending money on. At the moment accountability is done so randomly, what is entered in the study is not specified in detail or how it was spent. We would like to have access to the documents concerning the things that have been spent and bought. It must be made in detail in future." Author's field research: interviewee from Qocha (Severo).

Despite the adverse effects of material disadvantage and the effects of insecurity, anxiety and lack of social integration it is clear that the processes of accountability fall short of what they ought to look like.

One survivor describes the difficulties this now presents in the life of the community: "The voice of the people is not heard by the district authorities; we are not heard, we have no voice and that's one of the shortcomings of the authorities, the mayor is incapable, and has made no effective impact at all." Author's field research: interviewee from Qocha (Jorge).

In relation to the aftermath of the violence another survivor indicated that the difficulties this presents for the community are unending: "It is always the same because when we appeal to the local authorities, we receive no support. They don't pay any attention to us." Author's field research: interviewee from Qocha (Ofelia).

8.3 The Potential of Local Authorities to Channel Resentment

To feel safe, people need to know that their environment is secure. In the aftermath of violence this depends on the extent to which factors responsible for so much suffering and misery are being addressed. To this end people need to be reassured that local government institutions discharge their functions on a basis of accountability, responsiveness and receptivity. Unless people (and particularly survivors) can be persuaded of this point it is likely that they will remain "…in the status of powerless victims, making them vulnerable to ideological manipulation and in danger of becoming perpetrators."[22]

In these circumstances the role of local authorities is crucial. This is because they have a particular responsibility for rebuilding legitimate political authority after the violence. If they ignore this role it will obstruct any consolidation of viable local democracies and undermine the legitimacy of the government.

To enable people to engage as active citizens in the wider social-political community and public sphere the factors responsible for making their environment insecure have to be attended to. For survivors of the violence this involves improvements in their emotional safety as well as in their social, economic, cultural, and political safety. If this does not happen the state will lack legitimacy as a governing regime.[23] In this section the effects of corruption and discrimination will be discussed and how this affects the capacities for popular participation.[24]

Because of the political violence, the inherited goals, rules and boundaries of traditional Andean culture may no longer be viewed by people in the communities as that important in guaranteeing their personal and collective safety.[25]

The traditional support systems, with their core value: "…let's live with just one heart" have been offset by a more self-centred appraisal of how to live and survive, followed by a re-evaluation of the core values to live by.[26] The effects of this sea-change are being experienced at an individual and at a collective cultural level, and one of the main historical legacies of political violence in a context of poverty and vulnerability, remoteness and fear.

In the early years following the end of violence, the previous emphasis on unity and the importance of relationships shifted to a focus on the need to maintain indifference, the logic of apathy, selfishness and a preference for social isolation.[27] The idea that adversity in rural highland communities can only be confronted by survivors coming together, sharing their experiences and reflecting on solutions to their common problems, is no longer the preferred value for guiding daily living.

Instead, the normal systems of support that used to give people a sense of control, connection and meaning have been replaced by systems of self preservation that create individuals and communities that are in a state of permanent alert.[28] This

---

[22] Staub, E. et al. (2005: 300).

[23] Legitimacy refers to acceptance of a governing regime as correct, appropriate and right. See Brinkerhoff (2007a, b). See also Brinkerhoff (2005: 1).

[24] Other specific attributes of the legitimacy crisis in fragile settings (including the state's delivery of security to its citizens, the retention of a monopoly on the use of force and basic service delivery) have already been discussed in Chap. 5.

[25] Harvey (2015: 269–281) The Cultural Geography of Community Suffering in Anderson, R.E. (ed) *World Suffering & the Quality of Life*, Springer; Brinkerhoff, D. (2007a, b); McCAnn, I.L. & Pearlman, L.A. (1990a, b); Wilkinson, I. (2005a, b)

[26] In Quechua: *Jucshungulla cawashun.*

[27] Mills, C. & Zavaleta, D., (2015: 251–269) Shame, Humiliation and Social Isolation in Anderson, R.E. (ed) *World Suffering & the Quality of Life*, Springer.

[28] See Herman (1992).

insecurity has changed people's perception of one another, also altering how they see themselves. Instead of a strong sense of responsibility and attachment[29] towards something larger than their individual selves, people respond in ways that tend to further fragment a sense of shared community values, social ties and practices. Following the focus group discussions in the five communities studied these responses were organized into a series of damaging attitudes. They include the following:

1. The attitude that causes survivors to live from 1 day to the next under the expectation that at any one time everything may come to an abrupt end and that there is not much justification for making an effort.
2. The fatalistic attitude that changes everything is ruled by outside forces and what the individual thinks or plans is of no importance and which may inhibit the individual from taking the initiative.
3. The attitude that encourages survivors to blend in by being as inconspicuous as possible, even though this may be contrary to the needs, interests and priorities of the community.

The cumulative effect of this adoption of the previous 3 unhealthy attitudes gives rise to the belief that it is possible for people to excuse themselves from matters of moral/practical importance.[30]

Beneath this surface of frenzied reorganization and daily struggles for survival the individual survivors' memories from the violence remain blocked and unprocessed.[31] This has such a powerful impact on the individual's own identity and sense of belonging that the violence "...paradoxically becomes the basis for collective or personal identity, or both."[32]

In the following the effects of the destruction inflicted on people is discussed in relation to the life of the community and how this affects the bonds between individuals and groups. To understand the rising levels of self interest amongst people and its destruction of any empathic concern for others it is necessary to look more closely at the traditional support system. Before the violence the community and its

---

[29] Davidson and Cotter (1989).

[30] See for example Frankl (1985: 104ff) The four characteristics of social meaninglessness: (1) Ephemeral attitude: apparent in lack of aims and plans for life, making no efforts in reaching one's goals and being directed solely by wishes and impulses. This attitude is manifest in indecisiveness, lack of goals and lack of commitment. It leads to self indulgence, bitterness about life and hopelessness; (2) Fatalistic attitude: manifested in the assumption that everything is determined and that everything can be explained. No space for compassion; it is cynical and pessimistic, no empathy for others, irresponsible, inactive, seeking control and superstitious; (3) Collectivistic Attitude: observed in following the opinion of the majority to the extent of abrogating one's own individuality and personal responsibility; (4) Anticipatory anxiety is a symptom prompted by fear that the individual is fearful that the trauma will recur: flight from fear. See also Marshall and Marshall (2012).

[31] McCann and Pearlman (1990a, b); Pearlman and Saakvitne (1995).

[32] LaCapra (2001:81).

organizations were the medium through which basic needs were addressed. In the aftermath of the political violence this has all changed.

People's disillusionment with the traditional support system and its performance during the violence has brought about a level of destruction to the social environment that can be described as "…a blow to the tissues of social life that damages the bonds linking people-together and impairs the prevailing sense of communality."[33] To engage in non-negative thinking and the sort of coping activities that help to promote and maintain positive growth only tends to happen when individuals reconfigure their thoughts, beliefs and behaviours as the following statement indicates: "Before people were united and caring of each other; now they have a bit of money and move away and live their life as individuals. Everyone practically lives their lives, or what today matters which is money; even the children make you buy a meal by telling you how much to pay." Author's field research: interviewee from Unay (Reyes).

This interpretation underscores the shadow presence of the violence in the relationship between the individual and the life of the community: "Before the terrorism there was no progress and everything was in *ayni*. Now *ayni* is finished for us; with nothing more than *ayni* our land worked well, but no more." Author's field research: interviewee from Wamani (Marco).

Feeling powerless to change their situation so violates the belief system that gives meaning to human experience that it can make survivors want to avoid the overwhelming force of any further traumatic experiences or any initiative that might involve future planning and risk. Though this might not mitigate the effect of the traumatic experience itself, this might also open up new opportunities for successful coping and what is called post-traumatic growth.[34]

By altering their basic state of consciousness and by facing the limits of withdrawal from engagement as a solution, survivors may find that they are obliged to protest to ensure the public recognition they need in order to be able to start to rebuild their own sense of order and justice and repair some trust in social relations and the political authorities. In such reduced circumstances, survivors can only feel safe and protected if things change, and if there is growth in trust, social ties and honest local and national governance.

Most focus groups from all five communities studied identified feelings of fear and mistrust manifested in complaints about their situation as they perceive and cognitively construct it.

Participants said that because there is no interest in trying to resolve things within their community, relations between people became even worse. One said that he and his family were starting to plan the future – to seek escape from an impossibly difficult situation and had decided that things would be much better if they got out and left: "…the best thing to do is leave before SL comes back." Author's field research: interviewee from Unay (Honoré).

Participants in focus groups in Wamani said that people were no longer willing to stand for public office in the community, since they were afraid of what might

[33] Erikson (1976: 302–305); Davidson (1984: 555–572).

[34] See Herman (1992).

happen to them, should SL ever return. Consequently, many local political institutions were no longer functioning at all. Elected holders of public office in the community were also afraid of exercising the responsibilities they were expected to carry out, being unwilling to involve themselves in future-oriented planning and to take risks on behalf of others.

A survivor of the violence describes the difficulties this now presents in the life of the community: "The (community) authorities do not know enough about administrative procedures and the regulations in force and because of ignorance they exercise roles that are not within their jurisdiction. They also have no strategy for making links with other people to improve the community. They don't know how to go about tackling problems and conflicts when they happen. They have no political power; they are always being manipulated. Most people don't do anything, they just fill the position." Author's field research: interviewee from Wamani (Jerome).

Nearly all focus groups in Otoronco said that their situation was unlikely to improve unless they could obtain public recognition for the difficulties they were facing. However, they also recognized that improvements in their situation were also jeopardized by their own indifference, apathy, selfishness and isolation Participants said that "…there are no groups, no families, no individuals in the community that can confront government officials because we all feel incapable, we are all ignorant."[35]

This degraded sense of self-esteem makes post-traumatic growth an urgent necessity. The following statement is an illustration of the limits to the present pseudo-solutions adopted by local people to their own powerlessness: "Here there is no compassion, the people are just selfish, and no one listens to you. There is none of the unity that used to exist when I was little; then I saw it was not all money it was more, it was about mutual support, not now." Author's field research: interviewee from Qocha (Teófila).

Instead of a trusting social environment in which people are able to come together, share their experiences and reflect on their situation, reality has become so violated that there is nothing and no one left to identify with.

By depriving survivors of the normal symptoms of support the social environment is powerless to provide the very qualities needed to restore a sense of control, connection and meaning, something which the community will need to rediscover and reinvent in order to be able to become more forward-looking and goal-oriented. This perspective is conditional on the capacity to resist future stressors that occur whilst survivors are still struggling with the backlog of dangerous memories from the political violence.

The difficulties this presents are illustrated by the following statement: "For me, my people are poorly organized, like I said they are concerned with earning money. When we are in (community) meetings they don't attend because they are tired or (if they do attend) they just go to sleep in meetings. They are nothing but pawns that listen: others don't even listen, they are not interested; they just say the government will sort it out." Author's field research: interviewee from Qocha (Alvaro).

[35] Author's field research: Interviewee from Wamani (Samaria).

8.4 Moving Towards a More Trusting Social Environment

The characteristics of a relatively trusting social environment can be grouped together under two separate headings: internal and external, categories with some overlap and which are not mutually exclusive. Good community leadership, tight control of government handouts in relation to local capacity, improved trust of local officials are all issues that are seen as being essential and were frequently mentioned (usually in terms of their absence) across all five communities studied but were also variable and reflected contextually specific issues.

Deeply rooted in all of the problems with a trusting social environment is the conflict between the actual awfulness of human suffering and the lack of any emotional reaction to it. Here it is not just the experience of violence but the force of circumstances that feel so inescapable. Instead of any kind of emotional engagement at both the personal and collective level, the social environment (both within and outside the community) fall back on an acknowledgement of the facts without any acknowledgement of their existential and experiential impact. This is the central issue regarding the use of an objective attitude.

The debilitating effect of this breach of normative expectations not only makes survivors powerless to restore a sense of control, connection and meaning to their lives it also causes them to remain frozen in an unprocessed silence. This is demonstrated by the following statement: "At night, I have nightmares and am permanently scared, having suffered a lot of torture. Due to all these factors, I am very concerned about everything that is currently going on. No authority is bothered about us, and no one is sorry." Author's field research: interviewee from Wamani (Fabian).

This annulment of any emotional reaction to human misery does not destroy feelings of injustice. To the contrary: resentment about past injustices is likely to provide survivors with the only means by which they can challenge government indifference and detachment. For those subject to resurgence in violence resentment also provides a means by which the truth about government incompetence, negligence and corruption can be exposed. In this respect resentment has "…a constructive and positive role to play in the maintenance of social harmony and human relationships."[36] The effect of this highly aversive state therefore gives survivors a means by which they can strive to reduce their own powerlessness.

In recent years a CBO has been organised to represent the interests of the survivors of the political violence. This is the *Asociación de familias afectadas por la violencia política* (AFAVIP) (Association for Families who are Victims of Political Violence). Its purpose is to record the number of deaths, disappearances and torture; support the exhumation of mass graves, lobby for a public works budget and establish appropriate local government policies for those affected by political violence.

Its membership consists of people affected by violence, including victims of torture and rape, orphans, widows, and family members who have been killed or

[36] Brudholm (2008: 46–50).

disappeared. Some of its activities are organised in conjunction with local authorities and local NGOs working on human rights issues.

Having consulted the Ombudsman in Lima the AFAVIP organization for Qocha was told to standardize information about all of its victims. All the information has since been entered into the registry of victims' book, which is needed if the data is to be legally authorized by the Justice of the Peace. One member of AFAVIP in Yachaya said that the regular updating of human rights abuses represented one of the organization's most important responsibilities: "The extrajudicial killings (in this community) have been registered by the President of the AFAVIP. However, there are at least four other mass graves that have yet to be fully uncovered; no one is yet certain how many more bodies they will find. The registrar has informed the community (verbally) that at least 220 victims have been registered, which is more than the community registered. That currently stands at 185. The community requested a copy of the updated version of the registry but the local authorities have not given us one." Author's field research: interviewee from Yachaya (Guillermo).

Many of the focus groups said that they did not want to talk about what happened because they are afraid about speaking in public and are worried that they may not be able to express themselves clearly. Participants in Unay said that many survivors do not want to participate in the activities of AFAVIP because they feel ashamed about what happened to them and fear the ridicule of other people.

This perspective is more consistent with the idea that recovery from extreme experiences is dependent on the individual and not on organizations, including organizations such as AFAVIP, as the following statement indicates: "Decisions at a meeting are made by about 10–12 people, even though there are about 70 people belonging to the organization. The trouble is those affected (by the violence) cannot speak, or they cannot speak in public or they are afraid to express themselves." Author's field research: interviewee from Unay (Fulgencio). All focus groups in Unay said that although there had been many cases of rape during the violence it was impossible to find out more details because the victims felt ashamed and wanted to try and forget.[37] However, one was prepared to testify and said that threats, intimidation and the fear of reprisals were a regular procedure: "They told me that they had taken my husband away. Then they grabbed me and threw me into this room and locked me in. Later more women were brought in and at midnight the soldiers began to rape them. Then they grabbed me by the feet, hands and my head, and started to rape me. I haven't told my husband because I was afraid they would kill him." Author's field research: interviewee from Unay (Lidia).

[37] Mills and Zavaleta (2015: 251–269) Shame, Humiliation and Social Isolation in Anderson, R.E. (ed) *World Suffering & the Quality of Life*, Springer.

The lack of confidence in the government's promises to make reparations to individual victims is responsible for much cynicism and scepticism about AFAVIP and its activities.

Despite repeated attempts on the part of its board members, representatives said that it was almost impossible to find or interact with senior government officials, either because they were always travelling or involved with other arrangements: "The trouble is we are not perceived to have the same importance as more influential people. Any claims made by people like us are not heard by the rich and the powerful, but among themselves whether they steal or not they always have the chance to conceal, but here a poor man who steals the smallest thing is brought to justice. Just giving us collective reparations for what happened is a trick to make us believe that we will be given individual reparations, but this is business for them; it's still the same people who have power." Author's field research: interviewee from Qocha (Pastor).

Most focus groups in Yachaya said that people affected by violence did not participate in AFAVIP because they regard it as a waste of time. Participants said that they want to be left alone and want nothing to do with dubious promises from the government.[38] Survivors feel unsafe, in their emotions and in their thinking and in relation to other people, as the following statement demonstrates: "The AFAVIP directive meets fortnightly and with all associates on the last Sunday of each month; most of the meetings have never been attended by more than twenty to twenty-five." Author's field research: interviewee from Yachaya (Isandro).

Some of the focus groups in Unay said that even if the government was to make progress on individual reparations they would only be used for political purposes, such as regional and national political campaigns.[39]

Other reasons for survivor scepticism include the competence of AFAVIP board members and their level of knowledge concerning the law of reparations. One focus group in Wamani described this as "very superficial." Participants said that board members are ignorant of the documents relating to individual reparations because the only information available to them is culled either from the local newspaper or from occasional references made to them by the local authorities. The board also lacks a secretary and this makes it difficult for the organization to draft appropriate documents for presentation to the relevant authorities. People do not want the job

[38] Many people entitled to register (and participate) do not do so because they are travelling (for work as economic migrants) or because they no longer live in the community. Those who stay away also include widows from the political violence, people who have been tortured; orphans etc. Nevertheless, the principal deterrents to people's participation remains the scepticism people have about individual reparations. In spite of their own particular connection with the events of the political violence (either as orphans or because members of their immediate family had been killed or disappeared) attendance in AFAVIP meetings by young people is consistently low.

[39] Feelings of scepticism about state reparations began with collective mechanisms, which for many participants are seen as little more than mechanisms for the manipulation of the people at election time. People are also fearful that a change of government will change everything and lead to the cancellation not just of the reparations scheme, but of other government programmes and projects as well.

out of fear that they lack the necessary skills to make effective representations on behalf of the organization. Instead survivors have sought advice about individual reparations and the drafting of related documents from members of the health post or from schoolteachers.

For a senior member of APAVIF from Qocha loss of interest in the organization and poor attendance at meetings is explained by the fact that "...people are so accustomed to state handouts, such as the glass of milk programme, the soup kitchen program, JUNTOS that they want to stick with these things and nothing else. They don't want to talk about individual reparations, particularly since collective reparations arrived." Author's field research: interviewee from Qocha (Mario).

In these circumstances any idea of 'working through' the past is meaningless. To recover historical memory requires not only the appropriation of their experiences of the violence but a form of empathy that enables them "...to feel that their thoughts and feelings have been heard, acknowledged and respected."[40]

Here it is not just the experience of political violence but the hard struggle for satisfying everyday basic needs that feel so inescapable. One survivor thought that there was little prospect of survivors recovering the sense of their own identity, let alone the pride of belonging to a people, or of being able to rely on a tradition and culture: "I'm sure that the state intends to do away with the rural community of Peru so that they do not have any kind of hindrance in their efforts to continue delivering our land to foreign investors; then all we will be is poor trash. In years to come we will see more exploitation and mining pollution; worse we will see all the best green areas being used for mining, so say the great geologists and that hurts the population. The only people that are benefiting in this process are the entrepreneurs; they are not interested if the people die or not, of course they pretend that they are going to help put in a school, water, etc but that is a bargain for them." Author's field research: interviewee from Qocha (Tulio).

8.5 Towards a Politics of Resentment

To recover their historical memory, survivors need to re-establish some kind of meaningful control over their environment but the government decision to suspend financial and other forms of support for the *Ronda* and the CAD at the end of the violence has created a social environment that is perceived as both threatening and incapable of improvement. Being unable to live under conditions in which the basic psychological need for safety is fulfilled is a reminder that the experience of the political violence is not the absolute limit of all possible suffering. Establishing a safe living environment is always conditional on a component of social support, but in the aftermath of the political violence this has been largely unavailable as the following indicates:

[40] Baron-Cohen (2011: 13).

"The community is in a bad position. There is fear from attackers and *mochileros* [drugs mules] in the highlands where there is no police or military. People never feel safe. It's the same near the community as well. Security is very bad. Most military and police don't come this far (from the district capital)." Author's field research: interviewee from Unay (Manola).

Faced with the possibility of resurgence in violence brings the survivor into connection with the question of prevention. However, the idea that people can transform their experiences of extreme events by making them the basis for social action is inconsistent with the promotion of psychosocial resilience in an environment that is neither health-promoting nor safe. Being unable to control their environment produces psychological states such as disillusionment, hostility, depression, a sense of hopelessness, anxiety and feelings of not being valued. Feelings like these are important because they are at the centre of the subjective experience of the quality of life.[41]

Until the political violence people's lives were less bothered by events for which there could be no closure. In the aftermath of violence, the inability to make "…a gradual shift from unpredictable danger to reliable safety, from dissociated trauma to acknowledged memory, and from stigmatized isolation to restored social connection",[42] make the circumstances under which people live so different as to be unrecognizable.[43] Outwardly survivors' lives are not so different from those of their ancestors but the quality of 'otherness' about the events inflicted on them is such that the individual is no longer fully integrated with the present.

Instead of being self directed and intellectually independent not even the immediate demands of self preservation are sufficiently all-consuming as to separate survivors from the legacies of the past. In the past membership of a particular rural highland community used to define what the individual was. Like any other traditional agrarian society that lives within the cycle of nature the individual's identity was locally orientated and inseparably linked with the established economic system. Irrespective of fluctuations in the maintenance and production of arable crops and livestock people's expectations rarely went beyond previous experience. To survive people had always depended on their skills being passed from one generation to the next. If anything in the traditional economy ever changed, "…then it changed so slowly and over so long a time that the breach separating previous experience and an expectation to be newly disclosed did not undermine the traditional world."[44]

However, the political violence has brought fundamental changes to individual identity and people's horizon of expectations. *Never before has the idea that the individual's own sense of personal identity as something inextricably linked with*

---

[41] Wilkinson (2005a, b: 65); Dussaillant and Gonzalez (2015: 233–251) Lifetime Suffering and Capabilities in Chile in Anderson, R.E. (ed) *World Suffering & the Quality of Life*, Springer.

[42] Herman (1992: 155).

[43] Mills and Zavaleta (2015: 251–269) Shame, Humiliation and Social Isolation in Anderson, R.E. (ed) *World Suffering & the Quality of Life*, Springer.

[44] Koselleck (2004: 264).

membership of a given community been so powerfully challenged.[45] These changes have repercussions for the future of the traditional economy and for the individual survivor's relationship with their own past. Being unable to make the gradual shift from unpredictable danger to relative safety helps to channel attempts into social change as the following statement makes clear:

"Nowadays I see my community in the same way as the changes in the city; there are things happening that are changing our way of life; though the changes in behaviour are slow you can still feel them. Before the violence we felt enclosed, we did not leave the community; we didn't know much about things outside. Now it's not like that; it's all changed, it's not like before. Before I did not know what was happening outside our place." Author's field research: interviewee from Qocha (Tulio).

This can be seen as a sign of post-traumatic growth, resulting in new expectations which have so encouraged survivors to invest in making reality conform to their own immediate needs that memories of the past can appear irrelevant in the present. However, the memory of past events cannot be ignored, and these recollections militate against the mechanisms of repression that are sought out to find some means of moving forwards into the future.

Irrespective of how much effort is expended in addressing the possible benefits of the future, the prospects of violence being renewed, can sometimes bring back old practices of avoidance and denial. In this way survivors transcend their own overriding fear of any repetition of the political violence by simple expedients: "The people in authority tell us that there is nothing, but what we hear is that the violence is starting again in other places; we are worried because we think it will come here too, so when there is a meeting of those who were affected by the violence a lot of people no longer take part because they think it is better to stay quiet." Author's field research: interviewee from Qocha (Marisa).

Though survivors may want to prevent their memories from interfering with their present mental constructs the experience of extreme events is too powerful. Instead past crimes and atrocities continue to have "... priority over the attempt to shape the future."[46] One survivor describes the consequences of this situation as follows: "People are leaving here for reasons of education and employment, but we are also waiting for any attack that might happen so that the community can withdraw. If the violence starts again we would just leave everything: our farms, animals, homes; the only thing would be to save ourselves and run away with our family. We do not want to relive that excrement we have already suffered and lose our families, property, all over again. Now that we have had these experiences we know the ways out of the community to avoid being killed." Author's field research: interviewee from Qocha (Severo).

By *refusing to forget their experiences victims contribute to a cultural politics in which the memory of injustice helps to uphold the importance of questions about the very meaning of justice*. When brutalities inflicted on people result from acts of injustice outside the bounds of normal experience, "...they cannot be simply articu-

[45] Kakar (1996).

[46] Amery (1980: 191).

lated through representation or by our ordinary categories of justice."[47] Instead the cultural space that people occupy provides a means by which the memory of past events can be used to expose deficiencies in the ordinary understandings of the categories of justice. For example, when survivors consider the investigations and recommendations of the TRC to be a product of legal justice, what this implies is that the more profound type of justice that they are seeking, may be missing.[48]

To build resources for resilience in these circumstances is close to impossible, irrespective of how socially desirable it may be as the following illustrates: "There are people who still need to be recognized and the damage repaired. For example, we have several mass graves here which the truth commission has been unable to establish the facts about and we ask that these facts are clarified for the good of the country and their relatives from this community." Author's field research: interviewee from Qocha (Tulio).

In the present, the memory of past events is not always fixed, but can change according to the pressures and key events in the survivor's present. In this respect the resurgence of SL, of robberies, drug trafficking, extrajudicial killings (including murder), forced labour and torture can bring the memory of wrongs suffered back to the forefront of people's thoughts, making memory of trauma more central in their lives. One survivor describes how easily these memories of past brutalities can be revived by experiences of distress in the present: "People have asked for the police to come, but I wonder what good they will do, those locusts. I'm very afraid of them. I don't want there to be a police station, because if there are any problems and they show up acting *macho*, they will just start messing around with the young people like they used to. In those days, they would torture and rape." Author's field research: interviewee from Qocha (Pomposa).

In the immediate aftermath of violence, the problems facing people in rural highland communities were intensified by the institutionalization of impunity for repressive acts.[49]

Initially acts of impunity were restricted to the lack of co-operation by the police and the armed forces with the judiciary, but this was subsequently extended to general, unspecified governmental and legislative actions as well.[50] This situation was not brought to an end until the overthrow of the Fujimori Administration in late-2000. Since then efforts to overcome injustice and the lack of official recognition have come from a range of different actors from the government as well as national and international civil society organizations and NGOs. However, the decline of

---

[47] Spargo (2006: 25).

[48] For Agamben "...the concepts of responsibility, accountability, dignity and respect are irremediably contaminated by the consequences of de-contextualisation. Anyone who has tried to make use of these terms outside the juridical sphere knows this. To assume responsibility is to leave the territory of ethics and enter that of law. Whoever has made this difficult step cannot presume to return through the door he has just closed behind him." Agamben (1999: 20ff).

[49] These self-amnesty laws (Laws 26,479 and 26,492) were first adopted by the Fujimori administration in 1995.

[50] See Montoya Vivanco (2012: 167) in Almqvist and Esposito (2012).

political will together with the problems facing the institutions of criminal justice in the investigation, prosecution and sanctioning of serious human rights violations make any reconciliation with the past through criminal justice look increasingly doubtful.

Recognition can be one demand that arises from resentment, but this is only possible if there is a concerted willingness on behalf of officials and other powerful players, to listen to such demands and take them seriously. To keep the human dimension at the centre of the relationship between citizens and representatives of the state is the goal, but by depriving people of separate identities the state appears to be engaged in trying to sever the links between people's memories and the history of political violence. For survivors from the communities studied this constitutes a breach of their normative expectations of the state. It is also a source of deep frustration about a breach they feel powerless to bridge. In this respect objectification becomes an official vehicle for exculpation, the annihilation of memories and failing to recognise local knowledge about the recent past.

Local people said that in spite of many promises to help them the government never has. The following statement encapsulates the desperation people feel about their situation and the life of their community since the conflict: "It is urgent that the government rectifies the problem we have with them. It has all been just lies. They do not respect our rights; we live in total chaos." Author's field research: interviewee from Unay (Nestor).

8.6 Conclusions

To highlight the struggle against official silence and indifference this study shows how by refusing to forget their experiences survivors (and those they influence) contribute to a cultural politics in which the memory of injustice helps to uphold the importance of questions about the very meaning of justice.

The physical impact of location on the kind of lives people actually lead and the manner in which this affects interaction between them and outside organizations and institutions mean that few people end up being interested in public affairs. Popular concerns urgently need to be adequately articulated through channels that do not discourage the exercise of individual and community voice. For people in the communities studied (as Chaps. 4, 5, 6 and 7 and this chapter) have shown, such channels barely exist.

In the aftermath of the violence the political will of local authorities and the extent to which they are accessible to rural people has not improved. Instead, opportunities for participation in public life remain stunted and undeveloped.

This helps to preserve the idea that public affairs are somebody else's responsibility and that civic engagement is a waste of time.

In this way the unequal power relationship between rural communities and outside organizations, institutions and NGOs is preserved and the feeling that local government is ineffective and uncaring is retained. Being shut out of opportunities to participate in public life affects people's awareness and consciousness of potential issues and conflicts.

By internalising their own powerlessness people understand the unequal distribution of participation in public life as the natural way of things. This makes people, including survivors of the political violence, unaware of their rights, including their ability to express desires and interests, to have interests taken into account and to have access to services. People have become so accustomed to the aforementioned problems that they are inclined to think of it as unchangeable, and therefore not to be questioned. This encourages submissiveness towards local authorities, regardless of the perceived legitimacy of the response. In these circumstances the individual's own sense of personal identity as something inextricably linked with membership of a given community is powerfully challenged to a degree that is unprecedented.

This chapter explored how the legacies of violence has led people in the Andes – and very likely in many other post-conflict situations worldwide – to question the trustworthiness of others. It has also shown how the state and its officials have sought (usually ineffectively) to make repair, whilst denying the lived material experience that affects ordinary people, an effort doomed to failure.

Finally, this chapter has shown that effectively treating disillusion and resentment are likely to be the first (but vital) difficult steps towards achieving posttraumatic growth and more positive social change in the future.

Chapter 9
Lessons from the Peruvian Highlands: Ways Forward and Wider Implications

In this chapter I shall consider some of the issues raised by this study and identify ways in which things can be taken forward, both with respect to future improvement in rural Andean communities, and in the application of findings to other situations in other countries and to further studies). In the first section human and social suffering is considered from three distinct perspectives: (a) the government; (b) the powerless and (c) the effects of suffering and reparation and how they are understood. To counter the objectification of human and social suffering and promote greater analytical precision, the second section of this chapter looks at the need for new methodological concepts based around empathy and participation.

To show how the subjective reality of human and social suffering matter, future research directions are discussed based around the need for linking psychosocial approaches with the actual lived experience of individuals and groups.[1] In the third section of this chapter, the conclusions of the findings from this study are identified, briefly discussed and some wider implications are cautiously explored.

9.1 Interpreting Suffering and Reparation

The materials included in this study provide a detailed examination of the historical and social conditions of people affected by political violence and living in a context of daily survival. To get closer to understanding what human and social suffering does to people this study looks at the un-reconciled elements in their lives to challenge the authority of abstract subjectivity and the objectification of human and social suffering.

To better understand what we know about how survivors interpret suffering and reparation the findings from this study will now be discussed.

[1] Dussaillant, F. & Gonzalez, P. A., (2015: 233–251) Lifetime Suffering and Capabilities in Chile in Anderson, R.E. (ed) *World Suffering & the Quality of Life*, Springer.

T. J. Bowyer, *Beyond Suffering and Reparation*,
https://doi.org/10.1007/978-3-319-98983-9_9

1. Interpreting suffering and reparation: the government response

In recent years physical and mental suffering has become a subject of increasing importance in conflict studies and post-conflict studies; social and cultural anthropology; political studies; migration studies; social care; reconciliation and social justice studies; development studies, civic studies, medical anthropology, ethnography, and Holocaust studies. However, the influence of such suffering on the nature of social, political and institutional responses to human affliction and social need has been less evident. For the government impartiality, neutrality, tolerance and pluralism have such a hold on the concept of policy and programme making that any emotional capacities to engage with the context in which people live out the subjective experiences of physical and mental suffering has been blocked.

From this perspective the TRC investigation into the historical, social and economic causes and conditions of the political violence in Peru represents a significant step forward in "…our understanding of the implications of the cultural construction of knowledge and the evolving local and provisional character of all frames of reference and identifications."[2]

Through its analysis of economic social and cultural inequalities the TRC in Peru not only "…provides new guidance for future truth commissions in post-conflict recovery settings sharing similar demographics,"[3] it also highlights the interconnectedness between the individual's psychological suffering and the social, economic and political context in which they live.

These developments militate against the reductionist view of physical and mental suffering and the destruction of any emotional capacity to engage with its subjective experiences in their own context.[4] From this new perspective, it is possible to refigure human suffering so that the individual and the specific context in which they live are no longer regarded as redundant or inter-changeable. This way representations made by a specific individual from a particular context are no longer vulnerable to the distortions of generalization and inaccuracy. There is thus need for government to disengage from agendas of development that rely on an abstract and formal definition of the universal self. Instead of imposing theory that insists on the translation of the evidence into its own categories, the government needs to turn this around and make theory into the servant of the evidence. However, before a government is sufficiently motivated to replace reductionist views of physical and mental suffering with an emotional response based around empathic engagement, and a sense of solidarity, other factors need to be in place.[5] One thing stands out: it is the capacity to systematically process information about psychological distress when information about psychological distress is related to the needs, expectancies and

---

[2] Watkins, M. & Shulman, H., (2008: 26).

[3] LaPlante, L.J. (2007: 176).

[4] Dussaillant, F. & Gonzalez, P. A., (2015: 233–251) Lifetime Suffering and Capabilities in Chile in Anderson, R.E. (ed) *World Suffering & the Quality of Life*, Springer.

[5] Chouliaraki, L., (2017: 49–61) Suffering and the Ethics of Solidarity in Anderson, R.E. (ed) *Alleviating World Suffering,* Springer

objectives of any particular situation. In this way, emotional engagement with other people becomes possible, and the emotional pain of wrongs suffered through such unconscious strategies as disavowal, psychic numbing, splitting of consciousness, doubling and other dissociative states can be revealed.

By breaking apart these normalised assumptions the structural factors underlying economic and political suffering, and the common emotions and behaviours associated with people affected by violence and living in a context where their priority is daily survival, can be revealed. This restores the interconnections between the psychological, the historical, the socio-economic and the spiritual, and provides people with the assurance that their suffering is properly acknowledged, and that appropriate responsibilities will be assumed.

2. Interpreting suffering and reparation: the powerless

Though self-interest informs many public policies and programmes and directs the daily lives of survivors of political violence, the expectation of help for someone in distress, the certainty of help in moments of direst need is one of the fundamental experiences of life.[6] The idea that such behaviour requires no explanation is one of the most important assumptions we make about victims of violence and people struggling with daily survival. In the absence of any resources to contain the experience, the individual is backed into a corner from which there is no escape. This is a situation that forces people to confront nothing less than raw existence. It has no moral or emotional framework and holds out no prospect of change, or any protection from a situation of unceasing tragedy and misfortune. Because people feel powerless to change their situation, their lives are tormented by the pretence that immersion in the present and the resumption of routine and regular activity are enough to coordinate social life and move shared goals forwards.

This makes people more willing to concede to the desires of the government, irrespective of the perceived legitimacy of their demands. In a post-conflict context this includes their tacit agreement to the use of closure as a formal cut-off point from the haunting past. To help survivors rebuild a positive sense of self-government, reparations policies and programmes need to take an emotional interest in the human impact of the situation. But this does not happen. Though Truth Commissions, reparations schemes and other initiatives may help strengthen a government's commitment to a better future, it does not make it any easier for victims and their ability to detach themselves from past suffering and injustice. Instead this makes the past as much a breeding ground for the return of memories about what was done, as the individual survivor's own feelings of impotence, frustration and despair.

To rebuild a positive sense of self, survivors need to empathically project themselves into their own thoughts and memories of the past, but they cannot accomplish this alone; to integrate their experience of extreme events they need the assistance of others. The frustration of such a basic psychological need is morally damaging because it is incompatible with any normal person's expectations of how human suffering should be dealt with. The crucial question therefore involves the

[6] Amery, J. (1980: 28).

transformation of human detachment and objectivity into an emotional response based around empathic engagement and a sense of solidarity with others.[7]

3. Understanding the effects of suffering and reparation

This study set out to challenge the authority of abstract subjectivity and the objectification of human and social suffering, by examining un-reconciled elements in the lives of people affected by political violence and living in extreme poverty in Peru. To explore this idea the study undertook a locally informed analysis of the structural factors underlying economic and political suffering, and the common emotions and behaviours with which it is associated.

From this analysis it was shown that a breakdown in the relationship between context and its influence on human nature and responsibility, and the failure of the social capital discourse has helped to lower the onset of feelings of shame between human beings.[8] In particular, it was found that any feeling for the misfortune of others is atrophying because the memory of past suffering is being lost.

Instead of engaging with "…the social structures, discourses and ideologies that create subjects in states of 'marginalized dependency' and 'oppressive misery'",[9] memory is increasingly restricted to the recall of past events.

In this way, memory is losing its capacity to influence the present, and with it any sense of responsibility that people have both to themselves and to others. By failing to engage with the original experiences of human and social suffering, the government is able to revert to the idea of business as usual without regard for the past. To understand human and social suffering, people therefore need to overcome this resistance to acknowledgement, and become close to the past and stay close to it, and never again ignore it. For the survivors of political violence, this is important for no other reason than that any response should be one that properly recognises what happened, in order that appropriate responses can be assumed.

9.2 New Methodological Concepts Based on Empathy and Participation

1. The Question of Responsibility

With respect to memory the research presented in this study suggests that we are witnessing the erosion of any sense of responsibility for victims and perpetrators, as well as bystanders. Though direct responsibility for the actual situation rests with others, the survivor's not choosing to act to make a difference for the better only

---

[7] Chouliaraki, L., (2017: 49–61) Suffering and the Ethics of Solidarity in Anderson, R.E. (ed) *Alleviating World Suffering,* Springer.

[8] Mills, C. & Zavaleta, D., (2015: 251–269) Shame, Humiliation and Social Isolation in Anderson, R.E. (ed) *World Suffering & the Quality of Life*, Springer; Martin-Baro, I. (1994a, b, c, d).

[9] Martin-Baro, I., (1994a, b, c, d: 26) as cited in Watkins, M. & Shulman, H., (2008: 26).

serves to release new symptoms of injustice because blindness to the misfortune of others, lack of imagination and inner indifference toward what is happening are not the only thing that matter.[10]

It is a consequence of this way of thinking that the blank indifference of some people to the terrible suffering of others is responsible for exacerbating the scale of human misery. Such a failure of moral responsibility on behalf of all those who know about the suffering of others is ably facilitated by the danger of individual and cultural amnesia. In this respect, the idea that everything should just revert to business as usual is the most destructive attitude that can be adopted. Though this happens time and time again survivors should be encouraged to fight against the use of closure as a formal cut-off point from the haunting past.

Forgetting past suffering and injustice in a world overpopulated by images of human misery may strengthen the government's commitment to a better future, but it does not absolve anyone from "…an historical judgement about what is good and what is wrong, what is evil and what is not."[11] The fact that all too often people simply do not care or claim not to know about the suffering of others, is a threat to both memory and human dignity. In the face of massive injustice, the lack of mutual human support and help is responsible for a permanent loss of trust.[12] This has a profound effect on the survivor's perception of themselves and of the outside world. They feel diminished, disarmed and defenceless.

In recent years the values associated with the expectation of help from others have been so weakened that self-interest is no longer thought of as shameful or dishonourable. This increasing indifference to community responsibility for the safety and wellbeing of others has a profound influence on people ravaged by economic and all the other hardships, including social injustice and political oppression. Instead of acting out of concern for others this lack of sympathy and understanding has made the world increasingly incomprehensible, so that the bonds of belonging between a person and a particular environment have been irremediably weakened.

For people living with the consequences of violence in a world of hunger, deprivation, ill treatment, injustice and poor health this is no one-off violation of traditional norms and values, but an intrinsic part of an on-going world-view. Over time the use of old views to meet new situations or information in the rural highlands of Peru have performed so poorly that an inability to identify with the suffering of others is no longer stigmatised in the way it once was.[13]

[10] Jaspers, K. (1947: 69–70).

[11] Schuster, E. & Boschert-Kimmig, R., (1999: 90).

[12] Amery, J. (1980: 70) And cf. pp. 28, 40, 96.

[13] For Logstrup "…the hope of morality is reflected in its pre-reflexive spontaneity; mercy is spontaneous because the least interruption, the least calculation, the least dilution of it in order to serve something else destroys it entirely; indeed, turns it into the opposite of what it is, un-mercifulness." Logstrup, K. (2002).

Instead of any meaningful human interaction, traditional norms and values, including the expectation of help, increasingly lack authority and credibility, making highland villagers and farmers feel powerless, uncertain and fearful of the future.

This debasement of the future undermines reliance on traditional patterns and routines that normally guide such people's behaviour in the course of their daily lives. If it's not possible to contain this set of conditions, and there is no convincing moral framework within which the expectation of help can be re-established, the available social support (practical, instrumental or emotional) is likely to lack substance.

In these circumstances the frustration of basic psychological needs, such as security or safety, trust, esteem, positive identity, feelings of effectiveness and control, positive connections to other people, a comprehension of reality and of one's own place in the world, and transcendence (or spiritual needs) become increasingly threatened and responsible for a retreat from duty, loyalty, self-preservation, loss of face, and comradeship; social identity is no longer perceived as a life line, but as an obstacle to realistic behaviour. It is at this point that we need to return to the issue of human solidarity, and the idea that the expectation of help for someone in distress, the certainty of help in moments of direst need, is plausible and realistic.

Though the experience of shared suffering is an important factor in the contribution to feelings of community, its significance for victims and others impacted by political violence and who find themselves at the lowest level of existence, is circumscribed by more immediate biological needs. It therefore follows that human solidarity, and the expectation of help, will only flourish if these norms and values are able to affirm and protect the individual.

To retain such a reality in consciousness human solidarity needs to minimize the psychological impact of physical and mental suffering, and its adverse effects on traditional norms and values; it also needs to help survivors improve their understanding of the situation they find themselves in, and of their relationship with other people and the outside world. However, human solidarity is unable to flourish in the way it is able to when basic survival is not always the overriding concern.[14]

2. Intergenerational Continuity and its Breakdown

Drawing on these studies in highland Peru everything is devalued to the point that a breakdown in intergenerational continuity is inevitable. For people affected by unrest and violence and struggling for daily survival it was clear that in practice this compels them to make fundamental changes in how they allocate their time and energy. If people cannot fulfil their immediate needs and want to stay alive, they have no alternative but to accept the situation and bear the consequences. To this end survivors must come to terms with a set of conditions in which the basic rules underlying all social interaction have been rescinded. This brings about changes in how people perceive each other and how they see themselves; it was apparent that it may well not help to resolve the problems they are facing. Instead, it can stretch

[14] Chouliaraki, L., (2017: 49–61) Suffering and the Ethics of Solidarity in Anderson, R.E. (ed) *Alleviating World Suffering,* Springer.

their understanding of what is happening to breaking point. In these circumstances interpersonal relations become a source of immense frustration and resentment that are often responsible for outbreaks of conflict and other forms of anti-social behaviour. Discretion, understanding, consideration, self-control and a sense of responsibility are not so much caste aside as ignored, on the grounds that these things do not resolve the immediate problem of self-preservation. Not only does this undermine dignity and respect, it also signals the end of a life based around shared values, common humanity and shared responsibility.

In a context of daily survival, the idea that the individual should continue to look to traditional norms and values for support and guidance is unrealistic. For those dealing with social capital and rehabilitation this draws our attention to the importance of the context of the relationship between the social and the individual. It also highlights the need for the link between social relationships and responses to the workings of community activities to be historically and socially grounded. Being more alert to the psychological, cultural and social origins of responsibility, accountability and decisions makes any engagement with what happens to people who suffer from economic and all the other hardships, including social injustice and political oppression, more effective. By emphasizing the contextual opportunities and constraints that affect social relationships, existing assumptions about traditional norms and values can be broken open and the interconnections between the psychological, the historical, the socio-economic and the spiritual explored.

In the aftermath of the violence the values associated with responsibility for others have been so invalidated that every possible choice is an insult to human dignity and respect. It therefore follows that the individual can only act once they have accepted that the situation they find themselves in is unalterable. This means that the attitude of the individual to the situation they find themselves in is what matters. For people affected by violence the individual's attitude is likely to be unpredictable.

Though the situation only permits people to choose from the restricted range of choices available, it does not mean that everyone in the same situation will make the same choices. It therefore follows that the allocation of responsibility and matters relating to the results of reasoning are explained by how the individual chooses to act.

For the hungry and deprived, this will depend on the range of factors relevant to the situation. It is therefore incorrect to assume that individual behaviour simply reflects the wider values of the group, because to do so makes no allowance for individual freedom of thought and action. In this respect, the one-dimensional caricature usually used to depict the suffering of people is both inappropriate and unhelpful. Facing the pain and hardship of extreme circumstances may rule out many options, but this does not make factors such as culture, ethnicity, and political tradition, local notions of what is right and wrong, and other established social mores irrelevant. The point is that difficult life conditions make for a social context that is unable to respect and defend the individual and link one individual with another in a spirit of mutual collaboration and support.[15]

---

[15] Harvey, D. C., (2015: 269–281) The Cultural Geography of Community Suffering in Anderson, R.E. (ed) *World Suffering & the Quality of Life*, Springer.

In less extreme circumstances, there is a basic trust. This is because the interplay between the individual and the group is guided by shared norms and values that foster solidarity, cooperation, security and respect, and whose values are fortified by the activities of a range of grassroots organizations. Infused with history and tradition, these norms and values represent the boundaries that define what it is possible for the individual to be and to do. Over time they make up the local rules, patterns and traditions that people use to guide their own daily behaviour.

By linking people with significant individuals and group norms and values helps them solve common human problems for survival, through shared understandings, common goals and the perception of a common/mutual future. In more extreme circumstances the capacity for self-determination is so weakened that it disrupts peace of mind and undermines self-confidence.

Instead of mutual recognition, trust, equal consideration and solidarity the social context has become one in which feelings of effectiveness and control, positive connections to other people, a comprehension of reality and of one's own place in the world, and transcendence (or spiritual need) either function very badly or not at all.[16] This is an environment that does not inspire trust in long term investments of any kind. Instead it restricts the interplay between the individual and the group to such an extent that shared understandings, common goals and the perception of a shared future are rendered meaningless. It follows that assignment of responsibility and questions of judgement derive from how, in the end, the individual chooses to respond to the restricted range of options available.

To understand how the individual fulfils or violates their responsibilities we need to focus on how people in extremely stressed circumstances understand responsibility. The starting point for such a more nuanced understanding is taken from the idea that moral and religious judgements are in some way contaminated by decontextualisation and their association with the law.[17] To move away from the idea that this drains responsibility of meaning the account used here pays particular attention to the specific context in which issues of responsibility arise. This permits us to focus attention on the contribution responsibility makes to the interpersonal relations in and through which individuals live their lives.

3. The Importance of Context

Difficult life conditions affect individuals in different ways. In situations of near total insecurity, the interplay between material deprivation and psychological stress are the very essence of daily life. Intensely negative experiences over any protracted period produce psychological changes that require frequent personal behaviour adjustments if any relief is to be obtained.

These adjustments afford the individual some temporary protection, but frequent behavioural changes are an inadequate safeguard and cannot shield the individual

[16] McCann, I.L., & Pearlman, L.A., (1990); Pearlman, L.A., & Saakvitne, K.A., (1995); Saakvitne, K.W., et al. (2000); Staub, E., (1989, 2003).

[17] Agamben, G. (1999: 20ff); Staub, E. (2003); Folkman, S. & Lazarus, R.S. (1984); Lazarus, R.S. & Folkman, S. (1986); Lazarus, R.S. (1993); Sandin, I. (1995); Martin-Baro, I. (1989).

indefinitely.[18] In this respect, the on-going nature and accumulation of stressful situations require that the individual make a permanent readjustment. However, this is conditional on the individual's own construction of the situation and its likely repercussions for that person's own well-being. People differ in their sensitivity and vulnerability to a specific set of conditions, and in the interpretation and reaction to those conditions as well.[19]

In this respect, the individual's own development and life experiences are as important to their interpretation of the situation as the social and political environment, personal goals, self-beliefs, beliefs about the world and personal resources. In less extreme circumstances, the individual's reaction to a difficult situation would be to make an appraisal and decide if it is harmful. This normally results in some sort of emotional reaction, followed by further evaluation and an assessment of the individual's own resources for coping with the situation.[20]

In more extreme circumstances, such as highland Peru, the stressful situation is on-going, and so multi-faceted as to make conventional approaches dedicated to problem solving and finding a solution, inappropriate. This means that any appraisal of the situation requires the individual to address a set of conditions that exceeds their own resources and threatens their personal well-being.[21] In circumstances of hunger and deprivation, the very nature, scale and on-going impact of the situation is such that individuals find it difficult to assume responsibility for their own lives.

The interminable accumulation of stressful situations, and the psycho-physiological disorders this involves, have a powerful influence on the individual's interpretation of the world around them, and are responsible for maladjusted behaviour that can be both irrational and illogical.[22] The bias, prejudice and ineffectual information processing this produces is a powerful obstacle to the search for explanations and coping strategies. There is a need to recognise the deleterious effects of dangerous memories, depression, sleeplessness, nightmares and all the other symptoms associated with political violence, perpetual uncertainty, insecurity and misery and their effects on people's cognitive and deliberative capacities. Also, it is overlooked that survivors thinking for themselves and the implications of this for their self-respect are disregarded. Political violence has undermined their ability to assess how useful (or injurious) post-conflict conditions actually are. It also damages their ability to anticipate the type of emotion these conditions are responsible for.[23]

This has a detrimental effect on individual survivors and their ability to foresee the impact of stress on future well-being as well as individual and group behaviour.[24]

---

[18] Thoits, P., (1995).

[19] Folkman, S, Lazarus, R.S., Dunkel-Schetter, C., DeLongis, A., Gruen, R.J. (1986).

[20] See Lazarus, R.S., (1991).

[21] Folkman, S. Chesney, M. McKusick, L. Ironson, G. Johnson, D. & Coates, T., (1991) in Eckenrode, J. (ed); Lazarus, R., (1993) in L. Goldberger and S. Breznitz (Eds); Lazarus, R., (2000); Lazarus, R & Folkman, S., (1986).

[22] Harvey, J. H., Weary, G. (1981).

[23] Lazarus, R.S., (1991).

[24] Compas, B.E., Banes, G.A, Malcarne, V. & Worsham, N., (1991); Fontaine, K.R., Manstead, A.S.R., & Wagner, H., (1993); Maier, S. F., & Watkins, L. R. (1998)..

In these circumstances the frustration of such basic needs as safety, control predictability and self-respect become a significant influence on interpersonal relationships. Stress affects relationships with other individuals as much as it affects informal social practices involving communal and cooperative relationships or formal institutions like law and government.

This makes people less sure about the strategies they need to adopt in order to most effectively address their situation. Instead of approaching stressful situations in a focused, goal consistent manner people use strategies that tend not to be as situation specific, or subject to as much variation as those permitted in more optimal settings.[25]

This can be explained as the result of an individual's own confusion of ideas, poor clarity about future actions to take, depression and fear. It also serves to validate the individual's impression that traditional norms and values are ineffective and no longer able to address the psychological effects of difficult life conditions. In the absence of any strongly held values, the interplay between the individual and others becomes so distorted that the ideas of mutual recognition, trust, equal consideration and solidarity are rendered meaningless.[26] The relevance of these findings to such things as post-migration assistance, forced relocation, recovery from political stress, natural disasters, lawlessness and much more around the world is obvious.

4. Motivation and the Emergence of Individualism

Nearly all the survivors of the Peruvian violence underwent experiences that have degraded their relationships with other people, undermined social practices and contributed to forced migration. This has stifled any reason for continuing to believe in the idea that human solidarity is always right, and that existing relationships with other people are always beneficial.[27] To possess such a limited perception of control the individual survivor is less likely to search for and depend on instrumental social support because the benefits of human solidarity simply lack credibility.[28]

By failing to trust in traditional norms and values, the idea that obligations, responsibilities and accountability are an intrinsic part of life which do not change, even if a particular situation can seem insurmountable, has been seriously impugned. This makes people less sure about what is good, beneficial, important, useful, desirable, constructive, etc. Over time this growing uncertainty about the importance of traditional norms and values is no longer perceived as unnatural.

---

[25] Russell, A.M., & Fiske, S.T., (2010: 231ff in Guinote, A. and Vescio, T. (2010).

[26] Chouliaraki, L., (2017: 49–61) Suffering and the Ethics of Solidarity in Anderson, R.E. (ed) *Alleviating World Suffering*, Springer.

[27] McCann, I.L. & Pearlman, L.A., (1990); Pearlman, Laurie A., & Saakvitne, Karen W. (1995).

[28] Chouliaraki, L., (2017: 49–61) Suffering and the Ethics of Solidarity in Anderson, R.E. (ed) *Alleviating World Suffering*, Springer.

Instead the numbing effect produced by an environment of perpetual uncertainty removes the tendency for people to be accountable and take responsibility for their own shortcomings.

In such contexts, people cease to worry when others are in difficulties, or become agitated when others are in danger, fail to feel compassion for the suffering of others, and do not feel outrage when long-held beliefs about what should be valued and honoured are brought into question. It is possible therefore, to assert that the individual is not in a position to develop benevolent feelings of mutual recognition, trust, equal consideration and solidarity. Instead the fight for existence leads to a feeling of inevitability about the need to abandon all values and use all means available, no matter how reprehensible, in order to survive. By accepting the need to become more ruthless and more unscrupulous than everyone else, the individual is signifying their assent to conduct based on selfishness and indifference to others. It also amounts to an acknowledgement of the realities of this on-going struggle with some of the greatest psychological difficulties imaginable. In less extreme circumstances people do not usually have to stand alone emotionally to be effective, well-functioning human beings, but in a world where the patterns and routines of the past have failed to provide protection from ongoing misery and suffering no such ethical behaviour is possible.

This breakdown in human values has and continues to take place under conditions in which the identity and dignity of an individual is progressively weakened by the pain and harshness of reality including malnutrition, neglect, fear, social discrimination, depression, sleeplessness, nightmares and all the other symptoms associated with political violence. The resulting loss of dignity, self-respect and inability to depend on old certainties is responsible for such a state of confusion that the capacity to bear direct witness to ongoing misery and suffering is compromised.

In this way people are so unaffected by the reality in which they are living that they behave without any kind of emotional engagement. By 'anaesthetizing' themselves from the formidable burden of so many unpleasant and painful emotions survivors become vulnerable to psychological destruction. By accepting the need to use all means possible to sustain life the individual has rejected the importance of taking responsibility for their own actions and being accountable to others.

9.3 From Traditional Support Systems to New Routines of Self Preservation

By making people insensitive to the suffering of others the intrinsic value of mutual respect, liberty, and justice is largely blotted-out. This subordination of traditional norms and values to the immediate question of self-preservation is an inevitable consequence of the increasing distance between reality and people's awareness of their responsibility to others. In a context of dire need the struggle for survival is so overwhelming that the destruction of any shared experience of difficult life conditions, of any shared motivations that result from them, and of any shared inclinations for ways to satisfy motives, are all but inevitable.[29] To survive this collapse in traditional norms and values, the individual is forced to assume greater responsibility for their own future. If the individual is unable to count on other people for help and support, they must learn to rely on their own resources and personal coping strategies.

One lesson drawn from this study is that new situations and information make it imperative for the individual survivor to recognise that if they are to survive, they need to be tougher and more unscrupulous than everyone else, otherwise they will succumb. In this respect trust, compassion and solidarity are side-lined.[30]

However, the idea that people who suffer from economic and all the other hardships, including social injustice and political oppression can somehow make the psychological shift from passivity, fatalism and disempowerment into "…critical consciousness, an awakening of agency and the power to perform our roles differently, and a quickening of imaginations of desire"[31] is by no means straightforward.

To reduce the impact of lasting stressful events, the individual survivor needs to bring order and control to the situation. However, this is not always possible. Individuals and groups may be able to identify possible solutions to some of their problems, but lack of knowledge as to what to do and how to bring about a possible solution remains a powerful constraint. Adopting any coping action can make it difficult for survivors to control their own situation and meet their own needs and those of their dependents. It is, after all, much more difficult to work out what to do if the relationship between the individual and what is happening can no longer depend on empathy, compassion, shared judgement and other forms of connection with other people. This means that people may ultimately do nothing at all on the grounds that the solutions are too difficult, impossible to do, or likely to have negative consequences.

From this failure to make reality conform to their immediate needs, feelings of impotence, frustration and despair are inevitable. Instead of being self-directed and intellectually independent, people become overwhelmed by feelings of anxiety, shame, desperation, fear, confusion, withdrawal and self-loathing.[32]

---

[29] Staub, E. (1989:38ff).

[30] Chouliaraki, L., (2017: 49–61) Suffering and the Ethics of Solidarity in Anderson, R.E. (ed) *Alleviating World Suffering*, Springer.

[31] Watkins, M. & Shulman, H., (2008: 25).

[32] Mills, C. & Zavaleta, D., (2015: 251–269) Shame, Humiliation and Social Isolation in Anderson, R.E. (ed) *World Suffering & the Quality of Life*, Springer.

9.4 From Coping Strategies to Post-traumatic Growth

In highland Peru, trying to negotiate daily life where history remains an open wound undermines the individual's sense of responsibility for making up their own mind about the particular situation they find themselves in, and for their own overall conduct. The lack of comfort, comradeship and, shared destiny that people have to endure only serve to exacerbate this deficiency and the corrosive effect it has on any sense of responsibility and self-respect. In these circumstances the use of any available coping strategy is likely to be half hearted, unfocused and only a few steps away from the individual not being accountable for their own actions.[33] People are not just confused; they are overwhelmed by feelings of self-reproach and a profound sense of helplessness.

To combat the impact of so many negative emotions people tend to break the relationship between themselves and what is happenin, and physically withdraw from the situation. In this way people become insensitive to the suffering of others, to such an extent that the intrinsic value of mutual respect, liberty, and justice is simply blotted out. The fact that this cuts people off from any deep and living connections with their environment makes the outbreak of violence more likely as they seek to improve their situation by aggressive means without facing up to their own responsibilities. More commonly, but less obviously, this breakdown in the relationship between individuals and groups and what is happening will lead to a psychological as well as a physical withdrawal from the situation. This is tantamount to an admission of failure to find any rational solution to the broad range of continuous and lasting stressful events.

In these circumstances, survivors have little alternative but to make use of emotional and social support, not as a solution to the problems they face but as a form of relief.[34]

Though this may not change anything, it is still important because it may help to alleviate loneliness, fear, vulnerability, failure and uncertainty.[35] Using coping strategies that emphasize emotional and social support can provide opportunities for the transformation of the individual's own evaluation of the situation.

Instead of maintaining the belief that the current situation is hopeless and beyond their control, emotional and social support can produce fundamental changes to the individual's own perception of the situation. However, this potential for individual freedom of thought and action is conditional on the way in which the individual face up to their responsibilities in relation to others. Facing the pain and harshness of reality involves survivors having the courage not to abdicate their identity or capacity for initiative.

---

[33] Bugental, D.B., (2010: 209) in Guinote, A. and Vescio, T. (2010).

[34] Antonovsky, A., (1990), in M. Rosenbaum (Ed), (2000); Cederblad, M., Dahlen, L., Hagnell, O., & Hansson, K., (1995).

[35] Folkman, Chesney, Mckusick, Ironson, Johnson and Coastes, (1991); Folkman and Lazarus, (1984); Lazarus and Folkman, (1986); Sandin, (1995).

In this respect, no two survivors affected by the violence and struggling to survive react in the same way. It therefore follows that assignments of responsibility and questions of judgement derive from how, in the end, the individual chooses to respond to the restricted range of options available.

For any experience of positive change to emerge from their struggle with the violence and all of the other ongoing problems, survivors need to be able to respond to their situation in order to perceive challenges, and to recognize sufferings and conflicts. The first action then is critical self-reflection on the burden of the difficult conditions confronting the individual; a more difficult action is to interrupt "…how people prefer to think about the way things are and …reveal new and dangerous insights for the present."[36]

The starting point of this non-negative way of thinking therefore needs to focus on the feeling that no one is interested in allowing them to make sense of their situation, and that nothing can be done, and that further misery and suffering are inevitable.

To rediscover their devalued identity, people need to engage with what prevents them from acting with dignity, morality and principle. This involves the government and NGOs (as well as the survivors,) being open to the subversive memories of the survivors, and having a sense of the suffering of others, in order that human suffering can become the basis for responding to human problems. It is possible, therefore, to assert that non-negative ways of thinking can be nurtured only if victims *and* those who render assistance are sensitive to the subversive memories of the political violence, and the emotional intensity of the interruptions they make into how people think about the way things are.

Through an ability to share in the suffering of others the individual and outside help are able to look deeply into the debilitating effects of people's suffering and come to understand the situation as they perceive and cognitively construct it. From this perspective, victims and outsiders are in a position to challenge the way in which the government is able to neutralize the moral impact on the stressed, and impede the development of a democratic political culture.[37] This requires outside help, not only with the moral concerns of the survivors, but also with the determining influence of such concepts as power, culture, conflict, exploitation and hierarchy, and the meanings given to them.

By showing little remorse or regret for what happened, existing social structures, discourses and ideologies have created an environment in which outside indifference and objectivity about past injustices can only be challenged through resentment.

Though this is contrary to the fashionable idea "…that negative attitudes and emotions are detrimental to being truly human,"[38] continuing outrage and refusal to forgive, can be seen as a moral protest against what happened and a justifiable

[36] Metz, J.B., (1980: 171).

[37] Harvey, D. C., (2015: 269–281) The Cultural Geography of Community Suffering in Anderson, R.E. (ed) *World Suffering & the Quality of Life*, Springer.

[38] Brudholm, T., (2008: 49).

reaction to the disrespect shown to them in the aftermath of the political violence. Its capacity for exposing the deliberate concealment of particular memories also means that resentment is an invaluable resource for people continuing to live under the threat of resurgence in political violence. In this respect, resentment can be seen as "…the reflex expression of an honourable emotional response to inexpiable wrongs and legitimate moral expectations that have not been properly dealt with."[39]

9.5 Taking Things Forward

It remains to explore how progress might be made in highland Peru and how far lessons from the region are relevant elsewhere in the world. In recent years there have been new developments within the professions informed by the psychological wounding caused by war, violence, terror, rape, torture, disasters and poverty that address themes, such as historical memory and the importance of context. This provides a means by which people can begin to make sense of what happened to them, and their world, through the determining influence of context, culture and institutions (and the subjective nature that the individual brings to their situation).[40] In order to effect such changes, the overriding importance of such methodological concepts as empathy, compassion and participation is clear.

Much of the research for this study was based around the idea that an understanding of the adverse effects of material disadvantage, and the effects of insecurity, anxiety and lack of social integration would be critical to future development of wellbeing.

To describe these adverse effects with any confidence new methodological concepts are needed to counter the objectification of human suffering by the government and NGOs. To more fully explain human and social suffering and help survivors move from a position of detachment about their own past, to one that enables them to reclaim it, this section is organized around three areas of controversy that have arisen in the course of assessing fieldwork findings.

(a) **To conceptualise suffering and reparations in ways that account for the cultural and historical differences that shape the actual lived experience of individuals and social groups**

It is easy to lose sight of the meaning of physical and mental suffering discussed in the medium of academic prose, so it is important that every effort is made to provide as subtle an interpretation as possible. For human suffering to become as self-evident to others as it is to the sufferer, requires it to be brought into full view, together with all the various and intricate processes responsible for its unfolding

[39] Brudholm, T., (2008: 49).

[40] Dussaillant, F. & Gonzalez, P. A., (2015: 233–251) Lifetime Suffering and Capabilities in Chile in Anderson, R.E. (ed) *World Suffering & the Quality of Life*, Springer.

development. However, as with the body in pain, it is only when the experience of human suffering is externalised that it is possible to offer up the best opportunity for its being better understood.[41] To gain admission to the lives of the poor and vulnerable (and especially survivors of trauma and stress), and the physical and mental suffering that affects them, we need to look at the amount of access they have to basic resources including:

1. Physical resources such as food, water, shelter, safety;
2. Economic resources such as money, material goods, employment opportunities;
3. Social resources, such as acceptance, a sense of control, social support and a trusting social environment.

Since access to these resources is conditional on the capacity to influence others in psychologically meaningful ways, it is important that we start by looking at the sources of power that shape relationships between individuals, within groups and between groups.

In normal circumstances this would involve conventional coping mechanisms, such as popular mobilization, solidarity and grassroots organizations, but under difficult life conditions these are rarely strong enough for people to be able to coordinate social life and move shared goals forwards.[42] This compels people to re-appraise their situation, and if they are not too damaged, adopt new ideas and ways of thinking about the struggle for existence, and satisfying core self needs. Though this brings about changes in how people perceive each other, and how they see themselves, it does not automatically resolve the problems they are facing. This is a source of immense frustration and frequently leads to conflict and other forms of anti-social behaviour. These conditions make people less motivated, less engaged, less passionate and less resilient. In various situations the impact of hunger, deprivation, ill treatment, injustice and poor health might cause people to make use of scapegoats or form new groups and take up new ways of doing things. The impact this may have on accepted boundaries, the stability of people's identities, respect for traditional values and ideologies undermines support for established rules, fixed beliefs and practices, and can often render them meaningless. Physically weakened by malnutrition and other misfortunes, people delude themselves into thinking that they no longer have a moral duty to others as well as to themselves. Instead, they allow themselves to be persuaded that other motives take precedence and have greater importance. However, the idea that opting out from the challenges this situation presents is not so much unthinkable as fraught with the difficult problems that arise from having to live with its consequences.

Though memories of trauma, such as violence, kidnapping, murder, disappearances, torture, police brutality, drugs and rape may cause survivors to want to dispense with their past and abandon it in favour of a way of life more to their choice; this becomes not so much an act of liberation, as a death blow to the traditional

[41] Scarry, E., (1985: 52–3).

[42] Chouliaraki, L., (2017: 49–61) Suffering and the Ethics of Solidarity in Anderson, R.E. (ed) *Alleviating World Suffering*, Springer.

supports of social cohesion. By wilfully opening themselves up to the contradictory pressures of powerful outside forces, the poor and vulnerable become exposed to the horrors of abandonment, isolation, exclusion, rejection and helplessness. In these circumstances, meaningful interactions with other people can become so difficult as to make the loss of traditional safety nets (and the human contact they provide) only too apparent.[43]

To live under these conditions is daunting, but for the survivors of the political violence it means that there is even less opportunity for the development of non-negative thinking patterns to influence reactions to what happened. Once again, it is not so much the capacity to forget that is in question, as the ability to wilfully abandon the memory of what happened. In this way, and for all these reasons, human suffering is only likely to inspire sympathy, empathy and action for change if it is able to break through the system of defences that empty its meaning of all subjective content. If the subjective felt-experience borne out of the frustration of basic psychological and material needs is to influence social, political and institutional responses to human affliction and social need the attributes that belong to the individual's subjective felt-experience must be brought to the fore.[44] For many survivors the experience of the reparations schemes, and the problem of premature forgetting on behalf of the government, is reason enough to remain fearful and mistrustful that this will ever happen.

(b) **Social, political and institutional responses to suffering and reparations need to be conceptualised and examined in terms of the adverse effects of material disadvantage, insecurity, anxiety and lack of social integration instead of being assessed in terms of output-oriented legitimacy and service delivery**

Failing to come to terms with the problem of human and social suffering is a symptom of the post-Holocaust age. Out of sight is out of mind. If people are not linked to those that suffer in a meaningful way their capacity for empathy and compassion must always be in question. This failure to engage with the original experience of suffering by the government may be the result of its inherent complexity and because so much about it is irrational.

In addition, lack of consideration for the adverse effects of material disadvantage, insecurity, anxiety and lack of social integration can be because these things are of low importance for the government, and other elements from the dominant culture, especially if they concern the marginalised and other marginalised groups including Indigenous People.

To make the government and NGOs more alert to the consequences of human suffering, the experiences with which they are associated need to be brought into full view in all the various and unpredictable changes responsible for their unfold-

[43] Mills, C. & Zavaleta, D., (2015: 251–269) Shame, Humiliation and Social Isolation in Anderson, R.E. (ed) *World Suffering & the Quality of Life*, Springer.

[44] Dussaillant, F. & Gonzalez, P. A., (2015: 233–251) Lifetime Suffering and Capabilities in Chile in Anderson, R.E. (ed) *World Suffering & the Quality of Life*, Springer.

ing development. The notion that output oriented legitimacy and service delivery are the most important means of addressing suffering overlooks the human dimension of the situation. Because of its emphasis on impartiality, neutrality, tolerance and pluralism, the government has excluded any engagement with the social experience of suffering. By failing to regard survivors as individuals who have been unjustly treated, the government (and NGOs) have turned them into an abstract category, thereby blocking their own capacity for any meaningful engagement.

Through its use of an abstract and formal definition of the universal self, the government has effectively dissociated itself from the cultural and historical differences that shape the actual lived experience of people. To gain access to the subjective aspects of individual suffering, and the loss of meaning that accompanies it, new methodological concepts are needed to counter this objectification of human suffering.[45] Though the research presented in this study underscores the importance of a locally informed analysis, human and social suffering rarely has been studied using methods that involve the relationship between context and its influence on human nature and responsibility, and the failure of the social capital discourse. To that end, this study has sought to elaborate on the reaction and attitude of individuals and groups to the emotional consequences of human and social suffering.

Because suffering devalues people's identity it undermines their capacity to act with dignity, morality and principle, and forces them to internalise that which has been devalued. In this way the ability to identify with what those who directly experience suffering are thinking or feeling is made much harder, and consequently becomes even more important for suffering to be properly acknowledged so that appropriate responsibilities may be assumed.

(c) **To rescue suffering and reparations from a slow transmutation into efficiency and cost an addition of narratives, ethnographies and social histories need to be considered as a complement to economic indicators.**[46]

By restricting our understanding of suffering to economic indicators we lose sight of what it means for those who are most vulnerable to its effects. To restore dignity, morality and principle to our interpretation of human suffering a more powerful understanding of the subjective aspects of its individual effects, and the loss of meaning that accompanies it is needed.[47]

This means replacing the culture that insists on the exchangeability of one person for another with one in which the reality of each individual and their experience can be properly recognised.[48] To identify the structural and underlying causes of human

[45] Dussaillant, F. & Gonzalez, P. A., (2015: 233–251) Lifetime Suffering and Capabilities in Chile in Anderson, R.E. (ed) *World Suffering & the Quality of Life*, Springer.

[46] Kleinman, A. & Kleinman, J., (1997a), Kleinman, A. & Kleinman, J. (1997b: 15) in Kleinman, A., Das, V., and Lock, M. (eds.).

[47] Dussaillant, F. & Gonzalez, P. A., (2015: 233–251) Lifetime Suffering and Capabilities in Chile in Anderson, R.E. (ed) *World Suffering & the Quality of Life*, Springer.

[48] Harvey, D. C., (2015: 269–281) The Cultural Geography of Community Suffering in Anderson, R.E. (ed) *World Suffering & the Quality of Life*, Springer.

and social suffering and what fuels it, we need to understand the debilitating effects of prolonged exposure to psychological demands when the ability to control the situation is perceived to be limited. In this way, the long-term consequences of physical and mental suffering and their impact on people, can be demonstrated. This requires engagement not only with people affected by political violence living in conditions of extreme poverty, but with the policies and programmes responsible for the objectification of human suffering. From this perspective, we need to recognize that the particular situation people find themselves in is as significant for policy makers and programme planners as it is for individuals and groups affected by physical and mental suffering. Instead of a culture that insists on the exchangeability of one person for another, a shift from the universal to the particular is needed in order that the reality of the individual and their experience can be properly recognised.[49]

To advance our understanding of the integrated psychosocial nature of human beings and how they manage and shape the everyday world we need to gain access to the reality of what it is like to live in conditions of low trust, anxiety, high vigilance and low safety nets. This requires a reformulation of policy making and the tools used. If a new generation of policies and programmes cannot begin their interventions by means of a more focused and localised approach the government will never be able to find out more about the feelings, opinions and attitudes held by local people in relation to their situation, and how they have strived to adapt themselves to it. Initiatives are needed to develop mutual understanding, straighten out conflicts, build connections and construct meaningful partnerships and other relationships.

In this respect, the far-reaching psychological implications of suffering make empathy and participation a pre-requisite for improving the seriousness of the relationship between the government, NGOs, and the powerless. To reposition suffering in terms that respect the uniqueness of the individual narratives, ethnographies and social histories relating to people's perceptions of the main structural factors affecting them as individuals and as groups are needed. This is only possible if the culture that insists on the exchangeability of one person for another is dispensed with and replaced by one in which the reality of each individual and their experience can be properly recognised.[50]

9.6 Concluding Observations

Suffering is all too common. Suffering transcends time. It devalues the importance of planning for the future. It undermines the capacity to remember earlier past suffering. It puts an end to empathy and compassion. It undermines mutual respect,

---

[49] Harvey, D. C., (2015: 269–281) The Cultural Geography of Community Suffering in Anderson, R.E. (ed) *World Suffering & the Quality of Life*, Springer.

[50] Harvey, D. C., (2015: 269–281) The Cultural Geography of Community Suffering in Anderson, R.E. (ed) *World Suffering & the Quality of Life*, Springer.

liberty, and justice. And it is often misunderstood and misinterpreted. There is almost nothing it cannot affect. Being unable (or unwilling) to unify past, present and future aspects of their own lives makes people live in ways that are incompatible with their own particular situation. Sometimes people ignore this. Other times people deceive themselves about the importance of suffering or their own responsibility for it; or, people may feel crippled by feelings of loss, shame or guilt about it. In summary, suffering is inconsistent with relationships that give meaning to life.[51]

To make people more alert to the causes and consequences of human suffering, the experiences with which it is associated therefore need to be brought into full view.

In recent years suffering has attracted the interest of scholars, researchers and practitioners from a range of disciplines including medical anthropology, ethnography, psychology, philosophy, theology, media studies, development studies, migration studies, memory studies and holocaust studies. However, the impact of suffering on social, political and institutional responses to human affliction and social need has been more muted and restrained. This is damaging for the study of human affliction and social need, just as much as it is damaging for those affected by it. To sharpen our thinking and challenge existing modes of political decision making, professional practice and policy formation a new approach is needed.

To be effective future intervention will need to involve psychosocial approaches based around the adverse effects of material disadvantage and the effects of insecurity, anxiety and lack of social integration. To describe these conditions with any confidence new methodological concepts are needed to counter the objectification of human suffering by the government and other outsiders such as researchers and NGOs. Using results obtained from the fieldwork undertaken for this study these new methodological concepts were organised around three issues.

1. To conceptualise suffering and reparations in ways that account for the cultural and historical differences that shape the actual lived experience of individuals and social groups.
2. Social, political and institutional responses to suffering and reparations need to be conceptualised and examined in terms of the adverse effects of material disadvantage, insecurity, anxiety and lack of social integration instead of being assessed in terms of output-oriented legitimacy and service delivery.
3. To rescue suffering and reparations from a slow transmutation into efficiency and cost an addition of narratives, ethnographies and social histories need to be considered as a complement to economic indicators.[52]

Much of this study research was based around the idea that an understanding of the legacy of the political violence, the adverse effects of material disadvantage, insecurity, anxiety and lack of social integration would provide a useful contribution

[51] Mills, C. & Zavaleta, D., (2015: 251–269) Shame, Humiliation and Social Isolation in Anderson, R.E. (ed) *World Suffering & the Quality of Life*, Springer.

[52] Kleinman, A. & Kleinman, J., (1997a, b: 15) in Kleinman, A., Das, V., and Lock, M. (eds.) (1997a, b).

toward a more integrated conceptualization of suffering. By focusing on the determining influence of culture, context and institutions (and the subjective nature that the individual brings to their situation), this study seeks to bring a more holistic response to the subject.

By documenting the psychological, cultural and social origins of responsibility, accountability and decision making, this study set out to demonstrate what happens to people who suffer from economic and all the other hardships, including social injustice and political oppression. In effect, the study has sought to show how the combined impact of these various forms of suffering undermines motivation and leads to unprecedented levels of disconnectedness.

The findings from this study contain a range of issues that bring our attention to the reality of what it is like to live in conditions of low trust, anxiety, high vigilance and low safety nets, and are likely to provide useful insights for other places in the world where irresponsibility and a frivolous disregard for the value of other people are ignored and go unpunished. The findings also point to a range of important consequences for people losing their connections with the past, and how this is affecting their own integral place in the world.

If circumstances are such that they prevent people from being able to keep the experience of extreme events present in their mind as historical memory, they will be unable to bear witness as to what happened, and therefore in no position to work through their experiences of extreme events. From a psychoanalytic perspective, this has a particular significance because the originality and the irreplaceable value of their experiences is something that connects the content of what they experienced to a way of being and existing.

If people are denied the opportunity to attest to their own experiences of extreme events they will be unable to escape the constant re-run of their own traumatic memories. In these circumstances the differences between internal and external spaces and past and present are eroded and the power of memory for breaking the *status quo* is undermined, and with it any sensitivity to suffering and to morality. To escape from this situation people, need to re-establish their status as individuals by being able to speak of their experiences. In this way, people are better placed to recreate some type of link at the point where the break first took place and so begin the process of recovering their own lost dignity and self-respect.

From this perspective, it is appropriate to end this study by including some observations made by Martin-Baro regarding the relationship between suffering and reparation, and how this should be interpreted for the benefit of all concerned: "It is clear that no one is going to return to the imprisoned dissident his youth; to the young woman who has been raped her innocence; to the person who has been tortured his or her integrity. Nobody is going to return the dead and the disappeared to their families. What can and must be publicly restored [are] the victims' names and their dignity, through a formal recognition of the injustice of what has occurred, and, wherever possible, material reparation.

Those who clamour for social reparation are not asking for vengeance. Nor are they blindly adding difficulties to a historical process that is already by no means easy. On the contrary, they are promoting the personal and social viability of a new society, truly democratic."[53] Needless to say this has implications that extend far beyond rural highland communities affected by political violence in the south-central Andes of Peru.

[53] Martin-Baro, I., (1990) in Hassett, J. & Lacey, H., (1991: 138–140); Martin-Baro, (1990) in Hassett, J. & Lacey, H., (1991: 184–186).

Appendices

Appendix 1

T. J. Bowyer, *Beyond Suffering and Reparation*,
https://doi.org/10.1007/978-3-319-98983-9

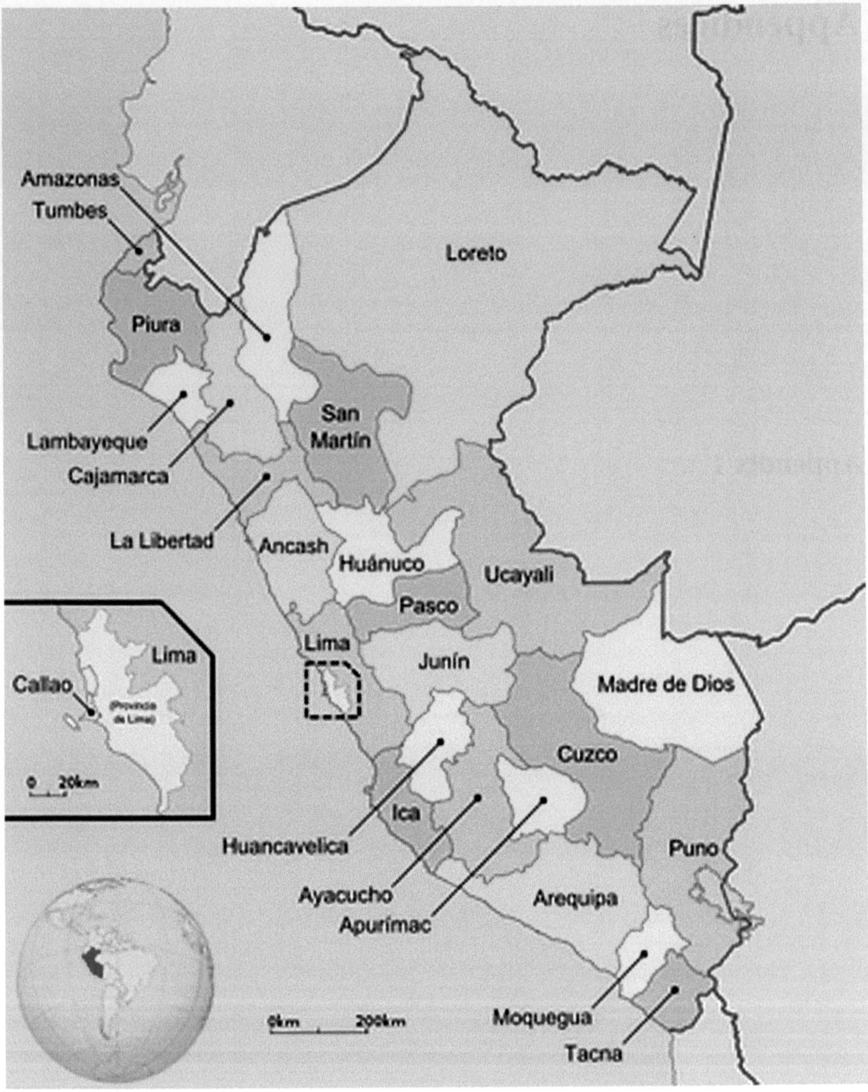

Map 1 Political Departments in Peru

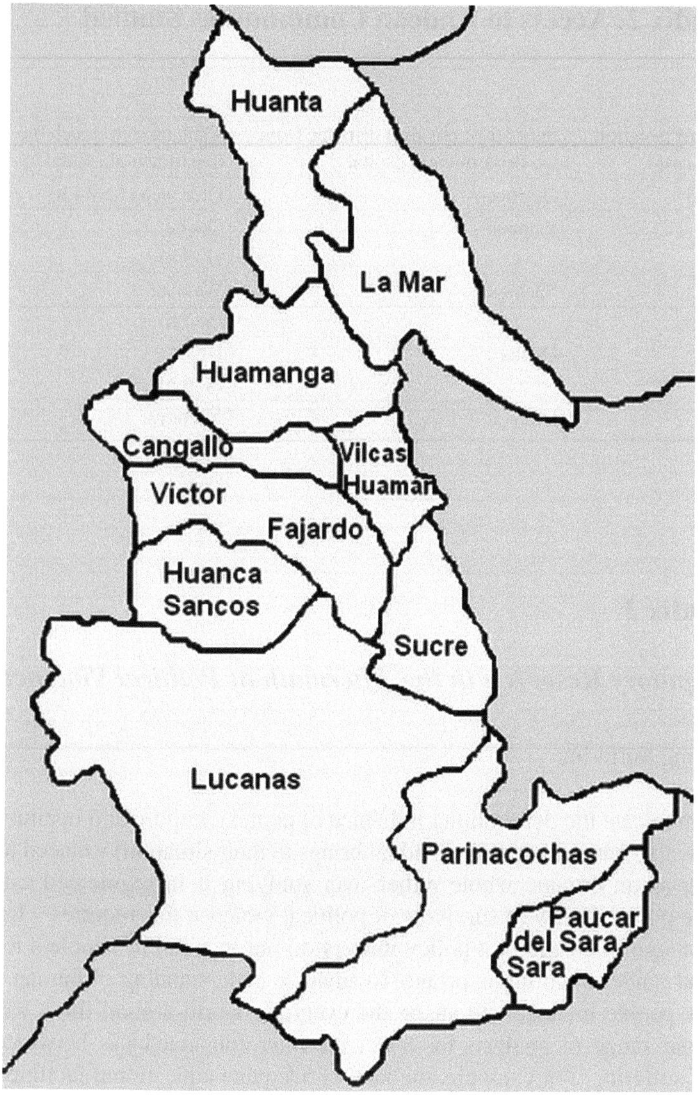

Map 2 Provinces of the Department of Ayacucho

Appendix 2: Access to Andean Communities Studied

In order of isolation (Road access)	In order of physical distance from the departmental capital	Time taken to reach the departmental capital by vehicle
Otoronco	Otoronco	Otoronco (12–14 h)
Wamani	Wamani	Qocha
		(7–9 h)
Yachaya	Yachaya	Wamani
		(5–7 h)
Qocha	Qocha	Unay
		(4–6 h)
Unay	Unay	Yachaya
		(3–5 h)

Appendix 3

Participatory Research in the Aftermath of Political Violence

Rethinking Suffering

To communicate the determining influence of context, culture and institutions (and the subjective nature that the individual brings to their situation) we need to explore suffering as an organic whole rather than studying it in segmented categories.[1] From the point of view of survivors of political violence this requires a framework broad enough to ensure that policy makers do not respond to people's feelings in ways that render them unimportant. To advance understanding of human suffering and how people manage and shape the everyday world around them we need to extend our range of analysis to reflect the inter-connectedness between specific types of suffering. For example, the lack of adequate educational facilities is often linked to delinquent behaviour, domestic violence and other forms of social disintegration within the community that encourage young people to leave both school and community in search of work in the local towns and cities or as drugs mules in the Amazon region. Such inter-connectedness is intended to assist policy makers to

[1] Kleinman, A. & Kleinman, J., (1997a, b: 8) in Kleinman, A., Das, V., and Lock, M. (eds.) (1997a, b); Dussaillant, F. & Gonzalez, P. A., (2015: 233–251) Lifetime Suffering and Capabilities in Chile in Anderson, R.E. (ed)*World Suffering & the Quality of Life*, Springer; Harvey, D. C., (2015: 269–281) The Cultural Geography of Community Suffering in Anderson, R.E. (ed) *World Suffering & the Quality of Life*, Springer.

view the causes and impacts of suffering in a holistic way and so move from individual reduction interventions towards more integrated, trans-disciplinary holistic study-based strategies.

To understand how people, perceive and cognitively react to their situation we need to examine what takes place within the community and in its exchange with outsiders. It is also important to avoid undue reliance on easily identifiable suffering.[2] To strengthen the analysis the framework needs to represent both the factors that accentuate and make more severe the underlying causes of suffering[3] as well as the nature of its structural and underlying causes.[4]

From the perspective of people in the Andean highlands this requires a trans-disciplinary and holistic approach able to capture the multiple links between the fields of psychiatry, politics, philosophy, sociology, anthropology and law (from a historical perspective).[5]

It should be stressed that communicating an accurate recognition of how people perceive and react to suffering in a manner that is sufficiently respectful of their experiences is not a precise science.[6] Nevertheless, by paying attention to the root causes that enhance or reinforce the effect of individual types of suffering it is possible to gain a better understanding of how people think, feel and act in relation to a socio-political environment that is as unpredictable as it is subject to almost indefinite revision. To this end the transformative effect of the post-conflict environment is examined from within a three-fold dialectic: (1) the *insider-outsider* dialectic, (2) that of emotion and rationality and (3) the dialectic of tradition and innovation.[7] This is critical to the success of any long-lasting effort to overcome the effects of the political violence and the consequences of living in a context of daily survival because it allows us to make a connection with other people's feelings.

---

[2] Easily identifiable occurrences comprise those aspects of suffering that are easily visible. Examples may be civil unrest, high unemployment, ethnic marginalisation, displaced people, delinquency, corruption, etc. See for example, Kleinman, A. & Kleinman, J. (1991a, b); (1997a, b); Wilkinson, I. (2005a, b); Prilletensky, I. (2008a, b).

[3] These comprise those aspects of suffering that can support or create the conditions for exacerbating the effects of individual types of suffering. They may change over time. Examples may be insecurity, fear, psycho-social stress, increase in the poverty level, sustained isolation and neglect, etc. See for example, Kleinman, A. & Kleinman, J. (1991a, b); (1997a, b); Wilkinson, I. (2005a, b); Prilletensky, I. (2008a, b).

[4] These are necessary, but not sufficient, causes of suffering, and tend to be well established and entrenched in the system. Examples may be poor governance, absence of the rule of law, lack of respect for fundamental rights, ethnic discrimination, marginalized history, etc.

[5] Pouligny, B., Chesterman, S. & Schnabel, A. (2007: 4).

[6] Schwartz, W., (2002); Schwartz W (2013).

[7] The need for a trans-disciplinary analysis of the impact of mass crime on the re-building of social and political relations using this three-fold dialectic was first put forward by Pouligny, B., Chesterman, S. & Schnabel, A. (2007: 4).

These are conditions that require participation and a willingness to imagine what it is like to be someone else, not detachment and objectivity. However, the use of narratives, ethnographies and social histories are at odds with the exclusion of the social experiences of suffering from the formulation of health and social policy.

Unless the economic measurement of suffering can be overturned as the only authorised construction of suffering the subjective felt experience of suffering will have no place in the lives of people affected by political violence.[8] For as long as this reductionist approach continues it will block any engagement with a world dominated by emotions, where behaviour is unpredictable and where it is possible to "…tolerate an inexact answer of what another person may feel."[9]

In this respect the limited impact of collective reparations for conflict affected communities, the policy of providing documentation for people and adding them to the civil registry and the registration of victims by the Truth and Reconciliation Commission (TRC)*Comisión de la Verdad y Reconciliación* (CVR) testify to the failure to engage with human suffering in a way that is meaningful to survivors.[10]

To better understand the emotional consequences of human suffering LaCapra developed an approach that involves feeling for another without losing sight of the distinction between one person's experience and the experience of the other. He calls this "empathic unsettlement" to denote the desired type of affective involvement and to distinguish it from what he calls "…self-sufficient, projective or incorporative identification."[11] Proper use of this approach can provide us with the opportunity to understand and anticipate the diversity of human experience because it engages with the subjective.

However, it is also likely to create problems for understanding how the past is remembered and interpreted as well as what the individual makes of a particular situation. This is because the reaction of one individual to the emotions being experienced by another can be interpreted in so many different ways.[12]

[8] Kleinman, A. & Kleinman, J., (1997a, b: 15); Dussaillant, F. & Gonzalez, P. A., (2015: 233–251) Lifetime Suffering and Capabilities in Chile in Anderson, R.E. (ed)*World Suffering & the Quality of Life*, Springer.

[9] Baron-Cohen, S. (2011: 83); Morris, D.B. (1991); Bryant, R.A., O' Donnell, M.L., Creamer, M,McFarlane, A.C., Silove, D. (2013); Buss, D.M. & Malamuth, N. (1996); McCann, I.L. & Pearlman, L.A. (1990a, b).

[10] *Comisión de la Verdad y Reconciliación* (Truth and Reconciliation Commission) installed in 2001, final report delivered in 2003.

[11] LaCapra, D., (2001: 40); See also Silverman, K. (1996).

[12] LaCapra, D., (2001: 78).

Psychological Dimensions of Suffering

To ground the determining influence of culture, context and institutions (and the subjective nature that the individual brings to their situation) it is important to begin by identifying some of the common feelings, emotions and behaviours associated with people affected by political violence and living in a context of daily survival.[13]

1. **Anxiety** is associated with feelings of nervousness and panic, especially when faced by reminders of the event; it is also associated with concerns about losing control or not coping. Post-Traumatic Stress Disorder (PTSD) may develop following exposure to any one of a variety of stressful events that involve actual or threatened death, or serious injury.[14] Traumatic life events are seen as the biggest cause of anxiety and depression and can also cause people to worry that the situation may recur. It is also linked to a fear of anxiety-related sensations. For example, anxiety-sensitivity.[15] Recent research demonstrates that how a person thinks about these events determines the level of stress they experience.[16]
2. **Hyper-vigilance** is an enhanced state of sensory sensitivity accompanied by an exaggerated intensity of behaviours the purpose of which is to detect threats. Hyper-vigilance is also accompanied by a state of increased anxiety, which can cause exhaustion. Other symptoms include: abnormally increased arousal, a high responsiveness to stimuli, and a constant scanning of the environment for cues of danger or seeing threat in things that would have appeared innocent before.[17]
3. **Sleep disturbance/insomnia**[18] are frequently associated with post-traumatic stress. It tends to manifest as a combination of insomnia and a higher-than-

[13] See Suarez, E., (2013); Charbonneau, B. and Parent, G., (eds) (2012); Justino, P., (2009); Srinisvasa Murthy, R and Lakshminayaranah, R., (2006); Brinkerhoff D. W., (2005); Moser, C., (1996); Moser, C., (1998); Dussaillant, F. & Gonzalez, P. A., (2015: 233–251) Lifetime Suffering and Capabilities in Chile in Anderson, R.E. (ed) *World Suffering & the Quality of Life*, Springer.

[14] Regel, S. & Joseph, S., (2010: 8) . A full list of the diagnostic criteria for PTSD is provided by the National Centre for PTSD (see http://ncptsd.kattare.com/ncmain/ncdocs/fact_shts/fs_dsm_iv_tr.html)

[15] Reiss, S. & McNally, R.J. (1985) in S Reiss & R.R. Bootzin (eds.); See also Shapiro, F., Silk Forrest, M.S. (1997).

[16] Kinderman, P., Schwannauer, M., Pontin, E. Tai, S., (2013).

[17] Zayfert, C. & DeViva, J., (2005).

[18] Cardena, E. & Spiegel, D. (1993; Sloan, P. (1988).

expected prevalence of Sleep-Disordered Breathing (SDB). In this model of complex sleep disturbance, the underlying sleep patho-physiology interacts with PTSD and related psychiatric distress.[19] The dreams, nightmares and other forms of sleep disturbance may be about the incident itself or the change but over time these can change to become less specific, but just as unsettling and generally disturbing.[20]

4. **Intrusive memories**[21] comprise stimuli that were present immediately before the traumatic event happened or shortly before the moments that had the largest emotional impact. For example, when the meaning of the event became more traumatic. Intrusive memories have acquired the status of warning signals, i.e., stimuli that if encountered again would indicate impending danger. Other intrusive thoughts and images include flashbacks of the traumatic incident, which appear out of the blue without any triggers or reminders[22]
5. **Guilt**[23] is a cognitive or an emotional experience that occurs when a person realizes or believes – accurately or not – that he or she has compromised his or her own standards of conduct or has violated a moral standard, and bears significant responsibility for that violation.[24] It is responsible for feelings of regret, about not having acted or coped as well as one would have wished, about letting oneself or others down, about being in some way responsible.[25]
6. **Sadness** is an integral part of post-traumatic stress. It involves feelings about having been victimized, about having developed a persistent mental disorder, about how few people understand what has happened, about how few people understand how the victim's life has been changed as a result, and about how difficult it is for these feelings to be effectively addressed. These are feelings of low mood and tearfulness that are associated with loss and horror and linked to a traumatic bereavement.[26]

---

[19] Krakow, B., Melendrez, D., Warner, T.D. Dorin, R., Harper, R., Hollifield, M. (2002).

[20] Brenneis, C.B. (1994); Mellman, T.A., David, D., Bustamente, V., Torres, J., & Fins, A. (2001).

[21] Ehlers, A., Hackmann, A., Steil, R., Clohessy, S., Wenninger, K., Winter, H. (2002).

[22] Frankel, F.H. (1994).

[23] See, for example, Lewis, H. B., (1971).

[24] Guilt, Encyclopaedia of Psychology 2nd ed. Ed. Bonnie R. Strickland Gale Group, Inc., 2001. eNotes.com. 2006. 31 December 2007; Wiseman, H.; Metzl, E.; Barber, J. P. (2006); Brudholm, T. & Cushman, T. (2009); Domhoff, G. (1998); Operario, D. & Fiske, S.T. (2001); Staub, E. (2003); Lynd, H.M. (1958: 20–26); Lewis, H. B., (1971); Morris, H. (1991: 59–63); Cheftez, J.S. (2008); Carr, S.C. & Sloan, T.S. (2008).

[25] Nishith, P., Nixon, R.D.V., Resick, P.A., (2005); Resick, P.A., Nishith, P., Weaver, T.L., Astin, M.C., Feuer, C.A., (2002).

[26] See Jacob, S., (1999); Prigerson, H.G., Shear, M.K., Frank, E., Beery, L.C., Silberman, R., Prigerson, J. et al. (1997); Sheer, M.K., & Smith-Caroff, K. (2002).

7. **Irritability and anger**[27] recognized as a feature of clinical disorders that result from trauma. It is commonly associated with PTSD, for which "…anger is considered a salient attribute of the arousal symptom cluster."[28] Irritability and anger manifest as a result of what happened and at the injustice of the event; it is directed at those who are thought to be responsible for the trauma and associated with feelings of wanting somebody to accept responsibility or blame. The frustration that this gives rise to can also result in irritability and other symptoms of incapacity that are often directed at loved ones, close family, friends or colleagues.
8. **Disappointment** for people affected by political violence can arise because they believe that people including members of their own family do not really understand how they are feeling. Disappointment can also arise from the amnesty process used by Truth Commissions in the aftermath of political violence. This is because Truth Commissions tend to give emphasis to 'restorative justice' as opposed to 'punitive justice.' This means that amnesty is granted to perpetrators. The lack of justice this produces is an inevitable source of disappointment for the survivors. Other sources of disappointment relating to the political violence are likely to include the failure to charge perpetrators for lack of evidence.

   People affected by political violence are also subject to disappointment as a result of the failure on behalf of the state to implement any effective reparations payments/compensation. This disappointment can apply to both and individual and collective forms of reparations. This is also responsible for keeping the victims of political violence and their descendants in poverty indefinitely.[29]
9. **Mental avoidance/concentration deficits** are associated with avoiding thoughts to do with trauma.[30] People affected by political violence try to push distressing thoughts out of their head, often unsuccessfully, and in the longer term this can result in further problems because it interferes with the person processing and making sense of their experience. Empirically identified responses to traumatic events include reduced awareness of the environment,

[27] Sloan, P. (1988).

[28] Novaco, Raymond W.; Chemtob, Claude M; Follette, Victoria M. (Ed); Ruzek, Josef I. (Ed); Abueg, Francis R. (Ed), (1998: 162–190).

[29] See for example: Reparations in Peru: From Recommendations to Implementation, (2013), International Center for Transitional Justice 5 Hanover Square. Floor 24, New York, NY USA 10004

[30] Cardena, E. & Spiegel, D. (1993); North, C.S., Smith, E.M., McCool, R.E. & Lightcap, P.E. (1989).

derealisation, depersonalisation, dissociative amnesia, avoidance behaviour, sleep disorders, narcolepsy, poor concentration, etc.[31]

10. **Behavioural avoidance**[32] In psychology, avoidance coping, or escape coping, is a maladaptive coping mechanism characterized by the effort to avoid dealing with a stressor – avoiding thoughts, feelings, activities that are reminders of the trauma. This is a symptom of behaviours that attempt to protect oneself from psychological damage. Variations of avoidance coping include modifying or eliminating the conditions that gave rise to the problem and changing the perception of an experience in a way that neutralizes the problem. PTSD symptoms are thought to be precursors to avoidance coping: PTSD sufferers draw into themselves, avoiding the trauma and partaking in cognitive or behavioural avoidance coping.
11. **Erratic behaviour** is associated with people who have experienced, witnessed, or confronted an event or events that involved actual or threatened death or serious injury, or a threat to the physicalintegrity of self or others may experience intense feelings and symptoms that include panic, trembling, trembling, agitation, rambling speech, sleep disorders and erratic behaviour.[33]

Communication of Suffering

It is not always possible for the nature, scale and on-going character of human suffering to be made as self-evident to others as it is to the sufferer. In the absence of any supra-individual quality that effectively represents the subjective felt-experience of the sufferer the only vehicle through which the subjective content of the lived experience may be communicated is language.[34] However, the difference between the experience of living in a context of absolute material want and the account that people are able to give of it can give rise to such despair that people may feel that it is beyond the power of language to communicate.[35]

---

[31] Bryant, R.A., et al., (2013).

[32] Friedman, H. S.; Silver, R.C., (2006: 124).

[33] Glick, R.L. Berlin, J.S. Fishkind, A., Zeller, S.L. (2008).

[34] "Suffering for Frank is "…the unspeakable as opposed to what can be spoken; it is what remains concealed, impossible to reveal…At the core of suffering is the sense that something is irreparably wrong with our lives, and wrong is the negation of what could not have been right." Frank, A.W. (2001: 355).

[35] Scarry, E., (1985: 13) argues that there is an "…inherent difficulty of accurately describing any event whose central content is bodily pain or injury."

Though the individual's subjective felt-experience may help to stimulate the actual exercise of people's emotional capacities it does not also mean that this will translate into action.[36] Even though human suffering has the capacity to inform critical thinking in ways that nothing else can, it also resists representation and destroys speech.[37] The communication of suffering is not a simple matter, and this can be demonstrated by ten key obstacles, each discussed in turn, as follows:

- Language as inadequate
- Pressures of daily survival
- Erosion of memory
- Hollowing out of language
- Scapegoating as diversion
- Decontextualized perceptions
- Failure to empathise
- Disillusionment and apathy
- Passivity legitimised understanding/acceptance
- Prioritising the self

1. Language as inadequate.

The experience of suffering is not easy to communicate because the actual use of words is inadequate; the subjective feelings of suffering do not translate effectively.[38] In a context of hunger, deprivation, ill treatment, injustice and poor health the idea of suffering has implications for how people think, feel and act that would not apply in other situations.[39] Such conditions force people to live in a world that is devoid of meaning; in which brutal circumstances impose themselves on people against their will.

And because the influence is anonymous and cumulative, it is also corrosive, which undermines people's identity and sense of dignity. Ill-treatment, injustice and condescension are so damaging and intrusive that they diminish the convictions of ordinary people and give rise to a pervasive paralysis and deadening of intellectual, mental and emotional life. Over time this can be so debilitating as to make people willing to abandon their sense of responsibility for what they do.

---

[36] Dussaillant, F. & Gonzalez, P. A., (2015: 233–251) Lifetime Suffering and Capabilities in Chile in Anderson, R.E. (ed) *World Suffering & the Quality of Life*, Springer.

[37] Geddes, J.L., (2009: 22), in Brudholm, T. & Cushman, T, (2009).

[38] Scarry (1985: 4–5): argues that "...suffering defies language and as an experience is utterly un-shareable."

[39] Geddes, J.L., (2009: 23).

This is suffering of an altogether different character to that associated with some sudden violent experience, which is why it is inappropriate to apply psychoanalytic categories from everyday life to extreme situations.

2. Pressures of daily survival.

The context of daily survival seriously compromises the sufferer's capacity to communicate complex thought and emotion.[40] This is because the immediate question of self-preservation makes such immense, unrestrained demands on the individual that subtle distinctions disappear.[41] Instead of a more nuanced appraisal the individual's assessment of their situation is governed by such dualistic categories as 'purity and danger', pain and relief from pain, victim and executioner, the edible and the inedible, a safe place to hide and an unsafe place to hide.[42]

However, this need to empty much of the subjective content of the lived experience from what is being communicated is not consistent with the idea of language as an effective medium for representing human suffering.[43] Instead of yielding up insights into the single lived subjectivity of an individual or group human suffering is compressed into the linguistic straightjacket of normalization and relativization.[44] This use of standard categories and concepts for describing the individual's subjective felt-experience does little to help reduce the distance between the inner world of the particular individuals who suffer in their daily lives and the perception and understanding of the other.[45]

3. Erosion of memory.

The power of language to communicate in a context of daily survival undermines the individual's relationship between past, present and future. For many people the incessant struggle to satisfy core self and group-serving needs will make it impos-

[40] For Caruth the physical condition of the human being may simply exacerbate the "…dilemma that underlies many survivors' reluctance to translate their experience into speech." In Caruth, C. (1996: 153–4). See also Bettelheim, B., (1960: 237) in reprinted Penguin Edition (1991).

[41] Geddes, J.L., (2009: 21).

[42] Alford, C. F. (2009: 37). Douglas, M., (1966).

[43] Geras, N. (1998: 131).

[44] For Agamben, "The concepts of responsibility, accountability, dignity and respect are also irremediably contaminated by the consequences of de-contextualisation. Anyone who has tried to make use of these terms outside the juridical sphere knows this." Agamben, G., (1999: 20ff).

[45] For the purposes of this study "distance" is particularly marked since people from the research communities are mainly mono-lingual Quechua speakers and most government officials speak Spanish only. See Geddes, J.L., (2009: 26) Religious Rhetoric in Responses to Atrocity, in Brudholm, T. & Cushman, T, (2009).

sible to create any distance between themselves and the present. Those who do go beyond the immediate exigencies of finding enough food for themselves and their family face other difficulties. Investigating other sources of information and knowledge may help improve access and control of future material and other necessities, but the time and energy this involves does not change real conditions, any more than it guarantees long term success. The likelihood that such a course of action will involve people in situations where they are powerless to influence the powerful is a source of anxiety that will deter many and defeat others. This disparity between what positive actions people are able to take and what they are actually compelled to live with is a source of immense frustration and resentment. In relational terms the psychological and social injuries of enforced passivity, debasement and the feeling that the situation is as unjustified as it is unwanted are an additional influence on the strategies people employ to deal with their situation.

This has a tendency to make people turn inwards and feel as though they have been cursed, leading to biases in information processing, potential conflict and a further erosion of respect, dignity and self-respect.

4. The hollowing out of language.

The tendency for post-conflict poor people to abandon traditional norms and values undermines the power of language to communicate suffering. This happens because impoverished survivors from political violence do not have access to any safe space in which they can reclaim their experience of extreme events. One consequence of this is for the memory of traumatic events to be recited as a series of facts without the accompanying of emotions. In a context of absolute material want the absence of any safeguards, security or stability make such people indifferent, apathetic and self-absorbed; they may give up hope, fail to take responsibility for their own lives and allow despair to overwhelm them. In this world of hunger, corruption, demoralization and despair mental abilities are damaged, sometimes extensively. Such relentless misery increases people's vulnerability to exploitation, making humiliation and inhumane treatment by other individuals and groups commonplace.[46] It also makes people defensive and wanting to block out painful or unpleasant emotions, even if this is at the expense of other people's feelings. Lifton has called this "psychic numbing" and the more stressful the situation the more likely it is for people to abandon their responsibilities, both to themselves and to others.[47] Over time such violations of social norms and behaviour causes the locus of power to shift from the group to the individual, generating increased friction and rivalries and obstructing solidarity. For people locked into a set of conditions where

[46] Mills, C. & Zavaleta, D., (2015: 251–269)Shame, Humiliation and Social Isolation in Anderson, R.E. (ed)*World Suffering & the Quality of Life*, Springer.

[47] Lifton, R.J. (1982).

the quality of life is poor the submergence of the individual into the group offers an escape from personalresponsibility and its attendant obligations.

This breakdown in respect for borders, positions and rules is an outright challenge to the idea that much of what human beings do is done out of a sense of belongingness.[48] Such an approach to social relationships and the workings of the social environment is therefore not about the individual's support for established rules, fixed beliefs and practices, but about their use of collective identity to disburden themselves of personal responsibility.[49] This subordination of personal responsibilities to those of the group makes it easier for the individual to adopt strategies that do not require them to take responsibility for themselves or their actions.[50] In such a situation the individual is able to become entirely passive and leave all decisions and responsibilities to others. It also makes it more difficult for the individual to distance themselves from the values of the group should a shift in beliefs and practices of the group occur. This increases the probability that people will use all means honest and otherwise, including brute force, opportunism, theft and betrayal of friends in order to save themselves.

5. Scapegoating as diversion

It is easy to lose sight of the particular individuals involved, each of whom experience and endure suffering and misery in different ways, with different degrees of resourcefulness and different consequences.[51] The frustration of basic psychological needs by social conditions means that different social contexts produce different ways of thinking about and experiencing the situation at both the individual and group level.[52] For many people the immediate question of sheer self-preservation will motivate people to seek refuge from harsh realities in a parallel universe in which it is possible to believe that problems are both manageable and predictable. Finding a scapegoat is not just a source of psychological comfort, but a means of avoiding the harshness of the situation and a means of evading self-knowledge as well.[53]

---

[48] Fromm, E., (1997).

[49] Simon, B. & Klandermans, B, (2001).

[50] See for example, Scott Peck, M., (1983: 214).

[51] See Greenberg, I., (1989: 327) in Roth, J.K., & Berenbaum, M. (1989) cited in Geddes, J.L., (2009: 23).

[52] See, for example, Geras, N. (1998: 86).

[53] Embedded in a group allows people to give up individual decision making to the group and its leaders See for example, Milgram, S., (1974); Zimbardo, P., (1969).

In these circumstances there are additional benefits from using the same scapegoat as other people entrapped in the same situation: it helps to sustain people in the belief that the old values, systems, rules and customs still have meaning, it helps people feel less alone and less vulnerable and it allows the individual to retain his identity without any of the burdensome responsibilities.[54] Over time the use of scapegoats undermines the individual's capacity for independent reasoning and judgement, making their behaviour increasingly passive and complicit in the social environment and the specific social conditions, institutions or relations that shapes people's lives.

6. Decontextualized perceptions

By failing to give consideration to the defining features of the lives of people outsiders ignore how people actually live and act out their lives. This happens because outsiders including organizations, institutions and governments make use of preconceived ideas and paradigms to understand and resolve the problems of human suffering. Instead of taking the particular facts into consideration the idea of human suffering is conceived in terms that are non-historical and non-specific. Such a conception of suffering reduces the complexities of human existence to a single category definition that is abstract, general and overtly simplistic. Adopting a non-historical and non-specific approach makes the concept easily transferable from one situation to another, but its indifference to the particular facts undermines its capacity to assess human suffering as it is experienced in practice. The power of language to communicate the actual subjective felt-experience of hunger, deprivation, ill treatment, injustice and poor health and their combined impact on the consciousness of reality is utterly compromised if human suffering is reduced to the status of *one way of life among others*.[55]

The idea that the context and the people in whom suffering arises are irrelevant makes for a lack of emotional connectedness that is morally offensive because it separates the outsider from the actual lived experience of people.[56] This disengagement from the uniqueness of human suffering is the *sine qua non* of the outsider's perspective. Out of this indifference to the suffering of others is borne the detachment from *prima facie* evidence that made the Holocaust possible[57] and which con-

[54] Staub, E., (1989: 17).

[55] For Des Pres., (1976) "To describe a situation of absolute material want in a neutral fashion is not to be objective. To write about terrible things in a neutral tone or with descriptions barren of subjective response tends to generate an irony risking either cynicism or despair." in Des Pres, T., (1976: vi).

[56] As Ervin Staub indicates, "States do not traditionally regard themselves as having moral responsibilities." Staub, E., (1989:158).

[57] Bauman, Z., (1989:18ff).

tinues to sustain the cool, rational observations of the postmodern voyeur.[58] In the absence of specific information about the particularity of the situation in which people live their lives and have their being universalizing the defining features of the lives of people becomes an empty and meaningless exercise. Such conditions make practical judgement and suitable action simply impossible and inappropriate. If human suffering is only interpreted according to a single category definition everything that fails to comply with it becomes invalid and irrelevant. This makes human suffering meaningful only insofar as it conforms to the preconceived stereotype.[59] For individuals and groups whose experience of suffering falls outside of this single category definition the imposition of a preconceived model of suffering results in humiliation, not help.[60] To avoid further trivialization recognition needs to be given to the fact that human suffering is incompatible with abstraction. This is evident from the implications that reductionist, single category definitions of human suffering have for people affected by hunger and deprivation. It is of paramount importance that the outsider should be clear that it is impossible for any individual or group to be granted recognition and respect from an abstraction. It is not logical to utilise an abstract and formal definition of the universal self as the basis for meaningful interaction if no consideration is given to the cultural and historical differences that shape the actual lived experience of people.

7. Failure to empathise

To bring the experience of suffering into full view so that it is as self-evident to others as it is to the sufferer requires a degree of empathy and understanding that is beyond the normal purview of the disinterested other here.[61] Powerful outsiders, such as institutions, organizations and the state resist any acknowledgement of what actually happens to the humanity of people who suffer by means of a highly structured environment that is not conducive to adaptability. This happens because rules and institutional procedures are used to eliminate uncertainty and reduce stress and anxiety in the face of ambiguity and misunderstanding.[62] Though use of rules and

[58] Sontag, S., (2003: 90f).

[59] Guinote, A. and Vescio, T., (2010: 97–155).

[60] "…The more bureaucracy is dehumanized the more completely it succeeds in eliminating from official business love, hatred, and purely personal, irrational and emotional elements which escape calculation." Weber, quoted in Doubt (2000: 78); Mills, C. & Zavaleta, D., (2015: 251–269)Shame, Humiliation and Social Isolation in Anderson, R.E. (ed)*World Suffering & the Quality of Life*, Springer.

[61] Krznaric, R., (2014: 5).

[62] Hickel, 2017: Addressing the structural causes of Suffering Jason in Anderson, R.E. (ed) *Alleviating World Suffering*, Springer.

procedures may help to eliminate uncertainty they do not promote the adaptability needed to engage with the subjective felt experience of daily survival. Instead familiar and manageable categories make pro-social behaviour including concern about others, tolerance of errors, being generous, being friendly, altruistic, caring for others, being fair, subordinate to a system in which rule-following and not empathy or compassion has become the moral good.[63]

Though this process is integral to any task and performance-oriented culture the subordination of interpersonal compassion to getting the job done, minimising errors and achieving high output levels rubs out the subjective content of the lived experience of other human beings. By failing to consider the historical and particular conditions under which people live their lives other human beings are perceived according to a form of reductionism that makes no concession to the available empirical evidence. From this perspective the lived experience of other people is defined by abstract and formal criteria that possess moral implications, which are both arbitrary and unpredictable.

By failing to reach out toward and relate to the emotional experiences of other people powerful outsiders deny themselves access to the human implications of a situation and its moral significance for suffering. This emotional and moral indifference to human reality makes any specific situation that is the focus of practical judgment subject to misrepresentation and inexactness. Though such an approach may rob powerful outsiders of any emotional bond with the human reality of the situation its lack of human attachment does mean that this definition of other people can be translated from one situation to another. However, the emphasis on the most universal aspects of human behaviour also means that specific elements about the human condition are either ignored or made subordinate to its most general characteristics. By excluding anything specific about the actual lived experience of misery and suffering the genuine voice of human people is replaced by a form of representation that is both formulaic and standardised. This one-dimensional approach to the lived experience of other human beings makes it impossible to contradict or confirm the subjective aspects of human behaviour. If the subjective content of the lived experience of other human beings is not important to the specific situation that is the focus of practical judgment it may not matter.

However, if the human implications of a situation and its moral significance for misery and suffering are important then the lack of an emotional bond with the human reality of the situation becomes the point at which the merits of this exclusion of anything specific about the actual lived experience of misery and suffering breaks down. In this respect the de-contextualisation of suffering keeps people locked into a situation of daily survival from which they feel they cannot escape.[64]

---

[63] See for example, Haas, P. J., (1988: 34).

[64] Amery, J. (1980: 62ff.)

From this position order-making, procedural rationality and the categorization of different human beings can be seen as the tools by which morality has fallen victim to expediency.

8. Disillusionment and apathy

The adverse effects of absolute material want seriously compromise the individual's capacity for self-assertion. In such conditions it is difficult for the individual to acknowledge and give due recognition to the intrinsic value of mutual respect, liberty and justice. Instead increasing scepticism about the value of human solidarity undermines the role of social norms, rules and procedures as a means of minimising the unpredictability of future events. In practice this discourages the individual from involving themselves in future-oriented behaviour such as delaying gratification, planning and investing in the future. This sort of irresolution makes people less sure about the strategies they need to adopt in order to most effectively address their situation. Instead of facing up to their responsibilities people are likely to respond with thoughts, feelings and actions that do not change their situation but help them cope with its psychological and emotional impact.[65]

To safeguard their capacity for self-assertion from the adverse effects of sustained negative emotions people are likely to approach information processing and problem solving in a non-situation specific manner and in language that is deliberately general and wide-ranging. However, the material and psychological benefits of such an approach are so uncertain that people tend to remain prisoners of their own strategies and of their own passivity.

Over time the adverse effects of indifference, apathy, lack of interest in the outside world, limited reaction to different types of stimuli are likely to result in the individual preferring to abdicate his condition as an individual by fully subjecting themselves to another. In such conditions the individual is so engulfed by passivity that they persuade themselves that the existing situation is sufficient and stop to want or expect anything else. This constitutes a rejection of the fundamental elements of self-assertive behaviour including the right to refuse, the right to request and the right to correct a wrong.

9. Passivity legitimized.

In a context of daily survival sustained exposure to negative emotions subverts the desire to communicate on account of the deeply held conviction that an outside audience is unable to understand or be interested in what people are going through. This psychic numbing leads to an inevitable reduction in the individual's capacity to think that his opinions and actions have any moral significance, making them insensitive to the suffering of others. Extreme long lasting negative emotions interfere

[65] For Agamben "…in many cases the peasant has moved into a zone of the human where not only conventional forms of help and support have become useless, but also dignity and self-respect as well." Agamben, G., (1999: 63); See also Chouliaraki, L., (2017: 49–61) Suffering and the Ethics of Solidarity in Anderson, R.E. (ed)*Alleviating World Suffering,* Springer.

with a person's ability to function to such an extent that they determine the human motivation to act.[66] In a context of daily survival these negative emotions derive from the frustration to satisfy such basic needs as safety, control, predictability and self-respect.

Though the failure to meet these needs on a regular or adequate basis may help to counteract feelings of apathy and indifference the inhuman conditions that have brought this situation about make it difficult for people to remain human. This undermines the motivation for communication because people no longer think of themselves as moral/thinking beings.

The failure to function effectively (in a psychological sense) means that people have little if any sense of control over their lives, no sense of purpose and is lacking in supportive and otherwise positive forms of relationship. In the absence of any positive emotional experiences all vitality and self-worth is stifled, making people dull and uninterested in the world around them.[67] This has a detrimental effect on the way people perceive and interpret social behaviours and how they initiate social interactions.[68] Sustained exposure to negative emotions leads vulnerable people to evaluate themselves and others more negatively, making them more self-centred and likely to behave in a less confident, pessimistic and selfish way in interpersonal relations.[69] The consequences of this process are arguably different for those who suffer injustices throughout their lives than for those who do not.

For people whose experience of enforced passivity arrives as an abrupt and unwanted interruption it is inevitable that the feelings it provokes are very raw. However, the feeling that enforced passivity is *illegitimate as well as unwanted* is less likely for people who have had to endure such conditions throughout their lives, and do not necessarily experience their vulnerability as a sharp transgression of the norm. This can explain the indifference, lack of empathy and unwillingness to make full use of the limited opportunities for being heard. These are not just moral injuries but psychological ones that fatefully damage the individual's motivation, ability and belief in the power of communication.

---

[66] Ervin Staub lists four primary kinds of motivation for human behaviour: personalgoals, biological needs, social customs, rules, and standards; and unconscious motivation. The key to understanding social interaction in the Andean context is seeing how these personal factors are shaped by greater social, political, and historical forces." Staub, E., (1989: 36).

[67] See, for example, Fromm, E. (1997: 397).

[68] Forgas, J.P. (Ed.) (2001); Forgas, J.P., Williams, K. R. & Wheeler, L. (Eds.) (2001); Ciarrochi, J.V., Forgas, J.P. & Mayer, J. D. (Eds.) (2001; Forgas, J.P. & Williams, K. D. (Eds.) (2001).

[69] Forgas, J.P. & Williams, K.D. (Eds.) (2002); Forgas, J.P. (Ed.) (2006); Sedikides, C. (1995).

10. Prioritising the self

Scepticism about the merits of human solidarity undermines the individual's motivation to communicate and has a powerful effect on what the individual makes of a particular situation and their attitude towards it.[70] Individual support and the principle of mutual aid and sharing on which the authority of human solidarity rests cannot operate effectively in conditions of extreme want. Instead, the idea of working together in a spirit of trust, compassion and mercy can seem so remote that it is likely to have other, more negative connotations.[71] The lack of tangible benefits arising from any support for traditional norms and values means that individual behaviour is increasingly driven by ruthless self-interest and a disregard for the other person. Operating from the idea that the only right that matters is that of the strongest, the individual tends to treat other people with suspicion and as a potential enemy, and not as a source of help and support and guidance. Though the seriousness of the situation helps to sharpen people's critical awareness so that they are better equipped to understand the available forms of social support, it also heightens people's appreciation of their shortcomings.

Over time these psychological interruptions call into question the idea that the social identity people acquire from their support for human solidarity is always right and that existing relationships with other people are always beneficial.[72] In the absence of reliable information any nurturing or supportive relationship is placed under such strain that it is devoid of any meaning compatible with ordinary life. The immediate question of self-preservation is so overwhelming that people use it to excuse themselves from any shared experience of difficult life conditions, of any shared motivations that result from them and of any shared inclinations for ways to satisfy motives.[73]

In these circumstances respect for the leaders, rules and culture surrounding human solidarity is so diminished that social support is able to make fewer and

[70] See for example, Abramson, Seligman, and Teasdale 1978; Seligman 1975). Furthermore, work has linked low power to feelings of general uncertainty (Anderson and Galinsky 2006) which itself is often aversive (e.g., Weary et al. 1993). Being powerless is also associated with less access to both physical (e.g., material wealth) and social rewards compared with being powerful (e.g., recognition; Buss and Malamuth 1996; Domhoff 1998; Operario and Fiske 2001); Chouliaraki, L., (2017: 49–61) Suffering and the Ethics of Solidarity in Anderson, R.E. (ed)*Alleviating World Suffering,* Springer.

[71] Chouliaraki, L., (2017: 49–61) Suffering and the Ethics of Solidarity in Anderson, R.E. (ed) *Alleviating World Suffering,* Springer.

[72] McCann, I.L. & Pearlman, L.A., (1990a, b); Pearlman, L.A. & Saakvitne, K.W. (1995); Chouliaraki, L., (2017: 49–61) Suffering and the Ethics of Solidarity in Anderson, R.E. (ed)*Alleviating World Suffering,* Springer.

[73] Staub, E. (1989:38ff).

fewer demands on those from whom it draws its support.[74] This failure to improve the individual's material situation deprives human solidarity of its importance and the values with which it is associated. Though people may make every effort to search for an interpretation and understanding of what they are going through the failure of human solidarity to improve the situation represents a fundamental threat to people's convictions and ultimately forces them into harder positions.[75]

In a context of daily survival, the demands of natural time influence the individual to fashion their own life course, even though it is without the guidance of the beliefs, meanings, values, valuations, symbols, myths and perspectives that normally underpin the foundations of action. This repudiation of traditional values and culture means that the individual has to accept a situation in which the struggle to construct a positive meaning out of the principle of mutual support and sharing has failed.

It is no longer possible to think that if the individual goes to the aid of someone in need of support that they would receive similar help from others whenever they are in difficulties. In a context of daily survival, the expectation of help has no place. Instead people are left to their own devices: the idea of people helping each other is at best superficial and more often simply moribund or just plain dead. The destruction of traditional norms and values is accompanied not by a sense of outrage and injustice, but by the silence of apathy and indifference. It is the loneliness of an individual whose normative expectations of human solidarity have been utterly invalidated.

In the face of such persistent unconcern by the state the individual has only one future, namely existence in abandonment.

Efforts to liberate themselves from this indifference and each become more integrated as a human being are frustrated by the overwhelming pressure from their own immediate needs. This inability to move from the biological and social sphere into the moral sphere mean that people are less clear about their needs, interests and priorities, causing the strategies they adopt to deal with their difficulties to not be as situation specific or subject to as much variation as those permitted people in more privileged situations.[76]

Instead of approaching problems in a focused, goal consistent manner people in this situation make use of detailed, controlled processes to drive judgement and

[74] Staub, E. (2012). in Anstey, M., Meerts, P. & Zartman, I. W. (eds.) (2012); Harvey, D. C., (2015: 269–281) The Cultural Geography of Community Suffering in Anderson, R.E. (ed) *World Suffering & the Quality of Life*, Springer; Chouliaraki, L., (2017: 49–61) Suffering and the Ethics of Solidarity in Anderson, R.E. (ed) *Alleviating World Suffering*, Springer.

[75] Chouliaraki, L., (2017: 49–61) Suffering and the Ethics of Solidarity in Anderson, R.E. (ed)*Alleviating World Suffering*, Springer.

[76] Staub, E. (2012).

behaviour.[77] This ignores other processes including associative, intuitive or experiential reasoning causing people to register half hearted, unfocused responses to acute stress.[78] Over time this is responsible for a decline in mental activities and the erosion of social relationships. For people having to face such adverse circumstances beyond their own control any capacity to protect themselves from anxiety, fear and mistrust is so diminished that people become withdrawn and increasingly indifferent to the world and their own situation. In these circumstances people cannot function properly, either in the society of others or by themselves. Instead, the unrelenting hardships borne out of social fragmentation, apathy and antimony are such that a person's autonomy and self-worth are in no position to withstand the pressure, making further disintegration of the personality inevitable.[79]

This is a life that is so close to losing all meaning that people are not always able to protect themselves from the onslaught of unremitting misery and the reality being lived. Unable to distance themselves from the present people lose the capacity to believe that they are able to do anything to change the situation.

Processing the Experience of Political Violence

Hidden under the surface of the daily struggle for survival in the Peruvian Andes is now the memory of trauma. This trauma causes attitudes that shatter the idea that human nature everywhere shares a fundamental core of humanitarian principles that can never be eroded.[80] The discovery that respect for human dignity cannot be assumed to be something characteristic of humans undermines the continuity of people from within.[81] In these circumstances efforts to keep the painful memories safely fixed in the past fail because nothing can ever measure up to what was done. To survive people, have no alternative but to normalize the past by separating themselves from it as much as they can.

This suspension of the past only increases the likelihood that it will re-establish itself in hidden form. Thus "…possession by the past may never be fully overcome

[77] See Fiske, S.T., (1993); Brewer, (1988); Fiske, S.T. & Neuberg, S. L. (1990); McCann I.L & Pearlman, L.A. (1990a, b); Pearlman, L.A. & Saakvitne, (1995); Saakvitne, K.W. et al., (2000); Staub, E. (1989; 2003).

[78] See Guinote, A. and Vescio, T. (2010: 154).

[79] Hallman, A.H. & Wandersman, W.K. (1992); Taylor, C. (1991); Pearlin, L.I. (1989); Pearlin, L.I. & Schooler, C. (1978).

[80] DePrince, A.P. & Freyd, J.J. (2002).

[81] LaCapra, D. (2001: 177).

or transcended."[82] For survivors who suffer as much from the harm caused by political violence as from poverty and social exclusion the violation of a fundamental core of humanitarian principles only serves to diminish how communities and individuals perceive their own suffering.

In the aftermath of political violence this inability to mourn and work through the memory of pain, suffering, grief and death undermines behaviour patterns and the most deeply held commitments become so weakened that people regress; they become more primitive, childish.[83] It also makes people believe that nothing can be done and that further misery and suffering is inevitable.

For survivors of the political violence the pressures of living in a context of daily survival make the suppression of the past overwhelmingly necessary, even though this tends to be almost impossible to achieve in practice. Outrage against past injustices inflicted on the individual is of little avail if the available resources are insufficient to meet daily needs. In these circumstances people are compelled to focus exclusively on the necessities of the present. To do otherwise is unthinkable because it would forfeit the opportunity to secure enough resources for themselves and their dependents. This devalues the past (and the future) to such an extent that it subverts traditional habits and behaviour, making people's attitude to time erratic and unpredictable.

Past injustices recalled in a context of struggle for daily survival have less practical value than concern for what will be tomorrow, no matter (perhaps) how terrible the memories. In this respect, sense of time has become twisted: it is not so much moral duty and the legacy of the past that guides present behaviour and decision making as rationality and self-preservation.[84]

Having no outlet means that feelings of injustice remain in the psyche and the cultural unconscious, trapped and unprocessed. As the following testimony illustrates: "I still have nightmares of violence now less than before but it has remained inside people's hearts; it is a psychosis of the people, they are not the same; they are not quiet any longer, not like before." Author's field research: interviewee from Otoronco (Paloma).

From my studies it is clear that the passage of time does not neutralise the traumatic impact of the past. Instead, lack of human connectedness helps keep the memory of past atrocities alive. To be able to make sense of pain and suffering, survivors need access to shared values, common humanity and shared responsibility. However, the persistence of a living past is not easily got rid of.

In the aftermath of political violence, the impact of SL and the armed forces and police still haunt survivors as the following testimony indicates: "When unknown

---

[82] LaCapra, D. (2001: 70).

[83] Scott Peck, M., (1983: 214).

[84] Bauman, Z., (1989: 207).

people come we weigh them up. When unknown people come here to know how we do things and come to find out; those things I think about a lot because we have been through such problems of violence, so we speak to these strangers but we do not talk at them, we talk with them only when we converse, I am scared of them." Author's field research: interviewee from Yachaya (Gaetan).

Wariness towards strangers is a potent example of how the political violence continues to violate ideas survivors have about the world and its norms and values. Before the political violence moral responsibilities were confined to the immediate realm of personal experience.

In the aftermath of the political violence the conditions for human connectedness and ultimately the victim's hold on the world have been placed in a state of extreme confusion and insecurity. One survivor reflected on the changes the political violence has brought to their lives as follows: "In earlier times people thought not only about bringing up their own family but also about helping the community and for that reason people were also coordinating and this usually meant with the local government of the day, but now this does not happen." Author's field research: interviewee from Qocha (Isabel).

It is a situation of helplessness that prevents the misery of conflict from being integrated into the story of the self. This means that most of the survivors live with psychological wounds that will never heal completely. If the origin of human suffering is to be found in a lack of empathy then it would be appropriate to suggest that the reality of survivors lies in an unrecognizable world of moral chaos and despair. Unless the system of defences that empties the meaning of human suffering of all subjective content can be broken down the reality of survivors seems unlikely to inspire sympathy, empathy and action for change.

The feeling that no one is interested in allowing survivors to make sense of their situation encourages them to believe that nothing can be done and that further suffering is inevitable.

This is exemplified by the following testimony: "I don't know if it is the fear talking, but I am nervous and I am afraid to walk in the streets at night. I always feel this way. When we see people, we don't know we ask ourselves who they are. Instead of asking them directly we ask ourselves what type of person he is because we are afraid the terrorists will come back; I do fear the possibility of the violence reoccurring." Author's field research: interviewee from Qocha (Pepita).

For survivors of the abuse of power, conflict, exploitation and hierarchy such indifference to human dignity and self-respect are a stimulus to feelings of anxiety, shame, desperation, fear, confusion, withdrawal and self-loathing. The combination of these feelings reinforces and further devalue the flow of time; in doing so they emphasize and make more severe the underlying causes of stress that devalue the importance of planning for the future.

To combat the impact of so many negative emotions survivors tend to break the relationship between themselves and what is happening and withdraw from the situation. In some cases, this leads to the outbreak of violence as survivors seek to improve their situation by aggressive means without facing up to their own responsibilities. More commonly, but less obviously, this breakdown in the relationship between individuals and groups and what is happening leads to a psychological and physicalwithdrawal from the situation. This is tantamount to an admission of failure to find any rational solution to the broad range of lasting stressful events. In these circumstances the only appropriate attitude is one of resignation and acceptance.[85]

Having to face truly unavoidable circumstances makes people less willing to help others.[86] It also makes them predisposed to expect bad faith and underhand behaviour, particularly if matters involving confidence, insecurity and fears of inadequacy are concerned.[87] This makes survivors distrustful, making it easier to harden their belief that others harbour only malign intent towards them.

The struggle to stand up to such a difficult environment is therefore not just about the objective circumstances; it is also about insecurity, fear, low self-esteem, social isolation and lack of control over work and home life and their impact on the internal resources of the individual. This state of mind is reflected in the following testimony: "Many people from the community leave for work in other places, but the only thing they bring back is money for themselves and their family. Other community members say that these people have no vision for the future, that they just live the present with a conformist mentality." Author's field research: interviewee from Wamani (Roberto).

This throws all traditional norms and values into doubt, thereby causing people to devalue other groups, make use of scapegoats, join new groups, and/or adopt new ideas. Not surprisingly, this emotional destruction of the norms and values of solidarity removes survivors from meaningful human interaction and ultimately prompts the abandonment of traditional norms and values altogether. This frustrates the basic needs for safety, control predictability and self-respect, making adaptation of and reduction in the old values of solidarity unavoidable.[88] It also weakens the relationship people have – not just with each other – but with the attitude they bring to their situation.

Instead of assuming full responsibility for themselves and thinking properly about the matter in hand survivors assume an attitude of acceptance and delude themselves with the feeling that the existing situation is sufficient and that it would be inappropriate to want or expect more. By failing to acknowledge the importance of thinking for themselves' survivors have moved into a position where there is no critical engagement and things are accepted at face value. This may have brought greater independence from other individuals and groups, but it has also brought the

[85] Smith C. Alford: 101).

[86] Smart, D., Sanson, A., Da Silva, L., & Toumbourou, J. (2000).

[87] Brewer, G. A. (2003).

[88] Staub, E., (1989: 45).

kind of fear, envy, violence, hatred and other features of social isolation normally associated with western cultures.

Human suffering may not be an illness, but accurate assessment of it is critical to a better understanding of how the immediate question of self-preservation can cause survivors to use it to excuse themselves of any shared experience of difficult life conditions.[89] However, this erosion of consciousness and any concomitant social isolation, apathy and subjugation with which it is associated are fundamental to understanding why survivors do what they do when they are unable to do what they want.

In circumstances where the workings of community activities, including access to services, communication, information, etc., no longer have the capacity to alleviate the material manifestations of suffering, the inability to coordinate social life and move shared goals forwards, plus the need to identify new understandings (slight though they may be) to help make the situation less unbearable becomes inevitable. However, if all the conventional coping mechanisms including popular mobilization, solidarity and grassroots organizations have failed it is very easy for survivors to give in to their situation and register half hearted, unfocused responses to acute stress.[90]

Insecurity, low self-esteem, social isolation and lack of control over their livelihoods not only dull the senses but it makes people blind and indifferent to the difficulties lying ahead. In these circumstances the damage done to the individual's capacity to think, feel and act makes the importance of planning for the future increasingly meaningless and the business of daily survival more important.

The typical response to these conditions are feelings of helplessness and fear leading to further erosion of the individual's sense of security and wellbeing. In this way the individual no longer experiences other people as a source of social support, comfort and self-realization. Instead other people become a source of anxiety and tension.[91] These responses are clear from the following testimony: "Yes, I get scared with unknown people. I've seen people killed, their throats cut like animals. There is always a level of mistrust with people you don't know; I scare easily, I've been too close to death too many times not to be anything else…If ever a stranger arrives with a weapon I plan to flee straightaway. Seeing strangers approaching the village always brings back memories." Author's field research: interviewee from Unay (Eurico).

By reliving the events of the painful past the individual survivor is returning to the feelings of helplessness and fear associated with the events being remembered.

---

[89] Staub, E. (1989:38ff).

[90] See Guinote, A. and Vescio, T. (2010: 209ff).

[91] "…For Freud anxiety had the quality of indefiniteness and absence or indeterminacy of an object; for Kierkegaard & Heidegger, it was the fear of something that is nothing." LaCapra, D., (2001: 57).

This increases the readiness to feel anxiety both towards the events themselves and towards the individual's relationship with the present.

Those who recognise that in spite of all that has happened they still have responsibilities that require them to find the right answers to the situation are most likely to survive their hardships.

In a context of daily survival this is most likely to involve the immediate question of the future survival of the individual and any dependents. By focusing consciously on positive, meaningful values and goals the individual is able to avoid the state of dejection that causes survivors to abandon the responsibilities they have to themselves and other people. This is reflected in the following testimony: "When unknown people come I am not afraid, I stay normal because my father taught me not to be afraid because years ago they did scare me more than I can say. It was to do with the military clothes; sometimes they walked about screaming, charging around with dogs until they brought people back bleeding; they shot them and they brought them back, dragging them along and seeing all that made us children scared." Author's field research: interviewee from Otoronco (Gala).

To live continuously with the knowledge that there is nowhere to go, no help to come, no interpersonal trust and no related practices of socialization and mutual help compels the individual survivor to endure conditions that are outside their control. Instead of a strong sense of responsibility and attachment[92] towards something bigger than themselves survivors respond to their social environment with feelings that encourage the adoption of unhealthy attitudes. These include: (1) the attitude that causes survivors to live from one day to the next under the expectation that at any one time everything may come to an abrupt end and that there is not much justification for making an effort; (2) the fatalistic attitude in which everything is ruled by outside forces and that what the individual survivor thinks or plans is of no importance and may inhibit the individual from taking the initiative; (3) the attitude that encourages survivors to blend in by being as inconspicuous as possible, even though this may be contrary to the needs, interests and priorities of the community.

The cumulative effect of these unhealthy attitudes is for people to believe that they can excuse themselves from matters of moral/practical importance.[93] However, failing to process painful memories has a corrosive influence on the living present that distorts perception and interferes with rational thought. In other words, the legacy of the past imposes itself on all aspects of the living present.

To bring the influence of the past into full view so that it is as self-evident to others as it is to the survivor requires a reassessment of the strict separation of the past

[92] Davidson, W. B., & Cotter, P. R. (1989).

[93] Scott Peck (1983: 214).

from the present.[94] First of all it is important to underscore how impossible it is for the survivors to forget any part of what their suffering means to them. Secondly, the legacy of the political violence is responsible for a violation of the individual survivor's familiar ideas about the world and its norms and values, putting the individual in a state of extreme confusion and insecurity. Thirdly, the pressures of daily survival make the suppression of the past overwhelmingly necessary. The motivation is strictly utilitarian.

Instead of making survivors more self-directed and intellectually independent this fictional oblivion is responsible for feelings of impotence, frustration and despair.

Unable to distance themselves from the immediate demands of survival the memory of pain and loss, suffering, grief and death lives on in their psyche, unprocessed and ignored. By using avoidance behaviour as a protective shield, the individual has sought to block any identification with their own painful experiences.[95] This is used by many of the survivors of the political violence to argue themselves away from the issue of moral duty because the post-conflict situation they find themselves in does not contain a good choice or renders such a good choice very costly.[96]

To succeed in bringing the influence of the past into full view so that it is as self-evident to others as it is to the sufferer therefore involves understanding how survivors come to terms with the shattering of their strongly held set of assumptions about the world, the self and others.[97]

For the families and communities studied political violence has done irreparable damage to the norms for social behaviour. In particular, respect for the core value that expects community members to share what they have and what they know and help others.[98]

To function effectively this requires the sharing of a set of beliefs that affirms acceptable behaviour and confronts deviant behaviour.[99] However, the traditional use of ridicule and public exposure of the person responsible for behaviour detri-

[94] Kleinman, A., & Kleinman, J., (1991a, b: 275–301).

[95] This type of emotional numbing is consistent with the symptoms of avoidance behaviour, one of the main categories of PTSD. It signifies a loss of the emotional capacity to develop respect for past suffering and the realization that these past experiences belong to them. The self-acquittal that underlies this kind of personaloblivion also impairs the emotional faculty for empathy, compassion and concern for others. See Frommberger, Ulrich (2014).

[96] Bauman, Z., (1989: 206).

[97] Janolf-Bulman, R., (1992).

[98] In Quechua society this is expressed as "Let's live with just one heart" (*Jucshungulla cawashun*).

[99] Skar, H. O. (1982: 93).

mental to these values has little impact on survivors of extreme psychological trauma.

For families and communities across the rural highlandstransgression of social norms by exposure in the public domain no longer has the significance it once had. Extreme psychological trauma significantly damages the social context that makes the control of behaviour through public embarrassment possible. Though this can make the social context feel so violated that there is nothing and no one to identify with, psychological trauma is not the only thing language and culture is being damaged by.[100] Inroads by the dominant *mestizo* culture into the attrition of traditional norms and values have been of overwhelming significance.[101]

In the years before the political violence individuals that chose to cross the cultural boundary into the *mestizo*domain would almost certainly incur the risk of being shamed in public.[102] In the aftermath of the political violence all this has changed. Though survivors often retain a deep sense of belonging to the land they farm, the *mestizo*culture imposes itself through the behaviour of the police and soldiers, land disputes, insults and humiliation as well as through more indirect routes, such as improvements in basic services including transportation, education, health and commercial opportunities. In practice this has led to the loss of much of their traditional cultural characteristics and values, sense of propriety, and their own self-respect; it has also made anomie, selfishness and other forms of social fragmentation commonplace.

Though this loosening of moralconstraints frees people from obedience more than ever before, it also undermines their consciousness of being able to resist, to cooperate, to participate in helping others.

In the aftermath of the political violence this has created a mental climate that in the rural highlands further impairs any capacity for self-determination. It is the overwhelming urgency of the aftermath of the political violence that shapes local reality and defines the meaning of normal behaviour, not respect for certain duties and the avoidance of shame. Individuals and groups feel resigned to this situation not through cowardice or weakness of will, but because of the perceived hopelessness of their situation.

---

[100] "Quechuas say the *mestizo* only looks on the external circumstances and insults them for not speaking Spanish, for not wearing shoes, and for being dirty. In the social stratification of Peru, the peasant farmers are often considered only slightly more civilized than the "jungle savages" (*chunchu*)." See Smith, Terry P. (2006).

[101] Quechua were originally known as *indio* but this term was banned by the Velasco military government in 1969 and replaced with *campesino* (peasant). Skar (1982:73) quotes Olien who described an Indian/*campesino* as "…a person who wears sandals, lives in a mud-walled, thatch-roofed house, maintains' pagan' beliefs and speaks Quechua or Aymara."

[102] For people who adopt the national language and culture the derogatory expression *mishtiyasha* is used by the community to refer to those who turn their back on their heritage.

This is clear from the following testimony: "Like I said people are concerned with earning money. When there are meetings people do not even attend or because they are tired they go to sleep in the meetings; they are nothing but pawns that listen, others do not even hear, and are not interested: they say that the government will bring everything from anywhere." Author's field research: interviewee from Qocha (Maximinio).

Beneath the veneer of this newly fashioned identity is to be found a fragile, indeterminate existence that resembles no previous version of their society. Instead of a place of safety and support rural life in the Andes has been transformed into one of loneliness, instability and danger. Survivors now adjust behaviour and respond to outside circumstances as individuals without reference to traditional routines and emotional support.

No longer beholden to traditional values and constraints survivors and all other people living in the research communities feel free to react to outside circumstances from a range of behavioural options not previously available. By accepting the need to use all means possible to sustain life people have rejected the importance of taking responsibility for their own actions and being accountable to others.

The impact this has on the community and its leadership is borne out by the following: "There are no active leaders within the community; only people who are meant to make decisions affecting the internal affairs of the community. The village leaders are farmers and the positions they occupy as community leaders are of secondary importance." Author's field research: interviewee from Otoronco (Fidele).

For survivors used to seeing misery around them all of the time and not thinking about it their reaction to outside circumstances tend to fall into two broad categories: (1) withdrawal responses or (2) attack responses.[103] Both responses reflect the belief that no one is concerned about what has happened to their world. For families and communities across the rural highlands this is less likely to find expression in feelings of outrage and injustice than through prolonged silence, apathy and indifference.

If old dominant values retain any influence it is in their capacity to intimidate people into silence and not from any ability to shape their beliefs.[104] These are conditions that condemn people to live in fear of ambiguity, fear of threat and loss, without order and structure. It involves living without the most basic aspects of human relations, namely trust, empathy and compassion. The impacts affect everyone's mental state. It empties the human condition of pride and dignity and encourages people to identify moraldespair as a source of vulnerability.

Unable to meaningfully respond to circumstances people internalise the threat posed to their way of life in the vain hope that this could somehow insulate them

[103] Miller, D. (2001). See also Weissmark, M.S., (2004: 19).

[104] Though as Langer points out: "…The concept of moralsurvival is too deeply embedded in the imagination to be surrendered without a struggle" Langer, L., (1983: 71).

from their situation. This is clear from the following: "If I see something violent and harmful I want to hide because I do not want to re-live what happened." Author's field research: interviewee from Unay (Olga).

For the survivors this reaction to outside circumstances is ethically defensible. In the rural Andes it is known as *conformismo.* It is used to describe the behaviour of people who have chosen to abandon the individual uncertainty that the collapse in traditional norms and values produces for the sake of collective identity.

It is regularly used to explain the behaviour of people in meetings with the local authorities, NGOs, GROs and Community Assemblies. The following testimony is typical: "Here the community leaders have a particular type of *conformismo* that we see in their plans for the community. They have no visions for the future; they don't plan their activities for the time they hold office. In the same way there are no plans for the community, no projects for the short term, middle term and long term. The only things they are worried about are their own interests; they aren't worried about us or the future of the community." Author's field research: interviewee from Wamani (Marco).

Through social interaction *conformismo* can appear deceptively like solidarity, but it is **not** the same; it lacks substance, it is more of a general orientation. Unlike solidarity *conformismo* does not link people to each other in a meaningful way, as the following shows: "The local people are *conformistas* because they do not speak; they never speak (in community/district authority meetings)." Author's field research: interviewee from Qocha (Hieronimo).

People find refuge in this type of collective identity because they are uncertain about what the collapse in traditional norms and values might ultimately signify. However, it does not represent a sanctuary from the effects of low self-esteem, loss of meaning, lack of goals, anger and hostility, loss of faith in the benevolence of the world or in legitimate authority. Instead it liberates people from responsibility for their actions and provides temporary relief from the feeling that no one takes their concerns seriously. In a context of daily survival this is highly desirable because resistance to such injustices as a weak political culture is no longer viable.

The feeling that nothing can ever get better makes it easier for survivors to merge their own particular personality into larger social structures because the structures provide a means by which some semblance of security, no matter how tenuous, may be regained. However, this changes the way in which people relate to each other.

By putting self-preservation above moral duty personal attachments, communal and cooperative relationships and inter-personal relationships lose much of their clarity and become a source of suspicion and mistrust.[105] When the individual is surrounded by ineffectual traditional values, "...proximity to suffering does not

[105] Bauman, Z. (1989: 206).

strengthen human ties but establishes a new priority of value whose sole aim is to strengthen the chances of survival."[106]

The uselessness of traditional values means that people are as likely to break entirely with this type of collective identity as they are to accept the situation. In this tangled situation the immediate question of self-preservation may give rise to the motivation for and diminish inhibition against harming others. These are circumstances in which social exclusion no longer carries the same stigma in the way that it used to. In the rural highlands this is known as *individualismo.*[107] It leads people to use all means honest and otherwise, even brutal force, theft and betrayal of friends to secure what they need. It involves selfishness, independence, resistance to peer pressure, indifference to democratic values, indifference/intolerance of others, indifference to opinions of others, selfish honesty, intimate relations with a few others, indifference to social justice, indifference to social awareness.

Individualismo is regularly used to describe people's attitudes to meetings with local authorities, NGOs, GROs and Community Assemblies. *Individualismo* is a symptom of people who have abandoned everything associated with the past for the sake of the present. One survivor seems well aware of this: "Before the people were united and now they have a bit of money so people move away and live their own life. Today everything is about money. Now there is no pity, just selfishness, no support for orphans or widows. Now there is no solidarity; when I was young there was mutual support, not now." Author's field research: interviewee from Qocha (Luna).

In combination with the erosion of old dominant values there is a corresponding increase in the frustration of basic psychological needs such as security or safety, trust, esteem, positive identity, feelings of effectiveness and control, positive connections to other people, a comprehension of reality and of one's own place in the world, and transcendence (or spiritual needs).[108]

However, this assault on the individual's self-awareness by the lack of connectedness to others, belongingness and community is of such an order that it also acts as a source of motivation for the recovery of self-worth and right to dignity. It is not an exaggeration to say that this is a process that begins where traditional authority and values end.

In a situation of such overwhelming powerlessness and helplessness the feeling that no one understands what people are going through or that there is anyone to turn to for help or advice compels them to fall back on their own resources.

---

[106] Langer, L., (1983: 108).

[107] For a discussion on the destructive aspects of individualism in Andean culture see Gonzalez, O.M., (2011: 103ff).

[108] McCann, I.L. & Pearlman, L.A. (1990a, b); Pearlman, L.A. & Saakvitne, K.W. (1995); Saakvitne K.W. et al., (2000); Staub, E., (1989, 2003).

However, these can be so limited that they may find it difficult to retain any hope in the future. Having no one to turn to inevitably causes people to think about why this is.

In a context of daily survival this involves revisiting particular structural, contextual and historical aspects of their situation time and time again.[109] It is a process directed against the thinking that it is possible to forget injustice, suffering, fear and misery and is responsible for feelings of anger and humiliation.

This keeps survivors in an abject condition because they are unable and unwilling to rid themselves of the sense of shame, loss of dignity and respect.[110] For the survivor the realities that comprise this abstraction include the loss of individuality, fear for one's life and one's family, the oppressive anxiety of an uncontrollable and unpredictable future and the disconnection among people who have lost their bearings in the world.

In conditions of extreme inhumanity and degradation these are things that make the denial of dignity permanent and unchanging. In these circumstances nominal, ill-considered initiatives intended to appease past survivors of injustice, suffering and misery only help keep these feelings alive and make resentment inevitable. For the survivors of the political violence this is a retrospective grudge which has to contend with the multiplicity of life's demands and the forgetfulness induced by the passage of time.[111]

Integrating Individual and Social Suffering

To ensure that the human significance of suffering is not "...trivialized to a point that is morally objectionable"[112] we need to create conditions in which individuals can reflect on and emotionally work through their relationship to the political violence and its aftermath.

But people struggling with unbearable memories do not willingly "...engage in public reflection on substantial matters of concern to them and also on the rules and norms of inquiry they customarily enact."[113] This is because people tend to dissoci-

[109] Herman, J. L., (1992: 41–2; 110–111).

[110] Kristeva, J., (1982: 4).

[111] Zolkos, M., (2007).

[112] See Wilkinson, I., (2005a, b: 18); Frank, A.W. (2001); Steiner, G. (1967).

[113] Argyris, C., Putnam, R., & Smith, D.M. (1985).

ate themselves from their own memories of fear, helplessness and rejection.[114] Daily survival is a hard struggle to satisfy basic needs. It follows that the stand people take towards their situation and the implications this has for an understanding of how they approach their future is dominated by a combination of the permanent psychological present and a "…dissociation from their own multiple and even unconscious understandings of the interrelatedness of suffering."[115]

In these circumstances the idea that the "…somatically lived experience of ripped flesh and disembowelled self-esteem ready for instant replay"[116] can be effectively subdued is unthinkable. Instead survivors feel unable to calm themselves whenever feelings about their situation intensify.

Having no access to formal treatment of any kind only strengthens the wall between self and others, thereby reinforcing feelings of worthlessness, impotence and utter despair about the situation ever changing.

This can be so overwhelming that memories of the political violence will be used by survivors to excuse themselves from matters of moral and practical importance.[117] In this dissociative mind what is remembered can be so difficult to tolerate that reflecting and emotionally working through their relationship to past events is likely to feel an abomination. This makes it impossible for survivors to process the images and memories of their trauma related experiences, and what is more important, to interpret those experiences in order that they may maximize their effectiveness as human beings. The negative image that survivors often have of themselves can be so deeply embedded as to make dissociation indispensable to any understanding of their relationship to the political violence and its aftermath.

It is dissociation that is responsible for disconnecting intense sensory and emotional experiences from the social domain of language and memory.[118] In this respect dissociation functions as an internal mechanism by which terrorized people can be kept silenced.[119]

However, this "…widespread survival strategy for the avoidance of painful emotional states" militates against the destruction inflicted on the fundamental assumptions of survivors.[120] Because their basic trust in the world has been violated the aftermath of the political violence has made people intensely vulnerable. In recent

[114] Janolf-Bulman, R., (1992: 101–103).

[115] Watkins, M. & Shulman, H. (2008: 283).

[116] Cheftez, R., (2008: 24).

[117] Prilleltensky, I. (2008a, b); Prilleltensky, I. 2008a, b in S.C. Carr & T.S. Sloan (Eds.) (2008); Scott Peck (1983: 214).

[118] Herman, J. L., (1992: 239).

[119] Van der Kolk, B.A. & Fisler, R., (1995).

[120] Watkins, M. & Shulman, H. (2008: 74).

years this has been exacerbated by endemic abuses of power, in particular the feeling that those responsible for widespread human rights abuses remain unpunished.

How to counter these processes of social amnesia and bring the experiences with which they are associated into full view? To begin the process of reflecting on and emotionally working through their relationship with what happened survivors need to re-establish links with their painful past. However, extreme levels of denial and dissociation do not always abate; in many cases they persist and remain adaptive throughout the life course.[121] In this way any confrontation with the subversive power of remembered suffering can be so psychologically devastating as to make it an enormously difficult undertaking for the traumatized survivor.[122] For people from the communities studied the utter isolation endemic to lifelong anxieties, doubts and fears is likely to aggravate this situation.

Being accustomed to conditions of high vigilance and intermittent chaos compels survivors to separate themselves from the past because they are unable to make the shift from unpredictable danger to reliable safety. Until a reasonable degree of safety has been established people will continue to feel unsafe in their bodies, their emotions, their thinking and in their relation to other people.[123]

Though physical isolation no longer constitutes the threat that it used to the lack of safety continues to affect everyone. This is reflected in the high level of crime, drug trafficking, teenage delinquency and other forms of anti-social behaviour. Though armed civilians and civilian self-defence still help to maintain social order, the exchange of information and the operation of joint patrols with the armed forces no longer operate as they used to during the political violence.[124]

This means that people have no real protection against the main sources of regional insecurity: drug traffickers, Shining Path terrorists[125] and the intrusion of

[121] Janolf-Bulman, R., (1992: 103).

[122] Metz, J.B., (1980: 110).

[123] Herman, J. L., (1992: 160).

[124] There were approximately 7226 *comités de auto defensa* as of 2005. Army of Peru (2005).

[125] Though the organization's numbers have considerably reduced, a militant faction of Shining Path called *Proseguir* (Onward) continues to be active. It is believed that the faction consists of three groups known as the North, or Pangoa, the Centre, or Pucuta, and the South, or Vizcatán. The government claims that *Proseguir* is operating in alliance with drug traffickers. United States Department of State (2005) Country Reports on Human RightsPractices: Peru: (2005).

oil and mining companies on indigenous land.[126] In these ways the lack of safety affects everyone and creates an environment of undiluted fear and insecurity that undermines confidence.[127]

For survivors of prolonged and repeated suffering these conditions obstruct the establishment of safety needed to confront the dissociative strategies that undermine "…the mind's motivation to confront, reconsider and integrate the traumatic experience."[128] In such circumstances any recollection of what happened is likely to be sterile and unproductive since an environment of undiluted fear and insecurity is not conducive to the accompanying emotions with which past suffering is associated.[129]

Because this makes the subjective felt-experience of another so difficult to determine with any precision the commonalities and differences in the experiences of researcher and participant need to be kept to a minimum. This makes it easier to give due attention to understanding how the past is remembered and interpreted as well as what the individual makes of a particular situation and their attitude towards it. Through such overlapping experiences participatory research becomes more of a collaborative undertaking.

For those affected by political violence and living in a context of daily survival this is absolutely vital since the damage inflicted on their capacity for basic trust has affected all subsequent stages of development as well. In this respect their factual accounts of what happened to them give a false impression of what it is that continues to affect them emotionally and psychologically.

Pushing such factors as overwhelming anxiety, abrupt changes between hope and desperation, self-preservation and self-abandonment to the side will only impede our understanding of the foundations of individual and group suffering.

To facilitate the recognition, understanding and management of a multiplicity of disconnected narratives and isolated events affecting another person therefore

---

[126] In the mid-1990s the Fujimori administration with World Bank and International Monetary Fund assistance, privatized and deregulated its traditionally state-owned mining sector. According to the Geological Mining and Metallurgical Institute of Peru this was responsible for 3100 mining permits being issued by the government in 2011 and 4668 mining permits in 2012. Despite this investment, many people in rural areas feel that they are not benefiting from mining on the grounds that it is responsible for environmental degradation and lack of benefits to local communities affected by mining. This has led to a 300% rise in social conflicts in Peru over the past 5 years, with 41.7% of conflicts related to social or environmental issues (*República del Perú*, 2012). These developments have been responsible for rural highland organizations to come together to form the *Coordinadora Nacional de Comunidades Afectados por la Minería* (CONACAMI) (National Coordination for Communities affected by Mining.).

[127] Economic safety is also a problem. It has a number of elements including lack of employment, job out-migration, poverty, lack of basic resources.

[128] Janolf-Bulman, R., (1992: 108).

[129] Herman, J. L., (1992: 177).

"...requires empathic imagination, the capacity to identify with another, and an effort to see and feel the questions that are essential to the other's being vis-à-vis the situation being studied."[130]

Participatory Research Used in Peru

This section outlines how participatory research was used to study the circumstances in which individuals can reflect on and emotionally work through their relationship to political violence and its aftermath. In contrast to most top-down research practices, the studies on which this study is based set out to find what the aftermath of the political violence looks like from the point of view of its survivors. The reason for this course of action derives from a moral sensibility that seeks to promote the recognition of the adverse effects of material disadvantage and the effects of insecurity, chronic stress, anxiety and lack of social integration.

By considering these problems from the perspective of the survivors of political violence this study is under an obligation to consider the relationship between an individual's psychological suffering and the social, economic and political contexts in which people live.

To get inside the perspective of the survivors of political violence it is therefore necessary to "...break with the culture of vitiated social relations and put other, more humanizing relations in their place."[131] In practice this made efforts to reduce the traditional distance between researcher and the researched particularly important.

To this end the 'participatory research' used for this study was fashioned around the creation and development of safe and protected spaces where people would be able to acknowledge "...the unspoken and unaccounted for" in their communities, histories and personalnarratives.[132]

By providing interaction with others this provides crucial inputs into the rebuilding of lives that had been shattered by the political violence. However, people from the communities studied are not used to the construction and use of safe and protected public spaces for the recovery of historicalmemory. Instead people have been accustomed to block any identification with their own painful experiences for so long that it has become habitual. Therefore, it was necessary for the research team to come to the study with cultural resources sensitive to the causes and consequences of the political violence across interpersonal, intra-group and inter-group levels of analysis; any empirical study of the nature of human and social suffering as a nego-

[130] Watkins, M. & Shulman, H. (2008: 285).

[131] Martin-Baro, I. (1994a, b, c, d: 120).

[132] Morrison, T., (2004) as cited in Watkins, M. & Shulman, H. (2008: 126).

tiated and contextually bound social force without these resources would, it was felt, be counter-productive. However, the construction and use of safe and protected public spaces is not enough without an effective collaborative partnership between researchers and the researched.

For people whose trust has been profoundly violated a process of inclusion is essential if they are to confront the dissociative strategies that undermine their capacities for self-reflection, dialogue, confrontation, reconsideration and integration of their traumatic experiences. To facilitate this aim participatory research was used to democratize the generation of understanding and so overcome "...barriers of shame and secrecy, making intolerable feelings bearable through connections with others, grieving the past, and coming to a new perspective with a more compassionate view of themselves in the present."[133]

To uphold the principles of participatory research enshrined in the work of Fals Borda (1988), Martin-Baro (1994a, b, c, d) and Watkins and Shulman (2008) "... every effort was made to respect, validate and help legitimize local knowledge and to listen attentively to how the survivors of the political violence understand their own situation."[134]

To best serve the needs of participatory research on people affected by the political violence and its aftermath a research team was selected and recruited from a pool of fluent Quechua-speakers with a good working knowledge of the general study area from local towns and suburbs situated within the Department of Ayacucho. Every person recruited for the investigation retains strong links with the countryside, either through family connections or from having grown up there. In addition, every member of the research team came to the study with first-hand experience of the political violence from having lived through at least parts of it either as teenagers or as young adults.

From this synthesis of cultural identity, experience and knowledge the research team was able to provide skills and competencies suited to the construction and use of safe and protected public space. To this end particular attention needed to be paid to the environment (especially 'safe area[s]') in which the in-depth investigation of the experience and aftermath of political violence was to be explored.

For people from the communities studied this was particularly important because the realities of power in their social situation are not consistent with the attributes of a sufficiently safe environment. In this case, creating a safe environment benefitted from the considerable overlap in background and life experiences of the researchers with those of the researched. This is because the researcher has an enhanced capacity to imagine how the researched subjects feel or how the researcher would feel if they were in the situation of the subjects researched.

[133] Herman, J. L., (1992: 276).

[134] Watkins, M. & Shulman, H. (2008: 278).

Though this type of empathic arousal may be the result of their own empathic feeling for the victim of injustice, it is highly probable that the moral issues responsible for the motivation of researchers involved in this study derive from their own experiences of injustice as well, either as a result of their own experiences or of what happened to members of their friends, family, or relatives.

From this beginning the study was well placed to open the investigation to the perspective of the research participants and their communities. Fieldwork began [in July 2008] with information collection on the long-term effects of insecurity, anxiety and lack of social integration, although this quickly became a route for understanding the context in which the research was taking place.

Because of the overlap in perspectives and life experiences the relationship between researchers and researched became increasingly participatory. By working alongside individuals and groups the researchers were able to forge relationships across conventional social boundaries.

In this way the research team was able to open up a series of social spaces in each research community and develop an atmosphere of trust and cooperation that continued to improve as the fieldwork progressed. For 3 years the participatory research that emerged from each of these social spaces became increasingly complex as the usual research formalities were dispensed with and replaced by a more open-ended relationship between researchers and researched. Over time this meant that the research process evolved from formal interviews, testimonies, semi-structured interviews, questionnaires, focus group discussions and field observation to a more collaborative relationship that was to become increasingly free-ranging and spontaneous.

In this way researchers and subjects became increasingly drawn to the notion that the far-reaching psychological implications of human suffering could only be effectively brought forward and reflected on through dialogue, mutuality and reciprocity. By working together people were able to increase their awareness of the psychological effects of the wider socio-economic context and begin to acknowledge and work through the "…anti-moral natural process of healing that time brings about."[135]

Because this process is conditional on an understanding of the traumatized "… way of being, of surviving, of resisting"[136] it became increasingly difficult to ignore specific aspirations, values, traditions, strengths and weaknesses.

---

[135] Amery, J., (1980: 72).

[136] Amery, J., (1980: 72).

This encourages the re-enactment of personal experiences as "...a genuine advent, an event in its own right."[137] In this respect the subjective felt-experience of human suffering is not about the actual facts of a particular historical event, but about the individual's "...way of being, of surviving, of resisting."[138]

These testimonials provide a vital counterweight to sweeping generalization about the nature of human suffering because the recall of the traumatized is "...not simply about the information, the establishment of the facts, but the experience of living through testimony of giving testimony."[139] For LaCapra, "...testimonies are significant in the attempt to understand experience and its aftermath, including the role of memory and its lapses in coming to terms with or denying and repressing the past."[140] In addition, testimony has general (non-personal) validity and consequences because it goes beyond the personal. This means that the purpose of testimony is no longer simply to obtain knowledge, but to keep the events before the eyes of the other.[141]

To ensure that "...the gap between the experience of the event and efforts to articulate that experience" are kept to a minimum, tape-recorded interviews were used on the grounds that spoken testimony is "...less reflexive and less mediated."[142] The value of this approach is further reinforced by the fact that all tape-recorded interviews were undertaken by individuals with first-hand experience of the political violence.

From this perspective the interview approach adopted included the participation and involvement of the researcher; to apply inflexible rules of research to interviews and testimonies would have been absurd and immoral. In this respect spoken testimony was found to have much greater value than fixed questions because it is not closed.

It also turns the interviewer into an active participant instead of a simple passive listener; it helps ensure that the person telling the story and the person listening make a joint effort to understand what it is all about; it makes it easier to ask the interviewee to expand on certain things without difficulty, including issues that are often personal and sensitive.

The authority with which people responded during this study derives from their own direct experiences. Their perception of themselves and of the world is a reflec-

---

[137] Laub, D. (1992: 62) in Felman, S. & Laub, D. (1992).

[138] Laub, D. (1992: 85).

[139] Laub, D. (1992: 85).

[140] LaCapra, D., (2001: 86–7).

[141] Kiss, E., (2000) in Rotberg, R.I. & Thompson, D. (2000: 72) (eds.), (2000).

[142] Chare, N., (2011: 137); Langer, L., (1999: xiv, 81ff).

tion of their own physical exhaustion, malnutrition, extreme mental distress and physical deprivation. It is the direct experience of the hard struggle for satisfying everyday basic needs that give these perceptions about the deadening effect of so much misery and suffering their authority. Just because the insights their testimonies offer and the contributions their actions testify to do not suffice to reverse conventional modes of political decision making, professional practice and policy formation is no reason to deny the importance of their opinions. This is because personalnarratives possess an enormous potential for raising psychological and ethical questions about the use of preconceived ideas and paradigms to understand and resolve the problems of human suffering.

To successfully challenge conventional modes of political decision making, professional practice and policy formation is a huge undertaking. However, the widely varied behavioural, emotional, cognitive, interpersonal, and spiritual adaptations that survivors make and which are recorded here retain their importance because they need to be recognised as normal responses to the consequences of human suffering.[143]

Limitations of the Participatory Research Adopted

Though a community unaffected by the political violence was included in the original participatory research studies were not sufficiently advanced by the end of the 3 years available for fieldwork to include the data.

Communities affected by the political violence were given overriding priority from the outset. The lack of sufficient data from a comparison community unaffected by the political violence therefore affects the interpretation of the information collected from the remaining five conflict affected communities. This is particularly important in relation to the causes and symptoms of psycho-social stress.

[143] Two papers based on the project's early findings were presented by the author in November and December 2008 respectively. The first paper was given at the Joint Initiative for the study of Latin America and the Caribbean (JISLAC) workshop 'Latin Americanists in Wales: New Perspectives on Latin America' held at the University of Aberystwyth 14 November 2008. The second paper was given as part of the Centre for Latin American Studies at Swansea (CLASS) seminar series organised by the Hispanic Studies department, Swansea University on 11 December 2008. A review of some of the work carried out by the project between June 2008–November 2009 was presented and discussed at a conference held between 24–27 November 2009 at the *Universidad Nacional San Cristóbal de Humanga,Ayacucho* (National University of San Cristobal of Huamanga, Ayacucho). The conference was entitled: "*Derechos Humanos y Medio Ambiente en un Contexto de Crisis": Experiencias y Desafios desde el Trabajo Social* (Human Rights and the Environment in a Context of Crisis: experiences and challenges in social work).

Selection and Credentials of Researchers

To give due attention to the human significance of suffering and what it actually does to people called for the selection of a research team with cultural resources sensitive to the causes and consequences of power across interpersonal, intra-group and inter-group levels of analysis; any empirical study of the nature of power as a dynamic, negotiated and contextually bound social force without these resources would, it was felt, be counter-productive. To this point, all team members came to the study with first-hand experience of the political violence having lived through at least parts of it either as teenagers or young adults. Every team member was a university graduate with degrees in sociology, anthropology, etc. and a minimum of 3–5 years' work experience with state-sponsored social development programmes in conflict-affected rural communities in the Andean region. Supervision of the day-to-day activities of the project was carried out by the local project manager assisted by an office secretary.

Both people are in their mid-late 30s and lived through most of the political violence in the area firstly as residents of rural communities and then as displaced people in Huamanga. Initial team training was carried out by the author in collaboration with two facilitators from a UK-based NGO specialising in mental health and psycho-social stress. Training comprised two theoretical and practical modules of 40-hours each.

This was followed by a 21-day pilot project (July–August 2008) held in four of the five rural communities selected for study by the author in consultation with the research team. In the pilot project each team member applied 10–15 interviews under the supervision of the local project manager. The field studies were undertaken between July 2008 and April 2011. At the end of the pilot project each team member was assigned a specific community and remained responsible for all participatory research from that community until fieldwork ended in April 2011. Fieldwork for the main study started in September 2008 and consisted of 3 weeks out of every 4 being spent by the research team in the communities they had each been assigned to.

At the end of every 3-week period the research team returned to the project office in Ayacucho to write up their reports, transcribe tape recordings of focus group discussions, interviews and plan the next stage of their fieldwork activities. To ensure maximum effectiveness the local project manager would make regular visits to each of the research communities to observe and provide advice. Additional training sessions were given to the research team by the author for the community work carried out by them in years two and three of the study.

Supervision of the day-to-day activities of the project was carried out by the local project manager assisted by an office secretary. Both people were in their mid-30s and had lived through most of the political violence in the area firstly as residents of rural communities and then as displaced people in Huamanga.

The Stages of Participatory Research

To conduct the research, I believe the only possible way is through participation and involvement on the part of the researcher and team. To apply inflexible rules of research to auto-narration would be absurd and immoral and make it impossible to obtain credible material. Using interviews, testimonies, semi-structured interviews, questionnaires, focus group discussions and field observation the research team began by asking randomly selected individuals to describe the issues that prevented them from obtaining sufficient access to basic resources and what the consequences of this were. The aim was to identify the main characteristics of human suffering by taking into consideration the experiences with which it is most commonly associated. In this way the research team was able to bring into full view all the particular facts about human suffering in terms that are both historical and specific.

By looking at the particular differences that shape the actual lived experience of local farmers, community leaders, householders, women, adolescents and the elderly it was possible to identify their reaction and attitude to the emotional consequences of suffering. To make their own assessment of their particular situation people were encouraged to describe their own perceptions of the coping strategies they used to address problems. The interviewees were adults of both sexes.

Though most took part as residents in their community of origin, a few participants were living as displaced people. To ensure that other perceptions of human suffering were represented interviews about state policies and programmes for rural services were also held with local officials, local and national institutions. This part of the study was carried out between September 2008 and December 2009 during which the research team completed between 40 and 60 semi-structured interviews and questionnaires and 25 focus group discussions per community.

From this basic survey of suffering and exposure to traumatic events it was possible to compile a list of key concepts and topics that local people had identified and which had been taken from their own subjective experiences of human suffering. This list was subsequently adapted and used by the research team as a framework and guide for more in-depth semi-structured qualitative interviews.[144] Prior to its use all of the guiding questions included in the framework were imported, trial tested, adapted, debated and discussed.[145]

Each interview was carried out in the participants' dwellings wherever possible. By the end of this part of the study an additional list of concepts and topics was compiled in order to examine the impact of traumatic events and the violence-

---

[144] Testimony based evidence about traumatic events are placed in five general categories and subcategories. The five general categories comprise: (1) Material deprivation (2) Bodily injury (3) Forced confinement and coercion (4) Disappearance, death or injury of loved ones (5) Witnessed violence to others. The five general categories are taken from the eight general categories used by the Harvard Trauma Questionnaire (HTQ) and (HSCL-25).

[145] To ground the determining influence of culture, context and institutions (and the subjective nature that the individual brings to their situation) a framework was built up around six major stressor domains comprising physical, social, economic, cultural, security and political.

related stressors to which people were exposed in greater detail. This focused on the experience of psychic wounds and their accompanying symptoms.[146] By the time fieldwork activities were brought to an end in April 2011 between 35 and 44 additional semi-structured qualitative interviews and 20 testimony interviews had been completed per community.

People who agreed to take part in the study were first informed in detail of the study procedures and consent requirements prior to their participation in any of the research activities. Trauma-related interviews and testimonies were held only if the interviewee reported at least one traumatic event and these were tape-recorded with the consent of the interviewee.

Every effort was made to find words in Spanish which reflected the realities local people would think about in Quechua on a day-to-day basis. Many of these difficulties were overcome thanks to the research team's specialist knowledge and skills, although it was not always easy to render semantic nuances and emotions to and from a language where no precise terms for these things existed.

The interviews/testimonies were translated from Quechua to Spanish by the same team member responsible for the interview. The final stages of the fieldwork involved transcribing the conversation from the tape-recordings for qualitative analysis and asking the interviewee to expand and explain on any issues that remained unclear. To protect their identity and ensure confidentiality the names of all those who agreed to take part in the study were removed and replaced with a pseudonym.[147]

Constraints Associated with Participatory Research Used

The development of a trusting relationship with the individuals, groups and communities included in this study was never going to be easy. However, the fact that every member of the research team was a fluent Quechua speaker with life-long links to the general study area was a tremendous asset for gaining confidence and acceptance. Nevertheless, additional confidence-building actions were needed.

To accustom people to the presence of outsiders (and win local confidence) community activities were organised by research team members. These included community-based games for the children, football matches, community haircutting (carried out by the relevant team member concerned) and distribution of gifts for the children of the community at Christmas time.

---

[146] Examples of guiding questions include: Were you living here during the political violence? Do you remember everything that happened during that time? How did it feel to live through an experience like this? Could you tell me a bit about it? How is your life now? Do you ever get nightmares?

[147] Examples of the semi-structured questionnaires and the guiding questions are to be found at Appendix Three.

Conclusions

Operating from the assumption that no individual corresponds to the overwhelming weight of the stereotype requires that we make use of ethnography to explain how people cope with the aftermath of the political violence and other types of suffering on a daily basis. To this end we need to be more attentive to the many different ways in which the traumatized encounter and give voice to their suffering.

This involves an assessment of the particular institutional settings, cultural formations and patterns of relationships and the influences they have on human and social suffering. To deepen our understanding of human suffering it is therefore necessary to underscore the importance of empathy and participation for the bringing forward of experiences that have been silenced. This means that the far-reaching psychological implications of human suffering can only be effectively brought forward and reflected on through dialogue, mutuality and reciprocity. By working together survivors were able to reveal the vulnerability of representations of human suffering to the distortion of generalization, over-simplification and superficiality; to find meaning "…in the psychological violation, physicaloppression and oppression and the marks this leaves on psyche, on the structure of its language, the staccato of its gaps and silences and the forms of its images."[148]

Appendix 4: Participatory Research in Practice

Focus Group Discussions

Summary of Purpose

The research team which undertook this study held FGDs between September 2008 and December 2009 involving people from the Andean communities studied including: teenagers (16+), householders, women, unemployed, local farmers, labourers, community leaders and the elderly. While not a true random sample there was an effort to get a representative sample and every effort was made to ensure that there was an even gender balance and that there were roughly equal numbers of young adults and the elderly as well as equal numbers of teenagers and middle-aged adults. It was understood that FGDs on security-related issues would only involve participants with relevant experience, either from the 1980s political violence or more recent troubles. Though most participants took part as residents in their community of origin, a few participants were living as displaced people.

[148]Watkins, M. & Shulman, H. (2008: 291); see also Denzin, N. K. (2004). in U. Flick, E. v. Kardorff, & I. Steinke (Eds.); Denzin, N. K., & Lincoln, Y. S. (Eds.). (2005).

Through the focus groups, the research team gathered information to identify the main characteristics of human suffering by taking into consideration the experiences with which it is most commonly associated. In this way the research team was able to bring into full view many particular facts about human suffering in terms that are both historical and specific. To make their own assessment of the situation people were encouraged to describe the coping strategies used to address these problems. By the time this part of the study was completed 25 FGDs had been carried out in each of the Andean communities studied in total 125 FGDs. From this basic survey of suffering and exposure to traumatic events it was possible to compile a list of key concepts and topics that local people had identified and which had been taken from their own subjective experiences of human suffering.

FGD Background

The FGDs explored a wide range of topics including: land issues, employment, economic migration, lack of investment, lack of state support, lack of reparations, low levels of education, etc. Participants provided information in two ways: individual responses and group discussion.

The FGDs were designed to gather information in relation to the following outcomes:

(a) To understand the role of physical factors (such as natural resources, agriculture, environment) in participants daily lives.
(b) To understand participants' experience of social factors (such as social cohesion and inclusion, traditional authorities and other forms of social capital at grassroots level).
(c) To understand the role of economic factors (such as degradation of natural resources and the environment, employment opportunities, social stratification and wealth differences).
(d) To understand cultural factors (such as mental health issues, socio-cultural perceptions of local authorities and other government officials, reparations and human rightsabuses relating to the political violence).
(e) To understand security factors (such as mental health problems relating to the political violence, personalsafety and welfare, fear of strangers, military, public service officials, etc.).
(f) To understand political factors (such as perceptions about the legitimacy of local and national government, links between the state and grassroots organizations, accountability, empowerment and political action).

Participant Demographics

There were between 5 and 12 participants in each focus group held in the five Andean communities studied.

Participant Perspectives

Outcome 1 To understand the role of physical factors (such as natural resources, agriculture, environment and ecology) in participants' daily lives.

What Are Participants' Perceptions of Physical Factors?

In general, land-related problems emerged as one of the single most important types of problems facing rural people. Within this category, specific types of land-related problems were endemic to all five communities studied. These include increasing population pressure on available land, land disputes, lack of sewerage, inadequate water supplies, environmental pollution, damage to biodiversity and ecological threats.

Positive Effects of Physical Factors

The two attributes mentioned by participants who we judged overwhelmingly positive are the activities of two relatively new grassroots organizations: NURAJ and JAAS.

Negative Effects of Physical Factors

The problems most frequently mentioned included inadequate sanitation, lack of drinking water, polluted rivers, soil and land erosion, climate change, illegal/damaging invasion of land by mining companies, intense competition for natural resources, lack of adequate drainage, lack of waste disposal, lack of basic infrastructure (including school buildings, teachers and teaching materials, inadequate health facilities health staff, medicines and drugs).

Outcome 2 To understand participants' experience of social factors (such as social cohesion and inclusion, traditional authorities and other forms of social capital at grassroots level).

What Are Participants' Perceptions of Social Factors?

In general, participants said that they feel increasingly threatened by the lack of solidarity. Within this category, specific types of social problems were found to be endemic in all five Andean communities studied. These include feelings of fear/anxiety and mistrust, fear of resurgence in political violence, fear of military/officials, etc., feelings of insecurity (lack of safety/social protection), fear of strangers, nervousness and tensions and poorly integrated personalities. Participants said that they feel powerless to change their situation and that this is forcing them to change the way in which they choose to carry on with their lives.

This is borne out by the feeling that the most frequent link between organizations, institutions and people is not active membership, but one-way delivery of public services and material assistance; and that any remaining grassroots organizations are closer to local people than any of the new NGOs.

Positive Influence of Social Factors

Though this highly aversive state encourages disillusionment and apathy it is also causing some participants to think about their lives in entirely new ways that are making them less dependent on traditional norms and values. It also reveals that people partly accept that there have been some structural improvements since the end of the conflict (drainage construction, school buildings, irrigation systems, road construction).

Negative Influence of Social Factors

The problems most frequently mentioned were feelings of fear, anxiety and intimidation. Increased violence in the form of terrorist resurgence, highway robberies, attacks on soldiers, drug trafficking, extrajudicial killings and deaths, delinquency, alcoholism and domestic violence contributed to a state of permanent vigilance. Participants also said that household fragmentation as a result of the violence is a commonplace. Many husbands were killed, especially if they held leadership positions within the community.

Other family members fled to the cities and have only recently returned or chosen to stay away, visiting only occasionally. There is now a high number of single parent, women headed households. In addition, low levels of control and access to basic resources with a range of adverse outcomes including withdrawal of effort and poor performance on cognitive tasks have brought participants into contention with the idea of effective cooperation. For example, participants said that the number and scope local collective actions have declined together with grassroots organizations and that this is linked to factors such as a decline in the skills of community leaders and the mobilization of local people. This was found to be endemic to all five research communities.

Finally, this section found that participants have a generally negative assessment of public services (low quality, high prices) and formal institutions (corruption, lack of commitment and professionalism).

Outcome 3 To understand the role of economic factors (such as degradation of natural resources and the environment, employment opportunities, social stratification and wealth differences).

What Are Participants' Perceptions of Economic Factors?

In general participants felt that unemployment, poverty and economic suffering are some of the single most important types of problems facing rural people. Within this category, specific types of economic problems were endemic to all five research communities.[149] These include land disputes, material assets, money, environmental and agricultural problems. Underlying the many overlaps between one type of economic problem and another is the future of subsistencefarming and a way of life that has remained relatively untouched for many generations.

Positive Influence of Economic Factors

By drawing attention to the long-term consequences of economic suffering participants also brought a badly needed focus to their own awareness of the social experience of suffering and its influence on internal migration and emigration from the rural highlands.

Negative Influence of Economic Factors

The problems most frequently mentioned by people were access to and distribution of adequate material resources necessary to sustain life including land, agriculture, foodsecurity, material assets, money and the lack of any assistance to ensure the reconstruction of physicalinfrastructure, to generate employment and open markets. Problems finding local work have led to extensive economic migration both for the young and for people with families.

Outcome 4 To understand cultural factors (such as mental health issues, sociocultural perceptions of local authorities and other government officials, reparations and human rightsabuses relating to the political violence).

What Are Participants' Perceptions of Cultural Factors?

In general participants felt that the political violence has contributed to a growing sense of disorientation, agitation and confusion and the feeling of being haunted by a past that intrudes into every aspect of their lives and beyond. In addition, the lack of emotional connectedness between the government and ordinary people was identified as the main reason for the emergence of particular types of attitude including

[149] *Some overlap with the negative features in relation to the outcomes for physical factors is inevitable.*

social withdrawal, hostility, estrangement, and isolation, feelings of meaninglessness, anticipation of betrayal, hyper-vigilance, and an inability to trust.

Positive Influence of Cultural Factors

Feeling powerless to change their situation has made participants distrustful of the belief system that used to give people a sense of responsibility and attachment.

However, the insights these changes give into their own situation have given participants the means to rescue themselves from past illusions about their way of life, including what can be trusted and what should be feared. By altering their basic state of consciousness and by facing the limits of withdrawal from engagement as a solution people are in a potentially better place from which to open up new opportunities for successful coping and what is called post-traumatic growth. It underlines the fact that both new and traditional grassroots organizations have the potential to contribute to the creation of social capital.

Negative Influence of Cultural Factors

The problems most frequently mentioned by people were lack of trust, lack of cooperation within the community, lack of participation, lack of leadership, lack of communication, loss of traditional culture, loss of traditional norms and values, lack of respect, discrimination against the indigenous. The effect of these problems is reflected in the waning authority of community assemblies, in people's attitude toward grassroots organizations, local authorities, formal institutions and organizations, increasing levels of economic migration, individualistic behaviour, conformity and dependency. In recent years the changes in people's behaviour has also led to declines in the use of traditional clothing and costumes, ceremonial occasions, festivities, the indigenous language, the import of western/urban customs and culture (as a result of economic migrants bringing back new ideas), and the expansion of medias.

Outcome 5 To understand security factors (such as mental health problems relating to the political violence; personalsafety and welfare, fear of strangers, military, public service officials, etc.).

What Are Participants' Perceptions of Security Factors?

In general, human suffering was more commonly associated with problems of security than any other type of outcome. The problems describe the practical opinions and attitudes about safety from the perspective of individuals and households and from the perspective of their community. Though important variations about the legacy of the political violence and the emergence of new forms of violence exist security is a continuing problem in all of the communities. It is associated with various types of abuse (rape, torture, etc) all of which live on in the form of delinquency, drug trafficking, economic migration etc. Other consequences of the violence, such as the corruption and inefficiency of the judiciary, the police and the armed forces (and the collapse in popular participation) – contribute to feelings of fear/anxiety and mistrust and insecurity.

Positive Influence of Security Factors

Though this highly aversive state encourages fear, anxiety and stress it is also causing some participants to think about their lives in entirely new ways that are making them less dependent on traditional norms and values.

Negative Influence of Security Factors

The problems most frequently mentioned were feelings of fear, anxiety and intimidation. Increases in delinquency, drugs, terrorism, kidnapping, highway robberies, attacks on soldiers, drug trafficking, extrajudicial killings and deaths and alcohol abuse, inefficiencies in the police, judiciary, armed forces, district and community authorities, the breakdown of the social fabric and the rise of individualistic and conformist behaviour.

Other security-related problems cited by participants include discrepancies between legitimate moral expectations and state-funded social programmes designed to 'mitigate' the effects of the political violence and the impact of extreme poverty have left participants with a feeling of powerlessness about their capacity to restore a sense of control, connection and meaning to their lives. Within this category, specific types of security-related problems were endemic to all five research communities including social withdrawal, hostility, estrangement, and isolation, feelings of meaninglessness, anticipation of betrayal, hyper-vigilance, fear of reprisal and an inability to trust. In the aftermath of the political violence participants said that this has led to a growing sense of disorientation, agitation and confusion and the feeling of being haunted by a past that intrudes into every aspect of their lives.

Outcome 6 To understand political factors (such as perceptions about the legitimacy of local and national government, links between the government and grassroots organizations, accountability, empowerment and political action).

What Are Participants' Perceptions of Political Factors?

In general, politically-related problems are a powerful source of stress and anxiety, both within the community and impacting from outside. They include specific problems with the public sector such as land disputes, education, health, water and sanitation, safety and social protection, the judiciary and state security. They also include more complex problems such as the legacy of the past, fear of resurgence in political violence, fear of military/officials, etc., lack of safety/social protection, fear of strangers, state reparations, other state programmes, NGOs. Other problems include lack of qualified staff, the high turnover of staff, the lack of basic equipment and the linguistic challenges as well as intermediate factors such as isolation, remoteness, transport difficulties and communication problems.

Within this category, feelings of isolation/solidarity, devaluing of other groups and violent reactions towards other groups were endemic to all five research communities.

Positive Influence of Political Factors

Participants said that there have been some structural improvements since the end of the conflict (drainage construction, school buildings, irrigation systems, road construction). Evidence of the emergence of new grassroots organizations in the aftermath of the political violence (NURAJ and JAAS) underlines the fact that both new and traditional voluntary associations retain the potential for being able to contribute to the creation of social capital.

Negative Influence of Political Factors

The problems most frequently mentioned are associated with discrimination against indigenous people by local authorities, regional and national government representatives as well as other organizations and institutions.

This is reflected not just in the attitudes towards people by school teachers and health post staff – but also in outside attitudes toward indigenous languages. Participants said that the abuse shown by the military towards local people during the political violence was unprecedented and that this was because they were treated as though they were terrorists rather than innocent bystanders.[150] In addition participants were found to have a generally negative assessment of public services (dependency, low quality, high prices) and formal institutions (including corruption, inefficiency, lack of commitment and professionalism). This was felt to be the result

[150] *This included material deprivation, bodily injury, forced confinement and coercion, disappearances, death or injury of loved ones, witnessing violence done to others.*

of policy makers and programme officials who do not treat people with respect and give them no opportunity for reciprocal exchanges of opinion and information.

FGDs: An Assessment and Taking Things Forward

It is clear from the responses and discussions that the understandings participants bring to bear on their appraisal of human suffering and on their expressions of distress and disruptions to the social and moral order are neither straightforward nor are they immediately reproducible elsewhere. To find out more about the feelings, opinions and attitudes held by people we therefore decided to explore the particular situation participants respond to in greater depth. From this perspective the individual subjective felt-experience is invaluable for the "...understanding of experience and its aftermath, including the role of memory and its lapses in coming to terms with or denying and repressing the past."[151] This made the interview/testimony method as the principle form of methodology essential.

Semi-Structured Interviews (SSIs) and Testimonies

Summary of Purpose

To counter the objectification of human suffering SSIs and Testimonies were used to explore the situation as people perceive and cognitively construct it. Its purpose was two-fold: to reveal the vulnerability of representations of human suffering to the distortion of subjectivity, generalization, over-simplification and superficiality; to find meaning in the experience of ordinary people.[152]

From this perspective the interview approach included the participation and involvement of the researcher; to apply inflexible rules of research to interviews and testimonies would have been absurd and immoral.

There was no discrimination amongst participants in the study but efforts were made to ensure that there was an even gender balance and that there were roughly equal numbers of young adults and the elderly as well as equal numbers of teenagers and middle-aged adults. In this respect spoken testimony was found to have much greater value than fixed questions because it is not closed. To give due atten-

---

[151] *LaCapra, D., (*2001*: 86–7)Writing History, WritingTrauma. The John Hopkins University Press: Baltimore 2715 North Charles Street, Maryland 21,218–4362.*

[152] *Denzin, N. K. (*2004*). Reading film: using films and videos as empirical social science material. In U. Flick, E. v. Kardorff, & I. Steinke (Eds), A Companion to Qualitative Research (pp. 237–42). London: Sage; Denzin, N. K., & Lincoln, Y. S. (Eds).* (2005*) The Sage Handbook of Qualitative Research (3rd edn) Thousand Oaks, CA: Sage.*

tion to the human significance of suffering and what it actually does to people information was gathered in relation to the following outcomes:

(a) Physical factors (such as natural resources, agriculture, environment)
(b) Social factors (such as social cohesion and inclusion, traditional authorities and other forms of social capital at grassroots level)
(c) Economic factors (such as destruction/degradation of natural resources and the environment, employment opportunities, social stratification and wealth differences).
(d) Cultural factors (such as mental health issues, socio-cultural perceptions of local authorities and other government officials, reparations and human rightsabuses relating to the political violence).
(e) Security factors (such as mental health problems relating to the political violence, personalsafety and welfare, fear of strangers, military, public service officials, etc.).
(f) Political factors (such as perceptions about the legitimacy of local and national government, links between the state and grassroots organizations, accountability, empowerment and political action).

Background

Between 2008 and 2011 in-depth interviews (SSIs) and testimonies were carried out with more than 500 informants including: teenagers (16 years plus), householders, women, unemployed, local farmers, labourers, community leaders and the elderly (60 yrs. plus).[153] Interviewees were not selected, although every effort was made to ensure that there was as even a gender balance as possible and that there were roughly equal numbers of the elderly, teenagers and middle-aged adults. It was understood that SSIs and Testimonies involving security-related issues would only involve people with relevant experience, either from the political violence or more recent unrest. Though most interviewees took part as residents in their community of origin, a few were living as displaced people. Through SSIs and Testimonies, the research team gathered information to identify the main characteristics of human suffering by taking into consideration the experiences with which it is most commonly associated. In this way the research team was able to bring into full view many particular facts about human suffering in terms that are both historically and locality-specific. To make their own assessment of the situation people were encouraged to describe the coping strategies used to address these problems.

During the first part of the study (between September 2008 and December 2009) the research team completed between 40 and 60 semi-structured interviews per community. From this basic survey of suffering and exposure to traumatic events it

[153] *This includes* multiple interviews with the same interviewee.

was possible to compile a list of key concepts and topics that local people had identified and which had been taken from their own subjective experiences of human suffering. This list was subsequently adapted and used by the research team as a framework and guide for more in-depth semi-structured qualitative interviews.[154] Prior to its use all of the guiding questions included in the framework were imported, trial tested, adapted, debated and discussed.[155] Each interview was carried out in the participants' dwellings wherever possible. By the end of this part of the study an additional list of concepts and topics was compiled in order to examine the impact of traumatic events and the violence-related stressors to which people were exposed in greater detail. This focused on the experience of psychic wounds and their accompanying symptoms.[156]

By the time fieldwork activities were brought to an end in April 2011 between 35 and 44 additional semi-structured qualitative interviews and 20 testimony interviews had been completed per community.

Subjects Covered in SSIs/Testimonies

1.Physicalfactors
Increases in socio-economic inequalities
Trends in access to social support and welfare
Social stratification and wealth differences
Competition for naturalresources
Degree of population pressure on the land
Disputes over land ownership
Distribution of water/land
Failure in agriculture
Natural disasters
Threats environmental, economic, etc.
Damage to biodiversity

(continued)

[154] Testimony based evidence about the traumatic events relating to the political violence are placed in five general categories and sub-categories. The five general categories comprise: (1) Material deprivation (2) Bodily injury (3) Forced confinement and coercion (4) Disappearance, death or injury of loved ones (5) Witnessed violence to others. The five general categories are taken from the eight general categories used by the Harvard Trauma Questionnaire (HTQ) and (HSCL-25).

[155] To ground the determining influence of culture, context and institutions (and the subjective nature that the individual brings to their situation) a framework was built up around six major stressor domains comprising physical, social, economic, cultural, security and political.

[156] Examples of guiding questions include: Were you living here during the political violence? Do you remember everything that happened during that time? How did it feel to live through an experience like this? Could you tell me a bit about it? How is your life now? Do you ever get nightmares?

Environmental pollution
Lack of sewerage
Malnutrition
Poverty: increases in socio-economic inequalities
Trends in poverty and food shortages
Links between the community and markets
Number of contacts between the community and markets
Channels for conflict management
Legitimacy or bias of traditional authorities
Evidence of violent and nonviolent protests
Presence of vertical and horizontal organizations
Socialcohesionand inclusion
Social unity and solidarity within the community
Social divisions within the community
Social exclusion as characterized by gender, age, type of activity
Evidence of vertical-type social interactions
Evidence of horizontal-type social interactions
2. Social factors
Mentalhealthissues
Social cohesion and inclusion
The perception of social unity and solidarity within the community
The perception of divisions within the community
Social exclusion as characterized by gender, age, type of activity
Evidence of vertical-type social interactions
Evidence of horizontal-type social interactions
Poverty: increased socio-economic inequalities
Trends in poverty and food shortages
Inequalities in the distribution of wealth
Links between the community and markets
Evidence of contacts between the community and the markets
Channels for conflict management/resolution
Legitimacy or bias of traditional authorities
Evidence of violent and nonviolent protests
Presence of vertical and horizontal organizations
Participation in groups and associations
Collective action and cooperation
Level of collective action
The type of collective action
Level of commitment to cooperate and participate in collective action
Comparison between cognitive social capital and structural social capital
Capacity of grassroots organizations
Capacity for decision making
Managing conflict
Sustainability

(continued)

Resource mobilization and management
Participation
Organizational culture
Level of satisfaction of its members
Representation and negotiation
Management of finance
Effectiveness/links
Communication/coordination
Accountability
Troubleshooting
Communal perceptions on ownership of the grassroots organizations
Individuals feel that they are owners or members of the organization
Level of the organization's financial sustainability
Level of independence
Level of vertical social capital for organizations involved in the markets
Level of vertical social capital for organizations involved in policy
Quality of relationships within the organization
Quality of relationships outside the organization
Alcoholism
Illiteracy
3. Economic
Mental health issues
Individual feelings about available employment
Increased socio-economic inequalities
Trends in access to social security and welfare
Social stratification and wealth differences
Economic migration
Competition for naturalresources
Degree of population pressure on the land
Disputes over land ownership
Distribution of water/land
Failure in agriculture
Natural disasters
4. Cultural
Mentalhealthissues
Loss/bereavement
Threats
Syndromes of depression and its symptoms
Do you trust government officials or members of other institutions? (NGOs)
What have you done for the development of the people in your village?
Socio-cultural factors
Political exploitation of cultural and other differences
Historical rivalries and other disputes remembered
Cultural discrimination

(continued)

Propaganda exclusionary
Defamation of certain social groups
The influence of negative stereotypes about the mutual perception
Social factors linked to conflict Article 45 (Integral Plan of Reparations)
Extrajudicial execution
Murder
Forced disappearance
Rape or sexual abuse
Torture
Kidnapping
Forced displacement
Forced recruitment
Violation of due process
Social factors linked to conflict Article 50 (Integral Plan of Reparations)
Evidence of the hierarchy of bosses and their workers
Level of inequality between citizens
Empowering the excluded
Establishing relationships that respect equality
Understandingby the individual on the responsibilities of the state:
The structure of government
The political system
The administrative system
Relevant policies
Relevant budgets
Money available to local services
Level of confidence in the state
The individual's ability to analyze and solve problems and provide regular feedback
Level of community consultation in resource management
Level of democracy at the community level
Level of appropriate organization at community level
Level of awareness on the part of the individual
Vertical investment planning
Investments without participation
Investment without accountability
Investment without feedback
Awareness of marginalized groups (women, elderly, etc.)
Understandingof the local government and its' responsibilities
Level of accountability by local government
Level of understanding by the local government on the rights of their workers.
Level of understanding by the local government on their own responsibilities as state officials.
5.Security
Mental health issues
Experiences of loss/bereavement

(continued)

Experiences of threats
Syndromes of depression and its symptoms
Experiences of life here during the political violence
Memories of the political violence in the community
Individual feelings about being a witness to the political violence.
Individual feelings about the new situation
Serious incidents that have affected you or any members of your family
Experiences of disturbed sleep patterns associated with the political violence
Fear of strangers
Feelings of nervousness, tension, anxiety and worry
Experiences of violent reactions to other people
Experiences of self-harm/hatred
Opportunities to confide in trustworthy people
Individual feelings about government officials or members of other institutions (NGOs)
Fear of the military
Individual feelings about the doctors and nurses
Experiences of how government officials treat people
Average daily income earnings
Access to local, national and international news
Level of job satisfaction
Individual feelings about the performance of basic services
Individual feelings about transportation services for the community
Legacy of violence
History of unresolved conflict at the community level
Levels of violent offenders, rape and kidnapping
Low intensity of political violence/political assassinations
Positive attitude towards violence in the community
Popular support and disillusionment with the security apparatus
Evidence of social reconciliation (vertical and horizontal)
Level of leadership in the community
The relationship between economic and political organizations within the community
Support for the establishment ofaccountability
Community members with links to the state
Level of feedback
Is there accountability inside the community
Is there accountability outside the community
Understandingby the individual ofhuman rightsin relation to:
Access to health services and education
Access to safe water
Access to basic sanitation
Trustandsolidarity
The extent to which there is trust between people
To what extent is trust possible between specific groups

(continued)

Confidence in other organizations
Confidence in the quality of organization members
Trust in government
6. Political
Mentalhealthissues
Trust in government officials or members of other institutions (NGOs)
Fear of the military?
Trust in the doctors and nurses?
Treatment by government officials
Access to information about a) community, b) province c) regional d) country e) world
Level of satisfaction with basic services
Confidence in transportation services for the community
Legitimate government and good governance
What do you think about the legitimacy of district/local government?
What do you think about political power?
Existence of abuse of power
Level of administrative centralization, strength of district/local government
Government ability to manage
Level of decentralization
Level of participation
Level of vertical planning
Level of accountability
Issues concerning the recommendations of the TRC
Effectiveness of the roundtables/multi-sectoral tables
Pluralismand participation
Popular approval or dissatisfaction with political leaders
Independence and political participation of civil society
Experience with a government official/programme (participatory, representative, democratic)
Procedures for elections (fraud, voter intimidation)
Channels for conflict management
Independence or institutional bias of the judiciary and the police
Respect for the law
Free speech
History of state repression
Repair and reconstruction (awareness of the law of reparations – including:
Repairs or Comprehensive Plan (IRP) Article 10 (b)[157]
Register of victims (RUV) Article 5[158]

(continued)

[157] Article 10 (b) State action to implement actions for restitution and full exercise of citizenship rights of the victims of the violence process).

[158] Article 5 State action on reparations is based on the concurrent action and express all the institutions of the state, aimed at promoting repair programs that allow victims the process of the return of violence to achieve their rights violated during the internal armed conflict, and guided by the Act, its rules, multi-year programming and annual operating plans.

Understandingby the individual on the responsibilities of the state:
Ownership level in initiatives or investments made by the state
Level of links between the state and grassroots organizations
Empowerment and political action
Level of involvement with the institutions that affect people in the community.
Feedback level institutions that affect people in the community.
Level of accountability institutions that affect people in the community.
Level of influence/control over the institutions that affect people in the community.
Level of government's commitment to the elimination of social barriers
Level of commitment by local government to increase social opportunity
Number (and type) of activities that increase empowerment (political, socio-economic, etc.)
Number of activities involving decision making that affects daily activities[159]
Comparison with empowerment and information access features, fear of violence, solidarity, etc

List of Interviewees (2008–2009)

Male/ Female	Age Approx.	Name [all names disguised]	Community	Interviews (2008–9) M = multiple interviews with same interviewee
M	46	Jose	Qocha	
F	40	Lidia	Unay	
M	44	Ramon	Otoronco	M
F	45	Clementina	Wamani	
M	46	Marcos	Yachaya	M
F	37	Agustina	Qocha	
M	48	Santos	Unay	M
F	40	Evita	Otoronco	
M	39	Sabino	Wamani	M
F	40	Eufemia	Yachaya	M
M	50	Valentin	Qocha	M
F	45	Maximo	Unay	M
M	43	Sanchez	Otoronco	M
F	46	Lorgio	Wamani	
M	45	Victor	Yachaya	M
F	45	Agustina	Qocha	
M	42	Julian	Unay	

(continued)

[159] This includes making requests, participating in public meetings, meetings with politicians, participation in multi-sectoral tables, voting in elections).

Male/ Female	Age Approx.	Name [all names disguised]	Community	Interviews (2008–9) M = multiple interviews with same interviewee
F	29	Luigi	Otoronco	
M	30	Palomino	Wamani	M
M	36	Alejandro	Yachaya	
M	34	Julio	Qocha	M
F	43	Grimalda	Unay	M
M	32	Carlos	Otoronco	
F	37	Julia	Wamani	
M	26	Eusebio	Yachaya	M
F	19	Felisa	Qocha	
M	38	Nestor	Unay	M
F	26	Maria	Otoronco	
M	24	Sabino	Wamani	M
F	35	Lupe	Yachaya	
M	38	Joaquin	Qocha	M
F	75	Alicia	Unay	
M	26	Esteban	Otoronco	
F	35	Rosa	Wamani	
M	25	Guillermo	Qocha	
F	33	Aline	Unay	
M	32	Miguel	Otoronco	M
F	31	Victoria	Wamani	
M	63	Guillermo	Yachaya	M
F	28	Paciencia	Qocha	
M	32	Jesus	Unay	M
F	20	Fidel	Otoronco	
M	29	Felix	Wamani	M
F	28	Vivian	Yachaya	
M	50	Marcelino	Qocha	M
F	26	Gracia	Unay	
M	36	Alvaro	Otoronco	
F	23	Gabriel	Wamani	
M	54	Faustino	Yachaya	M
F	25	Guadalupe	Qocha	
M	37	Fulgencio	Unay	
F	25	Paloma	Otoronco	
M	47	Herberto	Wamani	M
F	53	Rebecca	Yachaya	
M	30	Pastor	Qocha	
F	63	Gabie	Unay	
M	27	Ricardo	Otoronco	
F	31	Etalpalli	Wamani	
M	30	Tomas	Yachaya	

(continued)

Male/ Female	Age Approx.	Name [all names disguised]	Community	Interviews (2008–9) M = multiple interviews with same interviewee
F	43	Isabel	Qocha	
M	63	Reyes	Unay	
F	28	Gala	Otoronco	
M	32	Roberto	Wamani	
F	20	Regina	Yachaya	
M	29	Maximino	Qocha	
F	28	Olga	Unay	
M	51	Fidéle	Otoronco	M
F	26	Juana	Wamani	
M	36	Flavio	Yachaya	M
F	48	Luna	Qocha	
M	58	Juanito	Unay	M
F	30	Perla	Otoronco	
M	62	Marco	Wamani	M
F	27	Gaétan	Yachaya	
M	31	Hieronimo	Qocha	
F	30	Galetée	Unay	
M	30	Paulino	Otoronco	
F	26	Gildas	Wamani	
M	23	Florentin	Yachaya	
F	54	Margarita	Qocha	
M	25	Graciano	Unay	M
F	37	Jacinta	Otoronco	
M	25	Fabián	Wamani	
F	29	Luisa	Yachaya	
M	34	Godofredo	Qocha	
F	43	Lucita	Unay	
M	32	Guido	Otoronco	M
F	37	Mariangela	Wamani	
M	26	Fabricio	Yachaya	
F	19	Pepita	Qocha	
M	38	Eurico	Unay	M
F	26	Eva	Otoronco	
M	24	Ignacio	Wamani	
F	35	Amaranta	Yachaya	
M	38	Mario	Qocha	M
F	75	Amalia	Unay	
M	26	Gustavo	Otoronco	
F	35	Lola	Wamani	
F	25	Teressa	Yachaya	
M	33	Nacho	Qocha	
F	32	Yoyotli	Unay	

(continued)

Male/ Female	Age Approx.	Name [all names disguised]	Community	Interviews (2008–9) M = multiple interviews with same interviewee
M	31	Temotzin	Otoronco	
F	29	Jacquline	Wamani	M
M	30	Tonatzin	Yachaya	
F	26	Lina	Qocha	
M	34	Gregorio	Unay	M
F	43	Marisa	Otoronco	
M	32	Theodore	Wamani	M
F	37	Mora	Yachaya	
M	26	Ramiro	Qocha	
F	19	Joviana	Unay	
M	38	Tenyoa	Otoronco	
F	26	Verdad	Wamani	
M	24	Emilio	Yachaya	
F	35	Isolda	Qocha	
M	38	Honoré	Unay	M
F	32	Yolanda	Otoronco	
M	37	Nicanor	Wamani	
F	26	Liana	Yachaya	
M	29	Tiburcio	Qocha	M
F	38	Suniva	Unay	
M	26	Hipolito	Otoronco	
F	24	Susana	Wamani	
M	35	Tezcacoat	Qocha	
F	38	Laurelle	Unay	
M	45	Nahuatl	Otoronco	
F	63	Judit	Wamani	
M	27	Tenyoa	Yachaya	
F	31	Marisa	Qocha	
M	30	Severiano	Unay	
F	30	Salvadora	Otoronco	
M	26	Sabas	Wamani	
F	23	Imaculada	Yachaya	
M	54	Tulio	Qocha	M
F	25	Salud	Unay	
M	37	Victorino	Otoronco	M
F	25	Isbel	Wamani	
M	29	Nopaltzin	Yachaya	
F	34	Lina	Qocha	M
M	43	Ponce	Unay	
F	32	Marisol	Otoronco	
M	37	Theodore	Wamani	M
F	26	Mora	Yachaya	

(continued)

Male/ Female	Age Approx.	Name [all names disguised]	Community	Interviews (2008–9) M = multiple interviews with same interviewee
M	19	Ramiro	Qocha	
F	38	Manola	Unay	
M	26	Rufo	Otoronco	
F	24	Nelli	Wamani	
M	35	Isandro	Yachaya	M
F	38	Maritza	Qocha	M
M	51	Santiago	Unay	M
F	26	Ilhuitl	Otoronco	
M	35	Ismael	Wamani	M
F	25	Eufemia	Yachaya	
M	33	Valentin	Qocha	
F	32	Manauia	Unay	
M	31	Saturnin	Otoronco	
F	63	Martirio	Wamani	
M	28	Maximo	Qocha	
F	32	Tlacotl	Unay	
M	20	Icnoyotl	Otoronco	
F	29	Lurdes	Wamani	
M	28	Zolin	Yachaya	
F	51	Teófila	Qocha	
M	26	Sans	Unay	
F	36	Ofelia	Otoronco	
M	48	Jerome	Wamani	
F	58	Nohemi	Yachaya	
M	30	Julio	Qocha	
F	26	Momoztli	Unay	
M	19	Jeremias	Otoronco	
F	38	Rollande	Wamani	
M	26	Lino	Yachaya	
F	24	Necahual	Qocha	
M	35	Rafael	Unay	
F	38	Samaria	Otoronco	
M	55	Ordell	Wamani	
F	26	Raquel	Yachaya	
M	35	Severo	Qocha	
F	25	Rosalind	Unay	
M	33	Rubén	Otoronco	
F	32	Priscila	Wamani	
M	31	Marcelo	Yachaya	M
F	53	Rosa	Qocha	
M	28	Plinio	Unay	
F	32	Luna	Otoronco	

(continued)

Male/ Female	Age Approx.	Name [all names disguised]	Community	Interviews (2008–9) M = multiple interviews with same interviewee
M	20	Juanito	Wamani	
F	29	Perla	Yachaya	
M	28	Porfirio	Qocha	
F	51	Gaétan	Unay	
M	26	Flavio	Otoronco	
F	36	Prissy	Wamani	
M	48	Marco	Yachaya	
F	58	Pomposa	Qocha	
M	30	Orlando	Unay	
F	63	Ninon	Otoronco	
M	31	Rainerio	Wamani	

List of Interviewees (2009–2011)

Male/ Female	Age Approx.	Name [all names disguised]	Community	Interviews (2009–11) M = multiple interviews with same interviewee
M	26	Julian	Unay	M
F	23	Luigi	Otoronco	M
M	54	Palomino	Wamani	M
F	25	Alejandra	Yachaya	
M	37	Julio	Qocha	M
F	25	Grimalda	Unay	
M	29	Carlos	Otoronco	
F	30	Julia	Wamani	
M	30	Eusebio	Yachaya	
F	34	Felisa	Qocha	M
M	43	Nestor	Unay	
F	32	Maria	Otoronco	
M	37	Sabino	Wamani	M
F	23	Lupe	Yachaya	
M	23	Joaquin	Qocha	
F	51	Alicia	Unay	
M	25	Jose	Qocha	
M	37	Guillermo	Qocha	M
F	25	Aline	Unay	
M	22	Miguel	Otoronco	M
F	36	Victoria	Wamani	M

(continued)

Male/ Female	Age Approx.	Name [all names disguised]	Community	Interviews (2009–11) M = multiple interviews with same interviewee
M	43	Guillermo	Yachaya	M
F	32	Paciencia	Qocha	
M	37	Jesus	Unay	M
F	26	Fidel	Otoronco	
M	18	Felix	Wamani	
F	37	Vivian	Yachaya	M
M	29	Marcelino	Qocha	
F	26	Gracia	Unay	
M	39	Alvaro	Otoronco	
F	38	Gabriel	Wamani	
M	26	Faustino	Yachaya	
M	34	Felip	Qocha	
F	24	Guadalupe	Qocha	
M	35	Fulgencio	Unay	M
F	38	Lidia	Unay	
M	75	Ramon	Otoronco	M
F	26	Clementina	Wamani	
M	35	Marcos	Yachaya	M
F	25	Agustina	Qocha	M
M	33	Santos	Unay	M
F	32	Evita	Otoronco	M
M	31	Sabino	Wamani	
F	63	Eufemia	Yachaya	M
M	28	Valentin	Qocha	
F	32	Maximo	Unay	
M	20	Sanchez	Otoronco	M
F	29	Lorgio	Wamani	
M	28	Victor	Yachaya	M
F	51	Agustina	Qocha	M
M	26	Esteban	Otoronco	M
F	36	Rosa	Wamani	M
F	48	Paloma	Otoronco	
M	58	Herberto	Wamani	M
F	30	Rebecca	Yachaya	
M	63	Pastor	Qocha	M
F	27	Gabie	Unay	
M	31	Ricardo	Otoronco	
F	30	Etalpalli	Wamani	
M	30	Tomas	Yachaya	
F	26	Isabel	Qocha	M
M	23	Reyes	Unay	
F	54	Gala	Otoronco	M

(continued)

Male/ Female	Age Approx.	Name [all names disguised]	Community	Interviews (2009–11) M = multiple interviews with same interviewee
M	25	Roberto	Wamani	
F	37	Regina	Yachaya	M
M	25	Maximino	Qocha	
F	29	Olga	Unay	M
M	36	Fidéle	Otoronco	M
F	43	Juana	Wamani	
M	32	Flavio	Yachaya	
F	37	Luna	Qocha	M
M	26	Juanito	Unay	
F	19	Perla	Otoronco	
M	38	Marco	Wamani	
F	26	Gaétan	Yachaya	
M	24	Mario	Qocha	M
F	35	Amalia	Unay	
M	38	Gustavo	Otoronco	M
F	75	Lola	Wamani	
F	26	Teressa	Yachaya	
M	35	Nacho	Qocha	M
F	25	Yoyotli	Unay	
M	33	Temotzin	Otoronco	
F	32	Jacquline	Wamani	
M	31	Tonatzin	Yachaya	
F	63	Lina	Qocha	
M	28	Gregorio	Unay	M
F	32	Marisa	Otoronco	
M	20	Theodore	Wamani	
F	29	Mora	Yachaya	
M	28	Ramiro	Qocha	
F	51	Joviana	Unay	M
M	26	Tenyoa	Otoronco	
F	36	Verdad	Wamani	
M	48	Emilio	Yachaya	M
M	58	Hieronimo	Qocha	M
F	30	Galetée	Unay	
M	63	Paulino	Otoronco	M
F	27	Gildas	Wamani	
M	31	Florentin	Yachaya	
F	30	Margarita	Qocha	
M	30	Graciano	Unay	M
F	26	Jacinta	Otoronco	
M	23	Fabián	Wamani	
F	54	Luisa	Yachaya	

(continued)

Male/ Female	Age Approx.	Name [all names disguised]	Community	Interviews (2009–11) M = multiple interviews with same interviewee
M	25	Godofredo	Qocha	
F	37	Lucita	Unay	
M	25	Guido	Otoronco	
F	29	Mariangela	Wamani	
M	34	Fabricio	Yachaya	M
F	43	Pepita	Qocha	
M	32	Eurico	Unay	M
F	37	Eva	Otoronco	M
M	41	Ignacio	Wamani	M
F	37	Amaranta	Yachaya	
F	34	Isolda	Qocha	
M	51	Honoré	Unay	M
F	39	Yolanda	Otoronco	M
M	27	Nicanor	Wamani	
F	23	Liana	Yachaya	
M	42	Tiburcio	Qocha	M
F	24	Suniva	Unay	
M	32	Hipolito	Otoronco	
F	41	Susana	Wamani	M
M	45	Tezcacoat	Qocha	
F	30	Laurelle	Unay	
M	28	Nahuatl	Otoronco	
F	43	Judit	Wamani	
M	41	Tenyoa	Yachaya	M
F	26	Marisa	Qocha	
M	40	Severiano	Unay	
F	32	Salvadora	Otoronco	M
M	38	Sabas	Wamani	M
F	41	Imaculada	Yachaya	M
M	48	Tulio	Qocha	M
F	38	Salud	Unay	M
M	44	Victorino	Otoronco	M
F	39	Isbel	Wamani	
M	35	Nopaltzin	Yachaya	
F	39	Lina	Qocha	M
M	40	Ponce	Unay	M
F	35	Marisol	Otoronco	
M	47	Theodore	Wamani	
F	32	Mora	Yachaya	
M	40	Ramiro	Qocha	M
F	33	Manola	Unay	
M	31	Rufo	Otoronco	

(continued)

Male/ Female	Age Approx.	Name [all names disguised]	Community	Interviews (2009–11) M = multiple interviews with same interviewee
F	23	Nelli	Wamani	
M	21	Isandro	Yachaya	
F	40	Maritza	Qocha	
M	48	Santiago	Unay	M
F	37	Ilhuitl	Otoronco	
M	34	Ismael	Wamani	M
F	45	Eufemia	Yachaya	
M	49	Valentin	Qocha	M
F	33	Manauia	Unay	
M	35	Saturnin	Otoronco	
F	30	Martirio	Wamani	
M	54	Maximo	Qocha	M
F	27	Tlacotl	Unay	
M	31	Icnoyotl	Otoronco	
F	34	Lurdes	Wamani	
M	40	Zolin	Yachaya	M
F	34	Teófila	Qocha	
M	32	Sans	Unay	
F	42	Ofelia	Otoronco	
M	41	Jerome	Wamani	M
F	37	Nohemi	Yachaya	
M	47	Julio	Qocha	M
F	24	Momoztli	Unay	
M	43	Jeremias	Otoronco	M
F	46	Rollande	Wamani	M
M	49	Lino	Yachaya	M
F	46	Necahual	Qocha	M
M	46	Rafael	Unay	
F	32	Samaria	Otoronco	
M	41	Ordell	Wamani	
F	23	Raquel	Yachaya	
M	48	Severo	Qocha	M
F	34	Rosalind	Unay	M
M	45	Rubén	Otoronco	M
F	31	Priscila	Wamani	
M	37	Marcelo	Yachaya	
F	43	Rosa	Qocha	M
M	32	Plinio	Unay	M
F	24	Luna	Otoronco	
M	46	Juanito	Wamani	M
F	38	Perla	Yachaya	M
M	25	Porfirio	Qocha	M

(continued)

	Age	Name	Community	Interviews (2009–11)
Male/ Female	Approx.	[all names disguised]		M = multiple interviews with same interviewee
F	38	Gaétan	Unay	
M	46	Flavio	Otoronco	M
F	29	Prissy	Wamani	
M	32	Marco	Yachaya	M
F	27	Pomposa	Qocha	M
M	46	Orlando	Unay	
F	28	Ninon	Otoronco	
M	33	Rainerio	Wamani	M
F	37	Flora	Unay	
M	25	Percy	Otoronco	M
F	28	Frida	Wamani	
M	51	Jorge	Qocha	M
F	26	Carmelina	Unay	
M	36	Herminio	Otoronco	
F	23	Milca	Wamani	
M	54	Feliciano	Yachaya	M
F	25	Ofelia	Qocha	
M	48	Filomeno	Unay	M
F	58	Juna	Otoronco	
M	30	Mauricio	Wamani	M
F	63	Claudia	Yachaya	M
M	27	Teodoro	Qocha	
F	31	Lucia	Unay	
M	30	Feliciano	Otoronco	
F	29	Modesta	Wamani	
M	30	Ember	Yachaya	
F	36	Celestina	Qocha	
M	34	Jenry	Unay	
F	43	Rufina	Otoronco	M
M	32	Juan	Wamani	
F	37	Alfonsa	Yachaya	
M	26	Roger	Qocha	
F	19	Reyna	Unay	
M	38	Teodoro	Otoronco	M
F	26	Georgina	Wamani	
M	24	Yarner	Yachaya	
F	35	Aurora	Qocha	M
M	38	Vicente	Unay	M
F	75	Marisela	Otoronco	
M	36	Rildo	Wamani	

(continued)

F	35	Genoveva	Yachaya	M
M	25	Rolando	Qocha	
F	33	Fermina	Unay	
M	32	Damacino	Otoronco	M
F	32	Vanesa	Wamani	
M	20	Feliciano	Yachaya	
F	29	Juana	Qocha	M
M	31	Seberino	Unay	
F	63	Claudia	Otoronco	
M	28	Eugenio	Wamani	

F	37	Priscila	Unay	
M	25	Marcelo	Otoronco	
F	28	Rosa	Wamani	
M	51	Plinio	Qocha	M
F	26	Luna	Unay	
M	36	Juanito	Otoronco	M
F	23	Gaétan	Wamani	
M	54	Flavio	Yachaya	
F	25	Prissy	Qocha	
M	48	Marco	Unay	M
F	58	Juna	Otoronco	
M	30	Mauricio	Wamani	
F	63	Claudia	Yachaya	
M	27	Teodoro	Qocha	
M	41	Ordell	Wamani	M
F	23	Raquel	Yachaya	
M	48	Severo	Qocha	M
F	34	Rosalind	Unay	
M	45	Rubén	Otoronco	
F	31	Pomposa	Wamani	
M	37	Percy	Yachaya	M
F	43	Frida	Qocha	M
M	32	Jorge	Unay	
F	24	Carmelina	Otoronco	
M	46	Herminio	Wamani	
F	38	Perla	Yachaya	
M	25	Milca	Qocha	
F	38	Porfirio	Unay	
M	46	Feliciano	Otoronco	M
F	29	Ofelia	Wamani	
M	32	Orlando	Yachaya	
F	27	Flora	Qocha	
M	46	Rainerio	Unay	
F	28	Ninon	Otoronco	
M	33	Filomeno	Wamani	

Appendix 5: Reparations Programmes Established by Executive Decree 015-2006-JUS[160]

Programme	Services
Restitution of civil rights	Measures include declarations of absence due to enforced disappearance to allow the relatives of the disappeared to exercise their civil and inheritance rights; restitution of civil rights to those unfairly indicted or prosecuted for terrorism or treason; elimination of criminal records of victims; provision of civil records to those who became undocumented; regularization of property and inheritance rights of victims; and the waiver of fees and taxes imposed when initiating actions required to implement reparations, to be established by law in each case
Education	Directed at individuals whose schooling was interrupted as a result of violence, children of victims, and those forcibly recruited by self-defence committees,* these measures include adult education and literacy programs; access to primary education; access to vocational training; waivers of tuition and certificate and exam fees; student housing and meal stipends for qualified victims; and implementation of a full-scholarship program, covering tuition, books, transportation, and food for university and technical studies where victims could apply based on regional quotas to support students coming from the most affected areas
	* Some of these provisions were later modified by Decree 047-2011-PCM
Health care	Directed at victims suffering from physical or mental ailments resulting from the violence, these measures include delivering comprehensive health care services through the public network, with a priority on serving children, women, and the elderly; building comprehensive community health care programs, including rebuilding community support networks; recovery of historical memory about the conflict; and creating community programs for emotional support. These community programs also include clinical services according to the needs and of each area in the country as well as establishing education and outreach programs for promoting health and prevention and improving the health care network infrastructure
Collective reparations	Directed at assisting families, peasant communities, indigenous communities, settlements, and other communal organizations affected by the conflict, as well as at displaced families from conflict-affected communities that have resettled elsewhere, these measures—Aimed at strengthening the community—Include assistance for regularizing community property; human rights and conflict resolution training for communities and their leadership; communal participatory diagnosis for conflict prevention, peace education and promotion of a culture of peace; building of economic, productive, and commercial infrastructure; training to improve the capacity of community members to access economic opportunities; support for the return and resettlement of people displaced due to the conflict; rebuilding and improvement of the infrastructure of basic services, communal properties, and others to be identified by the communities

(continued)

[160] Table adapted from the report prepared for the ICTJ by Cristian Correa, Correa, C., (2013: 7–8).

Programme	Services
Symbolic reparations	Measures provide for public gestures, including apologies from representatives of the state, letters to victims, and public ceremonies to promote massive outreach of the *Comisión de la Verdad y Reconciliación* (CVR) (Truth and Reconciliation Commission) report. These actions must acknowledge the different types of victims. It also includes reconciliation gestures such as renaming symbols or places associated with violations; closing or reconditioning jails that symbolize human rightsviolations; and naming streets, squares, bridges, roads, districts, or regions after "heroes of peace." These symbolic measures should be implemented in consultation with victims' groups. Other gestures include the government declaration of August 28, the date on which the CVR report was delivered to the president, as the Day in Tribute to All Victims of Violence
Promotion and access to housing*	These measures are directed at individual or collective victims whose homes were destroyed or who experienced severe damage to their homes as a direct result of the violence. It creates a special program for building and assigning housing, to be implemented over time and in a decentralized way. This programme provides support for reconstruction of rural housing; support for the regulation of property rights; assistance in the resettlement of displaced persons and their preferential inclusion in public housing programs; and technical and financial assistance to displaced people living in provisional or precarious dwellings for self-construction of housing
	* This programme was not included in the recommendations made by the CVR but was included in the law
Economic reparations or compensation	Regulated by Decree 015-2006-JUS*, this programme includes as beneficiaries the following types of victims: Relatives of victims of murder, extrajudicial execution, and disappearance; those victims who are partially or totally disabled according to the evaluation made by the National Commission on Disability; and victims of rape. The CVR had recommended a lump sum, equivalent to US$ 10,000, to be distributed to families in a proportion of two-fifths to the widows or permanent partners, two-fifths to the children, and one-fifth to the parents of the non-surviving victims. This amount was based on the maximum amount received by members of self-defence committees as part of their demobilization programme. For victims over the age of 50, a pension equivalent to one-half of the minimum salary was recommended
	* The law creating the PIR did not explicitly reference this type of reparation, but did empower the *Comisión Multisectorial de Alto Nivel* (CMAN) (High Level Multisectoral Commission) to authorize other programs. This shows the reluctance of congress to expressly create a compensation programme, which was an important demand of victims' and human rights organizations and was included in the CVR's recommendations. The Toledo administration did not want to commit itself to this program either but accepted it on the condition of establishing certainty about the number of victims. That is why the executive decree regulating the (PIR) Law did not define the modality and amount, but established that they would be defined once the registration process was complete and that the process should be completed within 2 years of the establishment of the Reparations Council

Registration of Individual Victims for Economic Reparations or Compensation[161]

Type of crime	Direct victims	Relatives of victims	Total beneficiaries
Enforced disappearances	7,177	15,672	15,672
Summary execution or murder	22,071	58,075	58,075
Disability due to injury	734		734
Rape	2591		2,591
Total	**32,573**		**77,052**

[161] Table adapted from the report prepared for the ICTJ by Cristian Correa, Correa, C., (2013: 10).

Bibliography

Abadía-Barrero, C., & Castro, A. (2006). Experiences of stigma and access to HAART in children and adolescents living with HIV/AIDS in Brazil. *Social Science and Medicine, 62*, 1219–1228.
Abrahamson, P. (2004). Liquid modernity: Bauman on contemporary welfare society. *Acta Sociologica, 47*(2), 121–129.
Abramson, L. Y., Seligman, M. E. P., & Teasdale, J. D. (1978). Learned helplessness in humans: Critique and reformulation. *Journal of Abnormal Psychology, 87*, 49–74.
Abueg, Francis R. (Ed.) (1998). Anger and trauma: Conceptualization, assessment, and treatment, Cognitive-behavioural therapies for trauma. New York: Guilford Press, xii.
Acosta, A. M. (2011). *Analysing success in the fight against malnutrition in Peru* (May 2011 IDS Working Paper Volume 2011 Number 367).
Adimora, A. A., Schoenbach, V. J., & Floris-Moore, M. A. (2009). Ending the epidemic of heterosexual HIV transmission among African Americans. *American Journal of Preventive Medicine, 37*(5), 468–471.
Adorno, T. (1950). *The authoritarian personality*. New York: Joanna Cotler Books.
Agamben, G. (1999). *Remnants of Auschwitz: The witness and the archive*. Brooklyn: Zone Books.
Agger, I. (2001). Reducing trauma during ethno-political conflict: A personal account of psychosocial work under war conditions in Bosnia. In D. Christie, R. V. Wagner, & D. DuNann Winter (Eds.), *Peace, conflict and violence. Peace psychology for the 21st century*. Upper Saddle River: Prentice-Hall.
Agger, I., et al. (1999). *Evaluation of Norwegian support to psychosocial projects in Bosnia-Herzegovina and the Caucasus*. Oslo: Royal Ministry of Foreign Affairs.
Aguiar, C., Rosenfeld, J., Stevens, B., Thanasombat, S., & Masud, H. (2007). An analysis of malnutrition programming and policies in Peru; Dewey, K. G., & Begum, K. (2011). Long-term consequences of stunting in early life. *Maternal and Child Nutrition, 7*(3), 5–18.
Albo, X. (1972). Dinamica en la estructura intercomunitaria de Jesus de Machachaca. *America Indigena, 32*(3), 773–816.
Alcalde, M. C. (2010). *Peruvian lives across borders: Power, exclusion, and home*. Urbana: University of Illinois Press.
Alford, C. F. (2009). *After the holocaust: The book of job, Primo Levi, and the path to affliction*. New York: Cambridge University Press.
Almqvist, J., & Esposito, C. (2012). *The role of courts in transitional justice: Voices from Latin America*. London: Routledge.
Altamirano, T. (2014). *Refugiados Ambientales: Cambio climático y desplazamiento humano Fondo Editorial de la Pontificia Universidad Católica del Perú*, 2014 Av. Universitaria 1801, Lima 32, Perú.

T. J. Bowyer, *Beyond Suffering and Reparation*,
https://doi.org/10.1007/978-3-319-98983-9

Alonso, P. (2003). "*Programa de Mejoramiento de Acceso a la Justicia del Perú*". Paper presented at the VIII Congreso Internacional del CLAD sobre la Reforma del Estado y la Administración Pública, Panamá, October 28–31.

American Psychiatric Association. (2000). *Diagnostic and statistical manual of mental disorders* (4th ed.). Washington, DC: American Psychiatric Association.

Amery, J. (1980). *At the mind's limits. Contemplations by a survivor on Auschwitz and its realities*. Bloomington: Indiana University Press.

Amir, M., & Lev-Wiesel, R. (2001). Secondary traumatic stress, psychological distress, sharing of traumatic reminisces and marital quality among spouses of Holocaust child survivors. *Journal of Marital and Family Therapy, 27*(4), 297–308.

Anderson, C., & Galinsky, A. D. (2006). Power, optimism, and risk-taking. *European Journal of Social Psychology Special Issue: Social Power, 36*(4), 511–536.

Anderson, R. E. (2013). *Human suffering and quality of life, conceptualizing stories and statistics*. New York: Springer.

Anckermann, S., Dominguez, M., Soto, N., Kjaerulf, F., Berliner, P., & Mikkelsen, E. (2005). Psycho-social support to large numbers of traumatised people in post-conflict societies: An approach to community development in Guatemala. *Journal of Community & Applied Social Psychology, 15*, 136–152.

Anstey, M., Meerts, P., & Zartman, I. W. (Eds.). (2012). *The slippery slope to genocide: Reducing identity conflicts and preventing mass murder*. New York: Oxford University Press.

Antonovsky, A. (1990). Pathways leading to successful coping and health. In M. Rosenbaum (Ed.), *Learned resourcefulness: On coping skills, self control, and adaptive behaviour*. New York: Springer.

Appudarai, A. (2004). The capacity to aspire: Culture and the terms of recognition. In V. Rao & M. Walton (Eds.), *Culture and public action*. Stanford: Stanford University Press.

APRODEH. (2004). Violencia Contra Niños y Niñas: Hasta sus Menorcitos ahora Lloran. In Asociación Pro Derechos Humanos (Ed.), *Selección de textos del Informe Final de la Comisión de la Verdad y Reconciliación*. www.aprodeh.org.pe

Ardito and Lovatón. (2002). *Justicia de Paz Nuevas Tendencias y Tareas Pendientes*. Lima: Instituto de Defensa Legal (IDL). June 2002 (*Mimeo*).

Arendt, H. (1970:63). *On violence*. London: Allen Lane.

Arendt, H. (Ed.). (1999). *Illuminations*. London: Pimlico.

Argyris, C., Putnam, R., & Smith, D. M. (1985). *Action science*. San Francisco: Josey-Bass.

Ashley, J. M. (2014). In M. C. Bingemer & P. Casarella (Eds.), *Memory, mysticism and testimony in witnessing: Prophecy, politics and wisdom*. Maryknoll: Orbis Books.

Avelar, I. (1999). *The untimely present: Post-dictatorial Latin American fiction and the task of mourning*. Durham: Duke University Press.

Bachrach, P., & Baratz, M. (1962). Two faces of power. *American Political Science Review, 56*, 947–952.

Badiou, A. (2001). *An ethics on the understanding of evil*. London/New York: Verso.

Baehr, P. (2002). Identifying the unprecedented: Hannah Arendt, totalitarianism and the critique of sociology. *American Sociological Review, 67*(6), 804–831.

Bagilishya, D. (2000). Mourning and recovery from trauma: In Rwanda, tears flow within. *Transcultural Psychiatry, 37*(3), 337–353.

Balbi, C. R., & Callirgos, J. C. (1992). *Sendero y la mujer, Que hacer* 79, 50–53.

Bandura, A. (2001). Social cognitive theory: An agentic perspective. *Annual Review of Psychology, 52*, 1–26.

Baron-Cohen, S. (2011). *Zero degrees of empathy: A new theory of human cruelty and kindness*. London: Allen Lane.

Barnett, V. J. (1999). *Bystanders: conscience and complicity during the holocaust*. Westport: Praeger Publishers.

Bar-Tal, D. (2002). Collective memory of physical violence: Its contribution to the culture of violence. In G. Salomon & B. Nevo (Eds.), *Peace education: The concept, principle and practice around the world* (pp. 27–36). Mahwah: Erlbaum.

Bastien, J. (1978). *Mountain of the Condor: Metaphor and ritual in an Andean Ayllu, American Ethnological Society Monograph* (Vol. 64). New York: West Publishing.
Bauman, Z. (1989). *Modernity and the holocaust*. Cambridge: Polity.
Bauman, Z. (2004). *Identity: Conversations with Benedetto Vecchi*. Malden: Polity Press.
Baumeister, R. F., & Leary, M. R. (1995). The need to belong: Desire for interpersonal attachments as a fundamental human motivation. *Psychological Bulletin, 117*(3), 497–529.
Baumeister, R. F., Twenge, J. M., & Nuss, C. K. (2002). Effects of social exclusion on cognitive processes: Anticipated aloneness reduces intelligent thought. *Journal of Personality and Social Psychology, 83*, 817–827.
Becker, G., Beyene, Y., & Ken, P. (2000). Memory, trauma, and embodied distress: The management of disruption in the stories of Cambodians in exile. *Ethos, 28*(3), 320–345.
Ben-Sira, Z., (1991). *Regression, stress and readjustment aging: A structured, bio-psychosocial perspective on coping and professional support*. New York: Praeger.
Beneduce, R. (2007). Contested memories: Peace-building and community rehabilitation after violence and mass crimes – A medico-anthropological approach. In B. Pouligny, S. Chesterman, & A. Schnabel (Eds.), *After mass crime*. New York: United Nations University Press.
Benson, P. (2008). El campo: Faciality and structural violence in farm labor camps. *Cultural Anthropology, 23*(4), 589–629.
Berger, R. J. (2011). *Surviving the holocaust: A life course perspective*. New York: Routledge.
Berkman, L. F., & Kawachi, I. (Eds.). (2000). *Social epidemiology*. New York: Oxford University Press.
Bettelheim, B. (1960). *The informed heart,* The Free Press, in reprinted Penguin Edition (1991).
Bevernage, B. (2012). *History, memory and state-sponsored violence*. London: Routledge.
Biehl, J. (2005). *Vita: Life in a zone of social abandonment*. Berkeley: University of California Press.
Biehl, J. (2013). *When people come first: Critical studies in global health*. Princeton: University of Princeton Press.
Biehl, J., Good, B., & Kleinman, A. (Eds.). (2007a). *Subjectivity: Ethnographic investigations, Ethnographic studies in subjectivity*. Berkeley: University of California Press.
Biehl, J., Good, B., & Kleinman, A. (2007b). Introduction. In J. Biehl, B. Good, & A. Kleinman (Eds.), *Rethinking subjectivity in subjectivity: Ethnographic investigations*. Berkeley: University of California Press.
Biehl, J., & Moran-Thomas, A. (2009). Symptom: Subjectivities, social ills, technologies. *Annual Review of Anthropology, 38*, 267–288.
Bingemer, M. C., & Casarella, P. (Eds.). (2014). *Witnessing: Prophecy, politics and wisdom*. Maryknoll: Orbis Books.
Bittenger, J. N. (2004). On the uniqueness of trauma memories in PTSD. In G. M. Rosen (Ed.), *Post-traumatic stress disorder: Issues and controversies*. New York: John Wiley.
Bliese, P. D., & Britt, T. W. (2001). Social support, group consensus and stressor-strain relationships: Social context matters. *Journal of Organizational Behaviour, 22*(4), 425–436.
Bloch, M. (2009). *Heritage of our times*. Berkeley: Polity Press.
Blustein, J. (2003). On taking responsibility for one's past. *Journal of Applied Philosophy, 17*(1), 2000.
Blustein, J. (2008). *The moral demands of memory*. New York: Cambridge University Press.
Boehm, C., & Flack, J. C. (2010). The emergence of simple and complex power structures through social niche construction. In A. Guinote & T. K. Vescio (Eds.), *The social psychology of power* (p. 46). New York: The Guilford Press.
Boesten, J. (2007a). Marrying your rapist: Domesticating war crimes in Ayacucho, Peru. In D. Pankhurst (Ed.), *Gendered peace: Women's search for post-war justice and reconciliation*. London: Routledge.
Boesten, J. (2007b). Free choice or poverty alleviation? Population policies under President Fujimori of Peru. *European Review of Latin American and Caribbean Studies, 82*, 3–20.

Boesten, J. (2014). *Sexual violence during war and peace: Gender, power, and post-conflict justice in Peru, Studies of the Americas*. New York: Palgrave Macmillan.

Boltanski, L. (1999). *Distant suffering: Morality, media and politics*. Cambridge: Cambridge University Press.

Bolton, P. (2003). Assessing depression among survivors of the Rwanda genocide. In S. T. Krippner & T. M. McIntyre (Eds.), *The psychological impact of war trauma on civilians. An international perspective*. Westport: Praeger Publishers.

Bonanno, G. (2004). Loss, trauma and human resilience. Have we underestimated the human capacity to thrive after extremely aversive events? *American Psychologist, 59*(1), 20–28.

Bonilla Mayta, H., Fonseca Martel, C., & Hernandez, B. (1996). *Tradición y Conservadorismo en el área cultural del Lago Titicaca, Jesús de Machaca, Una comunidad aymara del altiplano andino*. Lima: Instituto del Estudio Peruanos.

Bourdieu, P. [1997] (2000). *Pascalian meditations*. Translated by Richard Nice. Stanford: Stanford University Press.

Bourdieu, P., et al. (1999). *The weight of the world: Social suffering in contemporary society*. Cambridge: Polity.

Bourgois, P. (2003). *In search of respect: Selling crack in El Barrio* (2nd ed.). New York: Cambridge University Press.

Bourgois, P. (2009). Recognizing Invisible Violence: A Thirty-Year Ethnographic Retrospective. In B. Rylko Bauer, L. Whiteford, & P. Farmer (Eds.), *Global health in times of violence*. Santa Fe: School for Advanced Research Press.

Bourgois, P., & Scheper-Hughes, N. (2004). Commentary on an anthropology of structural violence. *Current Anthropology, 45*(3), 317–318.

Bowlby, J. (1988). *A secure base: Clinical applications of attachment theory*. (Abingdon: Routledge). cited in Krznaric, R., (2014). *A handbook for revolution: Empathy*. Rider Books Ebury Publishing.

Brabeck, K. (2001). "*Testimonio*: Bridging feminist ethics with activist research to create new spaces of collectivity." *Bridging the Gap: Feminism and Participatory Action Research Conference Papers, Boston College*, June 22–24. http://ggsc.wamu.edu/gap/brabeck.htm

Bracken, P. J. (1993). Post-empiricism and psychiatry meaning and methodology in cross-cultural research. *Social Science and Medicine, 36*(3), 265–272.

Bracken, P. J. (2001). Post-modernity and post-traumatic stress disorder. *Social Science and Medicine, 53*(6), 733–743.

Bracken, P. J., & Petty, C. (Eds.). (1998). *Rethinking the trauma of war*. London: Free Association Books.

Bracken, P. J., Giller, J. E., & Summerfield, D. (1995). Psychological responses to war and atrocity: the limitations of current concepts. *Social Science and Medicine, 40*, 1073–1082.

Brady, D., & Burton, L. M. (Eds.). (2016). *The Oxford handbook of the social science of poverty*. Oxford: Oxford University Press.

Brandt, H.-J. (Ed.) (2013). Justicia comunitaria en los Andes: Perú y Ecuador cambios en la justicia comunitaria y factores de influencia. Serie Justicia comunitaria en los Andes: Perú y Ecuador, 9 Instituto de Defensa Legal, IDL, Lima.

Brehm, S. S., Kassin, S., & Fein, S. (2005). *Social psychology* (6th ed.). Boston: Houghton Mifflin.

Brenneis, C. B. (1994). Can early childhood trauma be reconstructed from dreams? On the relation of dreams to trauma. *Psychoanalytic Psychology, 11*, 429–447.

Brewer, W. F. (1988). Memory for randomly sampled autobiographical events. In U. Neisser & E. Winograd (Eds.), *Remembering reconsidered: Ecological and traditional approaches to the study of memory* (pp. 21–90). Cambridge: Cambridge University Press.

Brewer, G. A. (2003). Building social capital: Civic attitudes and behaviour of public servants. *Journal of Public Administration Research and Theory, 13*(1), 5–26.

Brewin, C. R., Andrews, B., & Valentine, J. D. (2000). Meta-analysis of risk factors for posttraumatic stress disorder in trauma-exposed adults. *Journal of Consulting and Clinical Psychology, 68*, 748–766.

Brickner, R. (1943). *Is Germany incurable?* New York: J. B. Lippincott Company.

Brinkerhoff, D. W. (2005). Rebuilding governance in failed states and post-conflict societies: Core concepts and cross-cutting themes. *Public Administration and Development, Special Issue: Rebuilding Governance in Failed States and Post-Conflict Societies, 25*(1), 3–14.

Brinkerhoff, D. (2007a). *Governance in post-conflict societies. Rebuilding fragile states.* London: Routledge.

Brinkerhoff, D.W. (2007b). *Good enough governance in fragile states: The role of center-periphery relations and local government.* Paper presented in Workshop No. 3: Making the good enough governance agenda realistic 4th International Specialised Conference "International Aid and Public Administration" International Institute of Administrative Sciences Ankara, Turkey June 23–27, 2008.

Brock, R. N. (1988). *Journeys by heart: A christology of erotic power.* New York: Crossroad Publishing Co.

Broucek, F. (1991). *Shame and the self.* New York: Guilford Press.

Brudholm, T. (2008). *Resentment's virtue: Jean Amery and the refusal to forgive.* Philadelphia: Temple University Press.

Brudholm, T., & Cushman, T. (Eds.). (2009). *The religious in responses to mass atrocities.* Cambridge: Cambridge University Press.

Brune, N., & Bossert, T. (2009). Building social capital in post-conflict communities: Evidence from Nicaragua. *Social Science and Medicine, 68*(2009), 885–893.

Bryant, R. A. (2003). Early predictors of post traumatic stress disorder. *Biological Psychiatry, 53*(9), 789–795. tłumaczenie angielskie University of California Press, 197.

Bryant, R. A., O'Donnell, M. L., Creamer, M., McFarlane, A. C., & Silove, D. (2013). A multisite analysis of the fluctuating course of posttraumatic stress disorder. *Psychiatry, 70*(8), 839–846.

Buber, M. (1958). *I and thou* (2nd ed.). New York: Scribner's Son.

Buckley-Zistel, S. (2006). Remembering to forget: Chosen amnesia as a strategy for local coexistence in post-genocide Rwanda Africa. *Journal of the International African Institute, 76*(2), 131–150. Published by: Cambridge University Press on behalf of the International African Institute.

Bueno-Hansen, P. (2015). *Feminist and Human Rights Struggles in Peru* (Dissident Feminisms). University of Illinois Press.

Bufacchi, V. (2007). *Violence and social justice.* New York: Palgrave Macmillan.

Bufacchi, V. (2009). Rethinking violence. *Global Crime, 10*(4), 293–297.

Bugental, D. B. (2010). Paradoxical power manifestations: Power assertion by the subjectively powerless. In A. Guinote & T. Vescio (Eds.), *The social psychology of power* (p. 209ff). New York: The Guilford Press.

Bullock, H. E., & Lott, B. (2010). Social class and power. In A. P. Guinote & T. K. Vescio (Eds.), *The social psychology of power* (pp. 408–427). New York: Guilford.

Bunge, M. (2004). How does it work? The search for explanatory mechanisms. *Philosophy of the Social Sciences, 34*, 182–210.

Burke, N. J., Joseph, G., Pasick, R. J., & Barker, J. C. (2009). Theorizing social context: Rethinking behavioural theory. *Health Education & Behavior, 36*(5), 55s–70s.

Burt Jo Marie. (2008). *Political violence and the authoritarian state in Peru.* Basingstoke: Palgrave Macmillan.

Burton, J. W. (1990a). *Conflict: Resolution and prevention.* New York: Macmillan/St. Martin's Press.

Burton, J. W. (Ed.). (1990b). *Conflict: Human needs theory.* New York: Macmillan/St. Martin's Press.

Business News Americas. (2008). *Los Militares #6191*, Las Condes, Santiago, Chile.

Buss, D. M., & Malamuth, N. (1996). *Sex, power, conflict: Evolutionary and feminist perspectives.* New York: Oxford University Press.

Byman, D. L., & Waxman, M. C. (2000). Kosovo and the Great Air Power Debate. *International Security, 24*(4), 5–38.

Camara, H. (1971). *Spiral of violence.* London: Sheed and Ward.

Calhoun, L. G., & Tedeschi, R. (Eds.). (2009). *Handbook of post-traumatic growth: Research and practice*. New York: Psychology Press: Taylor and Francis Group.

Cardena, E., & Spiegel, D. (1993). Dissociative reactions to the San Francisco Bay Area earthquake of 1989. *American Journal of Psychiatry, 150*, 474–478.

Caprara, G. V., & Cervone, D. (2000). *Personality: Determinants, dynamics and potentials*. New York: Cambridge University Press.

Carlson, N. (2012). *Physiology of psychology* (11th ed.). Boston: Pearson Education Inc.

Carnes, P. J. (1997). *The betrayal bond: Breaking free of exploitive relationships*. Deerfield Beach: Health Communications Inc..

Carr, S. C., & Sloan, T. S. (Eds.). (2008). *Poverty and psychology: From global perspective to local practice*. New York: Klewer Academic/Plenum Publishers.

Carrie, J. G. (2012). *A handbook of economic anthropology* (2nd ed.). Cheltenham: Edward Elgar Publishing Limited.

Caruth, C. (1995). *Trauma: Explorations in memory*. Baltimore: The John Hopkins University Press.

Caruth, C. (1996). *Unclaimed experience: trauma, narrative and history*. Baltimore: John Hopkins University Press.

Cassell, E. J. (1982, March 18). The nature of suffering and the goals of medicine. *The New England Journal of Medicine, 306*(11):639–645.

Cassell, E. J. (1991). The importance of understanding suffering for clinical ethics. *The Journal of Clinical Ethics, 2*, 81–82.

Cassell, E. J. (1992). The nature of suffering and the goals of medicine. *New England Journal of Medicine, 306*, 639–645.

Cassell, E. J. (2004). *The nature of suffering and the goals of medicine*. New York: Oxford University Press.

Cavell, S. (1996, Winter). Comments on Veena Das's essay "Language and body: Transactions in the construction of pain." *Daedelus Journal of the American Academy of Arts and Sciences, 125*(1), 193–208.

Cederblad, M., Dahlen, L., Hagnell, O., & Hansson, K. (1995 March). Intelligence and temperament as protective factors for mental health. A cross-sectional and prospective epidemiological study. *European Archives of Psychiatry and Clinical Neuroscience, 245*(1), 11–19.

Chapman, C. R., & Volinn, E. (2005). Narrative as a window on chronic disabling back pain. In D. B. Carr, J. Loeser, & D. B. Morris (Eds.), *Narrative, pain, and suffering* (pp. 73–86). Seattle: International Association for the Study of Pain Press as cited in Anderson, R. E., (2013:11). *Human Suffering and Quality of Life: Conceptualizing Stories and Statistics*, Springer Briefs in Well-Being and Quality of Life Research.

Charbonneau, B., & Parent, G. (Eds.). (2012). *Peace building, memory and reconciliation: Bridging top-down and bottom-up*. New York: Routledge.

Chare, N. (2011). *Auschwitz and afterimages: Abjection, witnessing and representation*. London/New York: I.B. Tauris & Co. Ltd.

Cheftez, J. S. (2008). *Handbook of the sociology of gender, Handbooks of sociology and social research*. New York: Springer Publishing.

Chorbajian, L., & Shirinian, G. (Eds.). (1999). *Studies in comparative genocide*. Basingstoke: Macmillan Press.

Chouliaraki, L. (2017). Suffering and the ethics of solidarity. In R. E. Anderson (Ed.), *Alleviating world suffering* (pp. 49–61). New York: Springer.

Christies, D. (2005). In D. Wagner (Ed.), *Peace, conflict and violence- peace psychology for the 21st century*. Upper Saddle River: Prentice Hall.

Ciarrochi, J. V., Forgas, J. P., & Mayer, J. D. (Eds.). (2001). *Emotional intelligence in everyday life*. Philadelphia: Psychology Press.

Cienfuegos, A., & Monelli, C. (1983). The testimony of political repression as a therapeutic instrument. *American Journal of Orthopsychiatry, 53*, 43–51.

Cittadini, R. (1995). La importancia de las redes locales de comunicación para una estrategia de extensión. *Visión Rural, 14*, 15–16.
Cohen, S. (2001). *States of denial: Knowing about atrocities and suffering*. Cambridge: Polity Press.
Cohen, H., & Lefebvre, C. (Eds.). (2005). *Handbook of categorization in cognitive science*. Amsterdam: Elsevier.
Coleman, J. S. (1989). Editors introduction: Rationality and society. *Rationality and Society, 1*(1), 5–9.
Colvin, C. J. (2006). Overview of the reparations program in South Africa. In P. De Greiff (Ed.), *The handbook of reparations* (pp. 176–215). Oxford: Oxford University Press.
Comisión de la Verdad y Reconciliación, Informe Final [CVR Final Report] (Lima, 2003). www.cverdad.org.pe/ifi nal/index.php
Compas, B. E., Banes, G. A., Malcarne, V., & Worsham, N. (1991). Perceived control and coping with stress: A developmental perspective. *Journal of Social Issues, 47*, 23–34.
Connolly, P., & Healy, J. (2004). Symbolic violence, locality and social class: The educational and career aspirations of 10-11-year old boys in Belfast. *Pedagogy, Culture and Society, 12*(1), 15–33.
Constance, P. (2003). "*One stop justice*", Magazine of the Inter-American Development Bank.
Constitution and Convention No. 169 concerning Indigenous and Tribal Peoples in Independent Countries.
Coronel, J. (1994). Comites defensa: un proceso social abierto. *Ideele, 59–60*, 113–115.
Coronel, J. (1996). Violencia politica y respuestas campesinas en Huanta. In C. I. Degregori (Ed.), *Las rondas campesinas y la derrota de Sendero Luminoso, Estudios de la sociedad rural*. Lima: IEP Ediciones.
Correa, C. (2013). *Reparative justice: Reparations in Peru: From recommendations to implementation*. New York: International Center for Transitional Justice.
Csordas, T. J. (Ed.). (1994). *Embodiment and experience: The existential ground of culture and self*. Cambridge: Cambridge University Press.
Dahl, R. (1957). Decision-making in a democracy: The supreme court as a national policy-maker. *Journal of Public Law, 6*, 279–295.
Dahl, R. (1961). *Who governs? Democracy and power in an American city*. New Haven: Yale University Press.
Das, V. (1994). Moral orientations to suffering: Legitimation, power and healing. In L. C. Chen, A. Kleinman, & N. C. Ware (Eds.), *Health and social change in international perspective* (pp. 139–170). Boston, MA: Harvard School of Public Health.
Das, V. (1995). *Critical events: An anthropological perspective on contemporary India*. Delhi: Oxford University Press.
Das, V. (1997a). Language and body: Transactions in the construction of pain. In A. Kleinman, V. Das, & M. Lock (Eds.), *Social suffering*. California/London: University of California Press.
Das, V. (1997b). Sufferings, theodicies, disciplinary practices, appropriations. *International Journal of Social Science, 49*, 563–572.
Das, V. (2000). The act of witnessing: Violence, poisonous knowledge, and subjectivity. In V. Das, A. Kleinman, M. Ramphele, & P. Reynolds (Eds.), *Violence and subjectivity* (pp. 205–225). Berkeley: University of California Press.
Das, V. (2007). *Life and words: Violence and the descent into the ordinary*. Berkeley: University of California Press.
Das, V., Kleinman, A., Ramphele, M., Lock, M., & Reynolds, P. (Eds.). (2001). *Remaking a world: Violence, social suffering and recovery*. Berkeley: University of California Press.
Davidson, S. (1984). *Human reciprocity among the Jewish prisoners in the Nazi concentration camps* (pp. 555–572). Jerusalem: Yad Veshem.
Davidson, S. (1992). In I. W. Charney New (Ed.), *Holding on to Humanity – The message of holocaust survivors: The Shamai Davidson papers* (p. 24). New York: York University Press.
Davidson, W. B., & Cotter, P. R. (1989). Sense of community and political participation. *Journal of Community Psychology, 17*, 119–125.

de Juristas, C. A. (1999). *Gente Que Hace Justicia – La Justicia de Paz* (p. 67). Lima: Comisión Andina de Juristas.

De Greiff, P. (2008). *The handbook of reparations*. Oxford: Oxford University Press.

Dean, C. J. (2010). *Aversion and erasure: The fate of the victim after the holocaust*. Ithaca: Cornell University Press.

Decreto Supremo de Peru, N° 065-2001-PCM., Art. 2(a), Available at http://www.cverdad.org.pe/lacomision/cnormas/normasOl.php

Defensoría del Pueblo, "Informe Defensorial No 140 – *Salud Mental y Derechos Humanos. Supervisión de la política pública, la calidad de los servicios y la atención a poblaciones vulnerables*," 225–54. www.defensoria.gob.pe/informes-publicaciones.php

Degregori, C. I. (1987). *Sendero Luminoso. I.Los hondos y mortales desencuentros. II.Lucha armada y utopía autoritaria*. Lima:IEP/CEPRODEP. (Documentos de Trabajo, 4 and 6).

Degregori, C. I. (1990). *El surgimiento de Sendero*. Ayacucho: Luminoso, 1969–1979 (Serie Ideología y política), Instituto de Estudios Peruanos.

Degregori, C. I. (1999). Reaping the whirlwind: The Rondas Campesinas and the defeat of Sendero Luminoso in Ayacucho, Kees Koonings and Dirk Kruijt Societies of fear: The legacy of civil war, violence and terror in Latin America (New York: Zed Books).

Degregori, I., Coronel, J., del Pino, P., & Starn, O. (1996). *Las Rondas Campesinas y la Derrota de Sendero Luminoso*. Lima: Instituto de Estudios Peruanos.

Degregori, C. I., Stern, S. J., & Appelbaum, N. (2012). *How difficult it is to be god: Shining path's politics of war in Peru, 1980–1999, Critical Human Rights*. Madison: University of Wisconsin Press.

De la Rey, C. (2001). Reconciliation in divided societies. In D. Christie, R. V. Wagner, & D. DuNann Winter (Eds.), *Peace, conflict and violence. Peace psychology for the 21st century*. Upper Saddle River: Prentice Hall.

De Lemus, Spears, & Moya. (2008). *Sexism with a smile – Just posturing? Complimentary conduct produces complementary contrast*. Paper presented at the symposium "Reducing and coping with intergroup bias" conveners: C. van Laar & K. Stroebe. 15th EAESP General Meeting. Opatija, Croatia

Del Vecchio Good, M. J., Brodwin, P. E., Good, B. J., & Kleinman, A. (1992). *Pain as human experience; An anthropological perspective*. Berkeley: University of California Press.

Demarest, A. A., & Conrad, G. W. (1984). *Religion and empire: The dynamics of Aztec and Inca expansionism*. Cambridge: Cambridge University Press.

Denzin, N. K. (2004). Reading film: Using films and videos as empirical social science material. In U. Flick, E. v. Kardorff, & I. Steinke (Eds.), *A companion to qualitative research* (pp. 237–242). London: Sage.

Denzin, N. K., & Lincoln, Y. S. (Eds.). (2005). *The Sage handbook of qualitative research* (3rd ed.). Thousand Oaks: Sage.

De Prince, A. P., & Freyd, J. J. (2002). The harm of trauma: Pathological fear, shattered assumptions, or betrayal? In J. Kauffman (Ed.), *Loss of the assumptive world: A theory of traumatic loss* (pp. 71–82). New York: Brunner-Routledge.

Desjarlais, R., Eisenberg, L., Good, B., & Kleinman, A. (1995). *World mental health: Problems and priorities in low-income countries*. London: Oxford University Press.

Desmond, M. (2014). How should we study suffering? *Ethnic and Racial Studies* Volume 37, Issue 10, 2014 Special Issue: *Ethnic and Racial Studies Review* pages 1761–1766.

Des Pres, T. (1976). *The survivor: An anatomy of life in the death camps*. Oxford: Oxford University Press.

Devenish, C., & Gianella, C. (2012). 20 years of Sustainable Mountain Development in the Andes: From Rio 1992 to 2012 and beyond, *Consorcio para el Desarrollo Sostenible de la Ecorregión Andina* (CONDESAN), 46.

De Waal, F. (2010). *The age of empathy: Nature's lessons for a kinder society*. London: Souvenir Press.

Dewey, K. G., & Begum, K. (2011, October). Long-term consequences of stunting in early life. *Maternal & Child Nutrition, 7*(3), 5–18.

Domhoff, G. W. (1998). The presentation of dreaming and dreams in introductory psychology textbooks: A critical examination with suggestions for textbook authors and course instructors. *Dreaming, 8*(3), 149–168.

Domhoff, G. W., & Zweigenhaft, R. L. (1998). *Diversity in the power elite: Have women and minorities reached the top?* New Haven: Yale University Press.

Douglas, M. (1966). *Purity and danger: An analysis of the concepts of pollution and taboo.* London: Routledge.

Doughty, K. C. (2016). *Remediation in Rwanda: Grassroots legal forums*. Philadelphia: University of Pennsylvania Press.

Dumezil, G., & Duviols, P. (1974). Sumaqw T'ika: La princesse du village sansa eau. *Journal de la Société des Americanistes, 63*, 15–198.

Dussaillant, F., & Gonzalez, P. A. (2015). Lifetime suffering and capabilities in Chile. In R. E. Anderson (Ed.), *World suffering & the quality of life* (pp. 233–251). Amsterdam: Springer.

Ehlers, A., Hackmann, A., Steil, R., Clohessy, S., Wenninger, K., Winter, H. (2002, September). The nature of intrusive memories after trauma: The warning signal hypothesis. *Behaviour Research and Therapy, 40*(9), 995–10002.

EM-DAT. (2011). *The OFDA/CRED International Disaster Database v12.07 Brussels*. Belgium: Université Catholique de Louvain. www.emdat.be

Eisenbruch, M. (2007). The uses and abuses of culture: Cultural competence in post-mass crime peace-building in Cambodia. In B. Pouligny, S. Chesterman, & A. Schnabel (Eds.), *After mass crime: Rebuilding states and communities*. Tokyo/New York: United Nations University Press.

Emmons, K. M. (2000). Health behaviours in a social context. In L. F. Berkman & I. Kawachi (Eds.), *Social epidemiology* (pp. 137–173). New York: Oxford University Press.

Erdinast-Vulcan, D. (2012). The Melancholy Generation: Grossman's Book of Interior Grammar. In J. Lothe, S. R. Suleiman, & J. Phelan (Eds.), *After testimony: The ethics and aesthetics of holocaust narrative for the future*. Columbus: The Ohio State University Press.

Erikson, K. T. (1976). Loss of communality at Buffalo Creek. *The American Journal of Psychiatry, 133*, 302–305.

Espinosa, O. (1995). *Rondas campesinas y nativas en la Amazonia peruana*. Lima: Centro Amazónico de Antropología y Aplicación Práctica.

Falk, R. (2006). Reparations, international law, and global justice: A new frontier. In P. de Greiff (Ed.), *The handbook of reparations*. Oxford: Oxford University Press.

Fals-Borda. (1988). *Knowledge and people's power: Lessons with peasants in Nicaragua, Mexico and Columbia*. New Delhi: Social Institute.

Farmer, P. (2003). *Pathologies of power: Health, human rights and the new war on the poor.* Berkeley: University of California Press.

Farmer, P. (2005). *Never again? Reflections on human values and human rights. The Tanner lectures on human values*. Salt Lake City: University of Utah.

Fassin, D. (2007). Humanitarianism as a politics of life. *Public Culture, 19*(3), 499–520.

Fassin, D. (2009). A violence of history: Accounting for AIDS in post-apartheid South Africa. In B. Rylko-Bauer, L. Whiteford, & P. Farmer (Eds.), *Global health in times of violence* (pp. 113–135). Santa Fe: School for Advanced Research Press.

Faundez, J. (2003). *Non-state justice systems in Latin America case studies: Peru and Colombia* (p. 30). Washington, DC: World Bank.

Feingold, H. (1981). The witness role of American Jewry: A second look. In M. Ryan (Ed.), *Human responses to the holocaust: Perpetrators and victims, bystanders and resisters* (p. 1981). New York: Edwin Mellen Press.

Feinstein, A. (1989). Posttraumatic stress disorder: A descriptive study supporting DSM III-R criteria. *American Journal of Psychiatry, 146*, 665–666.

Felman, S., & Laub, D. (1992). *Testimony: Crises of witnessing in literature, psychoanalysis and history*. New York: Routledge.

Fine, R., & Tuner, C. (2000). *Social theory after the holocaust*. Liverpool: Liverpool University Press.

Finkelkraut, A. (1980). *The imaginary Jew*. Lincoln: Bison Books.

Fiske, S. T. (1993). Controlling other people: The impact of power on stereotyping. *American Psychologist, 48*, 621–628.

Fiske, S. T., & Neuberg, S. L. (1990). A continuum of impression formation, from category-based to individuating processes: Influences of information and motivation on attention and individuating processes. *Journal of Experimental Social Psychology, 23*, 399–421.

Folkman, S., & Lazarus, R. S. (1984). *Stress appraisal and coping*. New York: Springer Pub. Company.

Folkman, S, Lazarus, R. S., Dunkel-Schetter, C., DeLongis, A., & Gruen, R.J. (1986, May). Dynamics of a stressful encounter: Cognitive appraisal, coping, and encounter outcomes. *Journal of Personality and Social Psychology, 50*(5), 992–1003.

Folkman, S., Chesney, M., McKusick, L., Ironson, G., Johnson, D., & Coates, T. (1991). Translating coping theory into an intervention. In J. Eckenrode (Ed.), *The social context of coping* (pp. 239–260). New York: Plenum.

Folensbee, R. (2008). The brain in psychotherapy: A framework. *Texas Psychologist, 58*(3), 17–21.

Fontaine, K. R., Manstead, A. S. R., & Wagner, H. (1993, October). Optimism, perceived control over stress, and coping. *European Journal of Personality, 7*(4), 267–281.

Food and Agriculture Organization. (1996). Rome Declaration on Food Security and World Food Summit Plan of Action.

Forgas, J. P. (Ed.). (2001). *Handbook of affect and social cognition*. Mahwah: Erlbaum.

Forgas, J. P. (Ed.). (2006). *Affect, cognition and social behaviour*. New York: Psychology Press.

Forgas, J. P., & Williams, K. D. (Eds.). (2001). *Social influence: Direct and indirect processes*. Philadelphia: Psychology Press. Isen, (1987).

Forgas, J. P., & Williams, K. D. (Eds.). (2002). *The social self: Individual, interpersonal and intergroup perspectives*. New York: Psychology Press.

Forgas, J. P., Williams, K. R., & Wheeler, L. (Eds.). (2001). *The social mind: Cognitive and motivational aspects of interpersonal behavior*. New York: Cambridge University Press.

Frank, A. W. (2001). Can we research suffering? *Qualitative Health Research, 11*(3), 353–362.

Franco, R., & Gonzalez, M. (2008). *Las mujeres en la justicia comunitaria: victimas, sujetos y actores*. Lima: Instituto de Defensa Legal.

Frank, A. W. (1992). The pedagogy of suffering: Moral dimensions of psychological therapy and research with the ill. *Theory & Psychology, 2*(4), 467–485.

Frankel, F. H. (1994). The concept of flashbacks in historical perspective. *International Journal of Clinical and Experimental Hypnosis, 42*, 321–336.

Frankl, V. (1985). (1955). *Man's search for meaning*. New York: Washington Square Press.

Frankl, V. (1994). *Logotherapy and existential analysis*. Munchen: Quintessenz.

Freire, P. (1980). (1972). *The pedagogy of the oppressed*, London: Sheed & Ward.

Freire, P. (1998). *Pedagogy of freedom: ethics, democracy and civic courage*. Lanham: Rowman & Littlefield Publishers Inc.

French, J. R. P., Jr., Caplan, R. D., & Harrison, R. V. (1982). *The mechanisms of job stress and strain*. London: Wiley.

Freud, S. (1962). *Civilization and its discontents*. New York: Norton.

Friedman, H. S., & Silver, R. C. (2006). *Foundations of health psychology*. New York: Oxford University Press.

Frommberger, U. (2014). Post-traumatic stress disorder – A diagnostic and therapeutic challenge. *Deutsches Ärzteblatt International*. https://doi.org/10.3238/arztebl.2014.0059.

Fromm, E. (1997). *Anatomy of human destructiveness*. London: Pimlico Press.

Fumerton, M. (2003). *From victims to heroes: Peasant counter-rebellion and civil war in Ayacucho, Peru, 1980–2000*. Amsterdam: Rozenberg.

Fumerton, M. (2001). Rondas campesinas in the Peruvian Civil War: Peasant self defense organizations in Ayacucho. *Bulletin of Latin American Research, 20*(4), 481.

Fumerton, M., & Remijnse, S. (2004). Civil Defence forces: Peru's Comites de auto-defensa Civil and Guatemala's Patrullas de Autodefensa Civil in comparative perspective. In K. Koonings & D. Kruijt (Eds.), *Armed actors: Organised violence and state failure in Latin America*. New York: Zed Books.

Galeano, E. (1993). *The book of embraces*. W. W. Norton & Company; New Edition.

Galtung, J. (1969). Violence, peace and peace research. *Journal of Peace Research, 6*(1), 167–191.

Galtung, J. (1996). *Peace by peaceful means peace and conflict, development and civilization*. Thousand Oaks: Sage Publications Ltd..

Galvez, M., Ansi6n, J., & Degregori, C. I. (1981). Lo individual y lo colectivo en la comunidad andina. *Ideología, 7*, 5–16.

Gautier, A., & Sabatini Scalmati, A. (2010). *Bearing witness: Psychoanalytic work with people traumatized by torture and state violence*. London: Karnac Books Ltd.

Gaventa, J. (1980). *Power and powerlessness: Quiescence and rebellion in an Appalachina Valley*. Urbana: University of Illinois Press.

Geddes, J. L. (2009). Religious rhetoric in responses to atrocity. In T. Brudholm & T. Cushman (Eds.), *The religious in responses to mass atrocity: Interdisciplinary perspectives*. New York: Cambridge University Press.

Geras, N. (1998). *The contract of mutual indifference: Political philosophy after the holocaust*. London/New York: Verso.

Gilbert, P., & McGuire, M. (1998). Shame, social roles and status: The psychobiological continuum from monkey to human. In P. Gilbert & B. Andrews (Eds.), *Shame: Interpersonal behaviour, psychopathology and culture* (pp. 99–125). New York: Oxford University Press.

Gilligan, J. (1997). *Violence: Reflections on a national epidemic*. New York: Vintage Books.

Glick, R. L., Berlin, J. S., Fishkind, A., & Zeller, S. L. (2008). *Emergency psychiatry: Principles and practice*. Philadelphia: Lippincott Williams and Wilkins.

Goldie, P. (2011). Empathy with one's past. *The Southern Journal of Philosophy Special Issue: Spindel Supplement: Empathy and Ethics, 49*(Supplements 1), 193–207.

Gonzales, O. M. (2011). *Unveiling secrets of war in the Peruvian Andes*. Chicago: The University of Chicago Press.

Gonzales, R. (1982, September–October). Ayacucho: ¿Por los caminos de Sendero? *QueHacer, 19*, 36–78.

Good, B. J. (1992). Culture and psychopathology: Directions for psychiatric anthropology. In T. Schwartz, G. White, & C. Lutz (Eds.), *New directions in psychological anthropology* (pp. 181–205). Cambridge: Cambridge University Press.

Good, M.-J. D. V., Hyde, S. T., Pinto, S., & Good, B. J. (Eds.). (2008). *Postcolonial disorders*. Berkeley: University of California Press.

Govier, T. (2002). *Forgiveness and revenge*. London: Routledge.

Grant, A. (2011, February). A critique of the representation of human suffering in the cognitive behavioural therapy literature with implications for mental health nursing practice. *Journal of Psychiatric Mental Health Nursing, 18*(1), 35–40.

Greenberg, I. (1989). Cloud of smoke, pillar of fire. In J. K. Roth & M. Berenbaum (Eds.), *Holocaust: Religious and philosophical implications*. St. Paul: Paragon House cited in Geddes, J.L., (2009: 23).

Green, L. (2004). Commentary on an anthropology of structural violence. *Current Anthropology, 45*(3), 319–320.

Grosh, M., del Ninno, C., Tesliuc, E., & Querghi, A. (2008). *For protection and promotion: The design and implementation of effective safety nets*. No 6582 in World Bank Publications from The World Bank.

Gruenfeld, D. H., Inesi, M. E., Magee, J. C., & Galinsky, A. D. (2008). Power and the objectification of social targets. *Journal of Personality and Social Psychology, 95*, 111–127.

Guillerot, J., & Magarrell, L. (2006). *Reparaciones en la Transicion Peruana:Memorias de un Proceso Incabado* as cited in Laplante, L. J. (2007: 14). "On the Indivisibility of Rights: Truth Commissions, Reparations, and the Right to Development," *Yale Human Rights and Development Journal*: Vol. 10: Iss. 1, Article 4.

Guinote, A., & Vescio, T. K. (2010). *The social psychology of power*. New York: The Guilford Press.

Gutiérrez, G. (1973). *A theology of liberation*. Edited and translated by Sister Caridad Inda and John Eagleson. Maryknoll: Orbis Books.

Gutiérrez, G. (1983). *The power of the poor in history*. Translated by Robert R. Barr. Maryknoll: Orbis Books.

Gutierrez, G. (2004). Memoria y profecia. In A. Gallego (Ed.), *Gustavo Gutierrez, textos esenciales: acordarse de los pobres* (p. 258ff). Lima: Fondo Editorial del Congreso del Peru.

Haas, P. J. (1988). *Morality after Auschwitz: The radical challenge of the Nazi Ethic*. Philadelphia: Augsburg Fortress Publishing.

Hague, E. (1997). Rape, power and masculinity: The construction of gender and national identities in the war in Bosnia-Herzegovina. In R. Lentin (Ed.), *Gender and catastrophe*. London/New York: Zed Books.

Hall, G., & Patrinos, H. A. (2006). "*Indigenous peoples, poverty and human development in Latin America: 1994–2004*." http://go.worldbank.org/RF879VREC0

Hallman, A. H., & Wandersman, W. K. (1992). Attribution of responsibility and individual and collective coping with environmental threats. *Journal of Social Issues, 48*, 4101–4118.

Hamburger, A. (Ed.). (2018). *Trauma, trust and memory: Social trauma and reconciliation in psychoanalysis, psychotherapy and cultural memory*. London: Routledge.

Hammergren, L. (1997). *The politics of justice and justice reform in Latin America: The Peruvian case in comparative perspective*. Boulder: Westview Press.

Hartman, G. (2002). *Scars of the spirit: The struggle against inauthenticity*. New York: Palgrave MacMillan.

Harvard Trauma Questionnaire (HTQ) and (HSCL-25). *Measuring Trauma, Measuring Torture* Harvard Program in Refugee Trauma.

Harvey, D. C. (2015). The cultural geography of community suffering. In R. E. Anderson (Ed.), *World suffering & the quality of life* (pp. 269–281). New York: Springer.

Harvey, J. H., & Weary, G. (1981). *Perspectives on attributional processes*. Dubuque: Wm C Brown.

Haslam, S. A. (1997). Stereotyping and social influence: Foundations of stereotype consensus. In R. Spears, P. J. Oakes, N. Ellemers, et al. (Eds.), *The social psychology of stereotyping and group life* (pp. 119–143). Oxford: Blackwell.

Hassett, J., & Lacey, H. (1991). *Towards a Society that serves its People: The Intellectual Contribution of El Salvador's Murdered Jesuits*. Washington, DC: Georgetown University Press.

Hatun Willakuy. (2004). *Version Abreviada del Informe Final de la Comision de la Verdad Y Reconciliacion*: 337 [hereinafter Willakuy].

Hayner, P. B. (2002). *Unspeakable truths: Facing the challenge of truth commissions*. New York/London: Routledge.

Heilman, J. P. (2010). *Before the shining path: Politics in rural Ayacucho, 1895–1980*. Stanford: Stanford University Press.

Henriquez, N. (2007). Genero y Poder en el conflicto armado. Verdades devaladas, verdades que rebelan. In M. Barrig (Ed.), *Fronteras Interiores, Identidad Diferencia y Protagonismo de los Mujeres*. Lima: IEP Ediciones.

Henry, P. J., & Pratto, F. (2010). Power and racism. In A. Guinote & T. Vescio (Eds.), *The social psychology of power* (pp. 341–362). New York: Guilford.

Hepner, T. R. (2011). *Soldiers, martyrs, traitors, and exiles: Political conflict in Eritrea and the diaspora*. Philadelphia: University of Pennsylvania Press.

Herman, J. L. (1992). *Trauma and recovery*. New York: Basic Books.

Hewstone, M., Stroebe, W., & Stephenson, G. M. (1996). *Introduction to social psychology: A European perspective*. Oxford/Cambridge, MA: Blackwell Publishers.

Heyd, D. (2004). Resssentiment and reconciliation: Alternative responses to historical evil. In L. H. Meyer (Ed.), *Justice in time. Responding to historical injustice* (pp. 185–197). Baden-Baden: Nomos.

Hickel, J. (2017). In R. E. Anderson (Ed.), *Addressing the structural causes of suffering, Alleviating world suffering*. Cham: Springer.
Hills, J., Le Grand, J., & Piachaud, D. (Eds.). (2002). *Understanding social exclusion*. Oxford: Oxford University Press.
Hinton, D., Ba, P., & Um. (2000, November–December). Panic disorder among Cambodian refugees attending a psychiatric clinic prevalence and subtypes. *General Hospital Psychiatry, 22*(6), 437–444.
Hinton, D. E., & Good, B. J. (2015). *Culture and PTSD, The ethnography of political violence series*. Philadelphia: University of Pennsylvania Press.
Hoffman, M. L. (2000). *Empathy and moral development: Implications for caring and justice*. Cambridge: Cambridge University Press.
Hoffman, M., & Grigera, A. I. (2013). *Climate change, migration, and conflict in the Amazon and the Andes: Rising tensions and policy options in South America*. Washington, DC: Center for American Progress.
Holland, T., & Martin, J. P. (2014). *Human rights education and peace building: A comparative study*. New York/London: Routledge.
Honneth, A. (1996). *The struggle for recognition: Moral grammar of social conflicts*. Cambridge: Cambridge University Press.
Horn, S., & Munafo, M. (1997). *Pain, theory, research and intervention*. Buckingham: Open University Press.
Hornberger, N. H., & King, K. A. (1998). Authenticity and unification in Quechua language planning. *Language, Culture, and Curriculum, 11*(3), 390–410.
Hornberger, N. H., & King, K. A. (2001). Reversing Quechua language shift in South America. In J. A. Fishman (Ed.), *Can threatened languages be saved? Reversing language shift, revisited: A 21st century perspective* (pp. 166–194). Clevedon: Multilingual Matters.
Hornberger, N. H., & King, K. A. (2006). Quechua as a lingua franca. *Annual Review of Applied Linguistics, 26*, 177–194.
Hromadžić, A. (2015). *Citizens of an empty nation: Youth and state-making in postwar Bosnia-Herzegovina*. Philadelphia: University of Pennsylvania Press.
Hudson, W. (2012). Historicizing suffering. In J. Malpas & N. Lickiss (Eds.), *Perspectives on human suffering*. Dordrecht: Springer Science & Business Media.
Iafrate, M. J. (2009). *We will never forget: Metz, memory and the dangerous spirituality of post-9/11 America (part II)*. Columbia: Vox Nova.
Ignatieff, M. (1996). Articles of faith. *Index on Censorship, 5*, 110–122.
Ignatieff, M. (1999). Human rights. In R. Post et al. (Eds.), *Human rights in transition: Gettysburg to Bosnia*. New York: Zone Books.
Illich, I. (1976). *Limits to medicine: Medical nemesis: The expropriation of health* (pp. 140–160). London: Penguin.
International Center for Transitional Justice. (2013). *Reparations in Peru: From recommendations to implementation*. New York: International Center for Transitional Justice.
Instituto Nacional de Estadística e Informática. (2011). *Evolución de la pobreza al 2010*. Lima: INEI.
Instituto Especializado de Salud Mental Estudio epidemiológico en salud mental. *Anales de Salud Mental* 2005; XXI (Nos. 1–2).
Inter-American Development Bank. (2000). *Acceso a la justicia y equidad. Estudio en siete países de America Latina*. Washington, DC: Instituto Interamericano de Derechos Humanos.
Isbell, B. J. (1985). *To defend ourselves: Ecology and ritual in an Andean village*. Prospect Heights: Waveland Press.
Jacob, S. (1999). *Traumatic grief: Diagnosis, treatment and prevention*. Philadelphia: Brunner/Mazel.
Jacoby, R. (1975). *Social amnesia: A critique of contemporary psychology from Adler to Laing*. Boston: Beacon Press.

Janolf-Bulman, R. (1992). *Shattered assumptions: Towards a new psychology of trauma*. New York: Free Press.

Jaspers, K. (1947). *The question of German guilt*. New York: Fordham University Press; 2 Rev Ed edition (31 Oct. 2000).

Jelin, E. (2002). *Los trabajos de la memoria*. Madrid: Siglo XXI. Cited in *Intimate Memories: Violence and Reconciliation in Peru* (2013: 30). Theidon, K., University of Pennsylvania Press. Philadelphia.

Jenkins, R. (1996). *Social identity*. London: Routledge.

Johnston, B. R. (Ed.). (2007). *Half-lives & half-truths: Confronting the radioactive legacies of the cold war*. Santa Fe: School for Advanced Research Press.

Johnston, B. R. (Ed.). (2011). *Life and death matters: Human rights, environment, and social justice* (2nd ed.). Walnut Creek: Left Coast Press.

Jones, E. C., & Murphy, A. D. (2015). Social organization of suffering. In R. E. Anderson (Ed.), *World suffering & the quality of life* (pp. 281–293). New York: Springer.

Journal of Community Psychology Special Issue.: The Assessment of Power Through Psychopolitical Validity March 2008 Volume 36, Issue 2.

Judt, T. (2000). *Writing history, facts optional*, New York Times (Op-Ed), April 13 2000 cited in Hartman, G. (2002). *Scars of the spirit: The struggle against inauthenticity*, Palgrave MacMillan.

Justino, P. (2009, May). Poverty and violent conflict: A micro-level perspective on the causes and duration of warfare. *Journal of Peace Research, 46*(3), 315–333.

Kabeer, N., & Haq, A. K. (2009). *Citizenship narratives in the absence of good governance: Voices of the working poor in Bangladesh* (IDS Institute of Development Studies Working Paper 331).

Kakar, S. (1996). *The colours of violence: Cultural identities, religion and conflict*. Chicago: University of Chicago Press.

Kang, S., & Meernik, J. (2005). Civil war destruction and the prospects for economic growth. *The Journal of Politics, 67*(1), 88–109.

Kaufman, C. (1996). Possible and impossible solutions to ethnic civil wars. *International Security, 20*(4), 5–34.

Kelman, H. C. (1990). Applying a human needs perspective to the practice of conflict resolution. In J. W. Burton (Ed.), *Conflict: Human needs theory*. New York: St. Martin's Press.

Keltner, D., Gruenfeld, D. H., & Anderson, C. (2003). Power, approach and inhibition. *Psychological Review, 100*, 265–284.

Keltner, D., Gruenfeld, D. H., Galinsky, A., & Krause, M. W. (2010). Paradoxes of power: Dynamics of the acquisition, experience, and social regulation of social power. In A. Guinote & T. K. Vescio (Eds.), *The social psychology of power*. New York: The Guilford Press.

Kilborne, B. (1999, December). When trauma strikes the soul: Shame, splitting and psychic pain. *The American Journal of Psychoanalysis, 59*(4), 385–402.

Kinderman, P., Schwannauer, M., Pontin, E., & Tai, S. (2013). Psychological processes mediate the impact of familial risk, social circumstances and life events on mental health. *PLoS One, 8*(10), e76564. https://doi.org/10.1371/journal.pone.0076564.

King, P. (2000). *Thinking past a problem: Essays on the history of ideas*. New York and London: Routledge.

Kipnis, D. (1976). *The power holders*. Chicago: University of Chicago Press.

Kipnis, D. (1990). *Technology and power*. New York: Springer-Verlag.

Kirk, R. E. (1995). *Experimental design: Procedures for the behavioural sciences* (3rd ed.). Pacific Grove: Brooks/Cole.

Kiss, E. (2000). Moral ambitions within and beyond political xonstraints: Reflections on restorative justice. In R. I. Rotberg & D. Thompson (Eds.), *Truth V. Justice: The morality of truth commissions, The University Center for Human Values Series* (Vol. 72). Princeton: Princeton University Press.

Klaren, P. (2000). *Peru: Society and nationhood in the Andes*. New York: Oxford University Press, Inc.

Kleinman, A. (1986). *Social origins of distress and disease: Depression, neurasthenia and pain in modern China*. New Haven: Yale University Press.

Kleinman, A. (1988). *The illness narratives: Suffering, healing and the human condition*. New York: Basic Books.

Kleinman, A., & Kleinman, J. (1991a). Suffering and its professional transformation. *Culture, Medicine and Psychiatry, 15*(3), 275–301.

Kleinman, A., & Kleinman, J. (1991b). Suffering and its professional transformation: Toward an ethnography of interpersonal experience. *Culture, Medicine and Psychiatry, 15*(3), 275–301.

Kleinman, A. (1992). Pain and resistance: The deligitimation and religitimation of local worlds. In M. J. DelVecchio Good, P. E. Brodwin, B. J. Good, & A. Kleinman (Eds.), *Pain as human experience; An anthropological perspective* (pp. 169–197). Berkeley: University of California Press.

Kleinman, A. (1995a). *Writing at the margin: Discourse between anthropology and medicine*. Berkeley: University of California Press.

Kleinman, A. (1995b). Pitch, picture, power: The globalization of local suffering and the transformation of social experience. *Ethnos Journal of Anthropology, 60*(3–4), 181–191.

Kleinman, A. (1996). Bourdieu's impact on the anthropology of suffering. *International Journal of Contemporary Sociology, 33*(2), 203–210.

Kleinman, A., & Kleinman, J. (1997a). The appeal of experience; The dismay of images: Cultural appropriations of suffering in our times. In A. Kleinman, V. Das, & M. Lock (Eds.), *Social suffering*. Berkeley: University of California Press.

Kleinman, A., & Kleinman, J. (1997b). Cultural appropriations of suffering in our times. In A. Kleinman, V. Das, & M. Lock (Eds.), *Social suffering*. Berkeley: University of California Press.

Kleinman, A., Das, V., & Lock, M. (1997a). Introduction. In A. Kleinman, V. Das, & M. Lock (Eds.), *Social suffering*. London: University of California Press.

Kleinman, A., Das, V., & Lock, M. (1997b). *Social suffering*. London: University of California Press.

Kleinman, A. (1999). 'Experience and its moral modes: Culture, human conditions and disorder, Peterson, G. B. The Tanner lectures on human values, Salt Lake City, University of Utah Press

Kleinman, A. (2009). Global mental health: A failure of humanity. *The Lancet, 374*(9690), P603–P604.

Kleinman, A., & Wilkinson, I. (2016). *A passion for society: How we think about human suffering, California Series in Public Anthropology*. Oakland: University of California Press.

Korsgaard, C. (1996). *The sources of normativity*. Cambridge: Cambridge University Press.

Koselleck, R. (2004). *Future's past. On the semantics of historical time*. New York: Colombia University Press.

Kotarba, J. (1983). *Chronic pain: Its social dimensions*. Beverly Hills: Sage Publications.

Krakow, B., Melendrez, D., Warner, T. D. Dorin, R., Harper, R., & Hollifield, M. (2002, October). To breathe, perchance to sleep: Sleep-disordered breathing and chronic insomnia among trauma survivors, *Sleep and Breathing*, *6*(4), 189–202.

Krause, K. (2009). Beyond definition: Violence in global perspective. *Global Crime, 10*(4), 337–355.

Kreimer, A., Arnold, M., & Scott, C. (1998). *The World Bank's experience with post-conflict reconstruction*. Washington, DC, World Bank.

Kristeva, J. (1982). *Powers of horror: An essay on abjection*. New York: Columbia University Press.

Kristeva, J. (1984). *Revolution in poetic language*. New York: Columbia University Press.

Krugman, P. (1991). Increasing returns and economic geography. *Journal of Political Economy, 99*(3), 483–499.

Krystal, H. (1995). Trauma and aging: A thirty-year follow up. In C. Caruth (Ed.), *Trauma: Explorations in memory* (pp. 76–99). Baltimore: John Hopkins Press.

Krznaric, R. (2014). *Empathy: A handbook for revolution*. New York: Random House.

LaCapra, D. (2001). *Writing history, writing trauma*. Baltimore: The John Hopkins University Press.

LaCapra, D. (2004). *History in transit: Experience, identity, critical theory*. Ithaca: Cornell University Press.

Lammers, J., & Stapel, D. A. (2009). How power influences moral thinking. *Journal of Personality and Social Psychology, 97*(2), 279–289.

Landini, F. (2011). Income and use of money in the peasant economy: Contributions to rural development psychology from a case study. *Journal of Alternative Perspectives in the Social Sciences, 3*(3), 674–703.

Lang, B. (2003, February 28). *Act and idea in the Nazi genocide. (Religion, Theology and the Holocaust)*. Syracuse University Press; New Ed edition.

Langer, L. (1983). *Versions of survival: The holocaust and the human spirit*. Albany: State University of New York: Albany State University of New York Press.

Langer, L. (1999). *Holocaust testimonies: The ruins of memory*. New Haven: Yale University Press.

Langer, L. (1980). The dilemma of choice in the death camps. *Centerpoint: The Holocaust, 4*(1), 54.

Langer, L. L. (1982). *Versions of survival: The holocaust and the human spirit* (SUNY series in Modern Jewish Literature and Culture). Albany: SUNY Press.

Langer, L. L. (1993). *Holocaust testimonies: The ruins of memory*. New Haven: Yale University Press Reissue edition.

Langer, L. L. (2008). The alarmed vision: Social suffering and holocaust atrocity. In A. Kleinman, V. Das, & M. Lock (Eds.), *Social suffering (1997)*. Berkeley: University of California Press.

Langle, A. (2008). Suffering – An existential challenge: Understanding, dealing and coping with suffering from an existential-analytic perspective. *International Journal of Existential Psychology & Psychotherapy, 2*(1).

Laplante, L. J. (2007). On the indivisibility of rights: Truth commissions, reparations, and the right to development. *Yale Human Rights and Development Journal, 10*(1), Article 4.

La Serna, M. (2012). *The corner of the living: Ayacucho on the eve of the Shining Path insurgency*. Chapel Hill: The University of North Carolina Press.

Laub, D., & Auerhahn, N. (1993). Knowing and not known massive psychic trauma: Forms of traumatic memory. *International Journal of Psychoanalysis, 74*, 287–302.

Lazarus, R. S. (1966). *Psychological stress and the coping process*. New York: McGraw-Hill.

Lazarus, R. S., & Folkman, S. (1986). *Estres y Procesos Cognitivos*. Barcelona: Martinez-Roca S.A.

Lazarus, R. S. (1993a). Coping theory and research: Past, present, and future. *Psychosomatic Medicine, 55*, 234–247.

Lazarus, R. S. (1993b). Why we should think of stress as a subset of emotion. In L. Goldberger & S. Breznitz (Eds.), *Handbook of stress: Theoretical and clinical aspects* (pp. 21–39). New York: Free Press.

Lazarus, R. S. (1991a). Progress on a cognitive-motivational-relational Theory of Emotion. *American Psychologist, 46*(8), 819–834.

Lararus, R. S. (1991b). *Emotion and adaptation*. New York: Oxford University Press.

Lazarus, R. S. (2000). Toward better research on stress and coping. *American Psychologist, 55*(6), 663–673.

Leatherman, T., & Brooke Thomas, R. (2008). Structural violence, political violence and the health costs of civil conflict: A case study from Peru. In *Anthropology (p. 70). and public health: Bridging differences in culture and society* (2nd ed., pp. 196–220). Oxford: Oxford University Press.

Leatherman, T. (2011). Health, human rights, and war: Structural violence, armed conflict, and human health in the Andes. In B. R. Johnston (Ed.), *Life and death matters: Human rights, environment, and social justice* (2nd ed., pp. 333–348). Walnut Creek: Left Coast Press.

Leder, D. (1990). *The absent body*. Chicago: University of Chicago Press.

Leinaweaver, J. B. (2008). Improving oneself: Young people getting ahead in the Peruvian Andes. *Latin American Perspectives, 35*(4), 60–78.

Lepore, S. J., & Revenson, T. A. (2006). Resilience and posttraumatic growth recovery, resistance, and reconfiguration. In L. G. Calhoun, & R. Tedeschi (Eds.), (2009), *Handbook of post-traumatic growth: research and practice*. New York/Hove: Psychology Press/Taylor and Francis Group.

Lever, J. P. (2008). Poverty, Stressful Life Events, and Coping Strategies. *The Spanish Journal of Psychology, 11*(01), 228–249.

Levinas, E. (1999). *Totality and infinity: An essay on exteriority* (L. Alphonso, Trans.). Duquesne University Press.

Levinas, E. (2006). *Entre Nous: Thinking of the other continuum*. London/New York: Continuum Press.

Loppie-Reading, C., & Wien, F. (2009). *Health inequalities and social determinants of aboriginal peoples' health*. Prince George: National Collaborating Centre for Aboriginal Health.

Lev-Wiesel, R., & Amir, M. (2006). *Growing out of ashes: Posttraumatic growth among Holocaust child survivors. Is it possible?* In L. G. Calhoun & R. Tedeschi (2009). (Eds.), *Handbook of post-traumatic growth: Research and practice*. Psychology Press: Taylor and Francis Group.

Lev-Wiesel, R., & Amir, M. (2000). Posttraumatic stress disorder symptoms, psychological distress, personal resources and quality of life in four groups of Holocaust child survivors. *Family Process, 39*(4), 445–460.

Lewis, H. B. (1971). *Shame and guilt in neurosis*. New York: International University Press.

Lewis, R. J. (2002). Beyond dominance: The importance of leverage. *Quarterly Review of Biology, 77*, 149–164.

Lickiss, N. (2012). *Perspectives on human suffering*. Springer.

Lifton, R. J. (1982). Beyond psychic numbing: a call to awareness. *American Journal of Orthopsychiatrics, 52*(4), 619–629.

Lifton, R. J. (1986). *The Nazi doctors: Medical killing and the psychology of genocide*. New York: Basic Books.

Lindner, E. G. (2001). Humiliation as the source of terrorism: A new paradigm. *Peace Research, 33*(2), 59–68.

Lira, E. (2001). Violence, fear and impunity: Reflections on subjective and political obstacles for peace. *Peace and Conflict: Journal of Peace Psychology, 7*(2), 109–118.

Literacy and Civic Education Program for Indigenous and Peasant Women, Peru. (1998). University of Pennsylvania/Graduate School of Education: *International Literacy Explorer*. www.literacy.org/Projects/explorer/peru_back.html

Logstrup, K. (2002). *After the ethical demand* (D. Susan, & N. Van Kooten, Trans.). Aarhus University Press.

Loux, M. J. (1998). *Metaphysics: A Contemporary Introduction*. New York: Routledge.

Loux, M. J. (2001). The problem of universals. In M. J. Loux (Ed.), *Metaphysics: Contemporary readings*. New York: Routledge.

Lukes, S. (1974). *Power: A radical view*. London: Macmillan (reprinted 2005, Basingstoke, Palgrave Macmillan).

Lykes, M. B. (2000). Possible contributions of a psychology of liberation: Whither health and human rights. *Journal of Health Psychology, 5*(3), 383–397.

Maier, C. S. (1997). *The unmasterable past: History, Holocaust and German national identity*. Cambridge: Harvard University Press.

Maier, S. F., & Watkins, L. R. (1998). Cytokines for psychologists: Implications of bidirectional immune-to-brain communication for understanding behaviour, mood, and cognition. *Psychological Review, 105*, 83–107.

Malpas, J., & Lickiss, N. (2012: 1–3) *Introduction: Human suffering* in Malpas, J., & Marcos, (2001: 209) *Our word is our weapon: Selected writings: Subcomandante insurgente marcos* (eds.) Juana Ponce de Leon. New York: Seven Stories Press.

Marcos, Subcomandante. (2001). *The speed of dreams: Selected writings 2001–2007: Selected Writings*. City Light Publishers.

Markle, G. E., et al. (1992). From Auschwitz to Americana: Texts of the Holocaust. *Sociological Focus, 25*, 179–202.

Margalit, A. (2002). *The ethics of memory*. Cambridge: Harvard University Press.

Marmot, M., & Wilkinson, R. G. (1999). *Social determinants of health*. Oxford: Oxford University Press.

Marshall, M., & Marshall, E. (2012). *Logotherapy revisited: Review of the tenets of Victor E. Frankl's Logotherapy*. Ottawa Institute of Logotherapy CreateSpace Independent Publishing Platform.

Martin-Baro, I. (1986). Hacia una psicologia de la liberacion. *Boletin de Psicologia, 5*(22), 219–231.

Martin-Baro, I. (1989). Political violence and war as causes of psychosocial trauma in El Salvador. *International Journal of Mental Health, 18*(1), Mental Health Aspects of Political Repression and Violence (II). (Spring 1989), pp. 3–20.

Martin-Baro, I. (1994a). *Writings for a liberation psychology*. Cambridge, MA: Harvard University Press.

Martin-Baro, I. (1994b). *The lazy latino: The ideological nature of Latin American Fatalism in writings for a liberation psychology*. Cambridge, MA: Harvard University Press.

Martin-Baro, I. (1994c). *Towards a liberation psychology in writings for a liberation psychology*. Cambridge, MA: Harvard University Press.

Martin-Baro, I. (1994d). *War and the psychosocial trauma of Salvadoran children, n writings for a liberation psychology*. Cambridge, MA: Harvard University Press.

Mathew Ashley, J. (2014). Memory, mysticism and testimony. In M. C. Bingemer & P. Casarella (Eds.), *Witnessing: prophecy, politics and wisdom* (p. 10545). New York: Orbis Books/ Maryknoll.

Mavila Leon, R. (1992). Presente y Futuro del las Mujeres de la Guerra. *Que Hacer, 79*, 44–49.

Mayer, E. (2009). *Ugly stories of the Peruvian Agrarian reform*. Durham: Duke University Press.

McCann, I. L., & Pearlman, L. A. (1990a). Vicarious traumatization: A framework for the psychological effects of working with victims. *Journal of Traumatic Stress, 3*(1), 131–149.

McCann, I. L., & Pearlman, L. A. (1990b). *Psychological trauma and the adult survivor: Theory, therapy, and transformation* (Brunner/Mazel psychosocial stress series, No. 21). Philadelphia: Brunner/Mazel.

McClintock, C. (1998). *Revolutionary movements in Latin America: El Salvador's FMLN and Peru's shining path*. Washington, DC: United State Institute of Peace Press.

McCullough, M., & Worthington, E. L. (2001). Religion and the Forgiving Personality. *Journal of Personality, 67*(6), 1141–1164 December 1999.

McIlwaine, C. (1999). Geography and development: Violence and crime as development issues. *Progress in Human Geography, 23*(3), 453–463.

McNulty, S. (2004 July, 8). Institutionalising Civil Society's Participation through Reforms of the State: The Case of Peru's Decentralization. Presented at the *Instituto de Estudios Peruanos* (IEP). 40th Anniversary Conference Lima, Peru.

Mellman, T. A., David, D., Bustamente, V., Torres, J., & Fins, A. (2001). Dreams in the acute aftermath of of trauma and their relationship to PTSD. *Journal of Traumatic Stress, 14*, 241–247.

Melzack, R., & Wall, P. (1965). Pain mechanisms: a new theory. *Science, 150*, 971–979.

Mendelson-Forman, J. (2002). Achieving socio-economic well-being in post-conflict settings. *The Washington Quarterly, 25*(2), 125–138 UNDP (2008: 4).

Metz, J. B. (1980). *Faith in history and society: Toward a fundamental practical theology* (p. 1980). New York: Seabury.

Metz, B., Mariano, L., & García, J. L. (2010). The Violence After 'La Violencia' in the Ch'orti' Region of Eastern Guatemala. *Journal of Latin American and Caribbean Anthropology, 15*(10), 16–41.

Meyerson, J. (1990). *Tambo: Life in an Andean village*. Austin: University of Texas Press.

Michailof, S., Kostner, M., & Devictor, X. (2002). *Post-conflict recovery in Africa – An agenda for the Africa Region* (Africa Region working paper; no. 30). Washington, DC: The World Bank.

Milgram, S. (1974). *Obedience to authority: An experimental view*. New York: Harper & Row.

Miller, D. (2001). Disrespect and the experience of injustice. *Annual Review of Psychology, 52*, 527–553.

Miller, K. E., & Rasmussen, A. (2010). War exposure, daily stressors, and mental health in conflict and post-conflict settings: Bridging the divide between trauma-focused and psycho social frameworks. *Social Science & Medicine, 70*, 7–16.
Mills, C., & Zavaleta, D. (2015). Shame, humiliation and social isolation. In R. E. Anderson (Ed.), *World suffering & the quality of life* (pp. 251–269). Cham: Springer.
Ministerio de Salud. Dirección General de Promoción de la Salud. (2001). Lima; Perú. Ministerio de Salud. Proyecto 2000.
Mischel, W. (1990). Personality dispositions revisited and revised: A view after three decades. In L. A. Pervin (Ed.), *Handbook of personality: Theory and research* (pp. 111–134). New York: Guilford Press.
Moeller, S. D. (1999). *Compassion fatigue how the media sell disease, famine, war and death.* Florence: Taylor and Francis.
Montoya Vivanco, Y. (2012). Responding to human rights violations committed during the internal armed conflict in Peru: The limits and advances of Peruvian criminal justice. In J. Almqvist & C. Esposito (Eds.), *The role of courts in transitional justice*. New York/London: Routledge.
Moodie, E. (2010). *El Salvador in the aftermath of peace: Crime, uncertainty and the transition to democracy*. Philadelphia: University of Pennsylvania Press.
Morgan, K., & Bjorkert, S. T. (2006). *'I'd rather you'd lay me on the floor and start kicking me': Understanding symbolic violence in everyday life. Women's Studies International Forum, 29*, 441–452.
Morgan, D., & Wilkinson, I. (2001). The problem of suffering and the sociological task of theodicy. *European Journal of Social Theory, 4*(2), 199–214.
Morrill, B. T. (2000). *Anamnesis as dangerous memory: Political and liturgical theology in dialogue*. A Pueblo Book published by The Liturgical Press.
Morris, D. B. (1991). *The culture of pain*. Berkeley: University of California Press.
Morrison, T. (2004). *Beloved.* New York: Vintage Press.
Moser, C. (1996). Confronting crisis: A comparative study of household responses to poverty and vulnerability in four urban poor communities (Environmentally Sustainable Development Studies and Monograph, Series No. 8). Washington, DC: World Bank.
Moser, C. (1998). The asset vulnerability framework: reassessing urban poverty reduction strategies. *World Development, 26*(1), 1–19.
Moser, C., & McIlwaine, C. (2000). *Violence in a post-conflict context: Urban poor perceptions from Guatemala*. Washington DC: The World Bank.
Moser, C., & McIlwaine, C. (2004). *Encounters with violence in Latin America: Urban poor perceptions from Colombia and Guatemala*. New York/London: Routledge.
Muller, A., et al. (2017). Digitized suffering reconciliation. In R. E. Anderson (Ed.), *Alleviating world suffering*. Cham: Springer.
Murphy, J. (2003). *Getting even: Forgiveness and its limits*. New York: Oxford University Press.
Murphy, J. T. (2011). The socio-spatial dynamics of development: Geographical insights beyond the 2009 World Development Report. *Cambridge Journal of Regions, Economy and Society, 4*, 175–188.
Murray, C. J. L., King, G., Lopez, A. D., Tomijima, N., & Krug, E. G. (2002). Armed conflict as a public health problem. *British Medical Journal*, 324 4(7333), 346–349.
Nielsen, J. (Ed.). (1990). *Feminist research methods: Exemplary readings in the social sciences.* Boulder: Westview Press.
Nishith, P., Nixon, R. D. V., & Resick, P. A. (2005). Resolution of trauma-related guilt following treatment of PTSD in female rape victims: A result of cognitive processing therapy targeting comorbid depression? *Journal of Affective Disorders, 86*, 259–265.
Nordstrom, C. (2004). *Shadows of war: Violence, power, and international profiteering in the twenty-first century*. Berkeley: University of California Press.
Nordstrom, C. (2009). Fault lines. In B. Rylko-Bauer, L. Whiteford, & P. Farmer (Eds.), *Global health in times of violence* (pp. 63–87). Santa Fe: School for Advanced Research Press.

North, D. (1990: vii). *Institutions, institutional change and economic performance*. Cambridge: Cambridge University.

North, C. S., Smith, E. M., McCool, R. E., & Lightcap, P. E. (1989). Acute post-disaster coping and adjustment. *Journal of Traumatic Stress, 2*, 353–360.

Nuñez-Palomino, G. (1996). The rise of Rondas Campesinas in Peru. *Journal of Legal Pluralism, 36*. http://www.jlp.bham.ac.uk/volumes/36/nunez-art.pdf

Olick, J. K. (2007). *The politics of regret: On collective memory and historical responsibility*. New York: Routledge.

Operario, D., & Fiske, S. T. (2001). Effects of trait dominance on powerholders' judgments of subordinates. *Social Cognition, 19*(2), 161–180.

Ozer, E. J., Best, S. R., Lipsey, T. L., & Weiss, D. S. (2008). Predictors of posttraumatic stress disorder and symptoms in adults. *Psychological Trauma Theory Research Practice and Policy, 8*(1), 3–36.

Pan American Health Organization. (2002). Peru. *Health in the Americas, 2*, 454–470.

Pan American Health Organization. (2012). *Health in the Americas Peru*.

Panter-Brick, C. (2010). Conflict, Violence, and Health: Setting a New Interdisciplinary Agenda. *Social Science and Medicine, 70*(1), 1–6.

Pearlman, L. A., & Saakvitne, K. W. (1995). *Trauma and the therapist: Counter-transference and vicarious traumatization in psychotherapy with incest survivors*. New York: Norton.

Pawelczynska, A. (1979). *Values and violence: The outline of the sociological problems of Auschwitz,* English translation University of California Press, 1979 and 1980 *Zarys socjologicznej problematyki Oświęcimia* , PWN, Warszawa 1973 (nagroda Polskiego Towarzystwa Socjologicznego im. Stanisława Ossowskiego), PWN, Warszawa 1995 , Test, Lublin 2001.

Pearlin, L. I., & Schooler, C. (1978). The Structure of Coping. *Journal of Health and Social Behaviour, 19*(1), 2–21.

Pearlin, L. I. (1989). The sociological Study of Stress. *Journal of Health and Social Behaviour, 30*(3), 241–256.

Pedersen, D., Tremblay, J., Errazuris, C., & Gamarra, J. (2008). The sequelae of political violence: assessing trauma, suffering and dislocation in the Peruvian highlands. *Social Science & Medicine, 67*, 205–217.

Pedersen, D., Kienzler, H., & Gamarra, J. (2010). Llaki and Ñakary: Idioms of distress and suffering among the highland Quechua in the Peruvian Andes. *Culture, Medicine and Psychiatry, 34*(2), 279–300.

Peña, A. (1998). *Justicia Comunal en los Andes del Perú*. Lima: Fondo Editorial, Pontificia Universidad Católica del Perú.

Peña, A., Cabedo, V., & López, F. (2002). *Constituciones, Derecho y Justicia en los Pueblos Indígenas de América Latina* (p. 197). Lima*: Pontificia Universidad Católica del Perú.* tłumaczenie angielskie University of California Press

Peña, D. G. (2011). Structural Violence, Historical Trauma, and Public Health: The Environmental Justice Critique of Contemporary Risk Science and Practice. In L. M. Burton, S. P. Kemp, M. C. Leung, S. A. Matthews, & D. T. Takeuchi (Eds.), *Communities, neighborhoods, and health: Expanding the boundaries of place* (pp. 203–218). New York: Springer.

Peru. http://education.stateuniversity.com/pages/1188/Peru-EDUCATIONAL-SYSTEM-OVERVIEW.html

Pervin, L. A. (1984). *Personality: Theory and research*. New York: Wiley.

Poole, D. (2015). *Companion to Latin American Anthropology*. Wileyblackwell.

Poole, D. (1997). *Vision, race, and modernity: A visual economy of the Andean Image World* (Princeton Studies in Culture/Power/History). Princeton: Princeton University Press.

Poole, D., & Renique, G. (1992). *Peru: Time of fear*. London: Latin America Bureau.

Poole, D., & Das, V. (2004). *Anthropology in the margins of the state*. Oxford: James Currey.

Polsby, N. W. (1963). *Community power and political theory*. New Haven: Yale University Press.

Pouligny, B., Chesterman, S., &Schnabel, A. (Eds.). (2007). *After mass crime: Rebuilding states and communities*, United Nations University Press.

Prigerson, H. G., Shear, M. K., Frank, E., Beery, L. C., Silberman, R., Prigerson, J., et al. (1997). Traumatic grief: A case of loss induced trauma. *American Journal of Psychiatry, 154*, 1003–1009.
Prilleltensky, I. (2008a). The role of power in wellness, oppression, and liberation: the promise of psychopolitical validity, *Journal of Community Psychology Special Issue: The Assessment of Power Through Psychopolitical Validity, 36*(2).
Prilleltensky, I. (2008b). Poverty and power. In S. C. Carr & T. S. Sloan (Eds.), *Poverty and psychology: From global perspective to local practice* (pp. 19–44). New York: Kluwer Academic.
Programa de las Naciones Unidas para el Desarrollo (PNUD). (2005). (United Nations for Development).
PRU: Peru-UNICEF. (2004). *Country programme evaluation UNICEF NYHQ*.
Putnam, H. (1973). Reductionism and the nature of psychology. *Cognition, 2*(1), 131–146.
Putnam, R., Leonardi, R., & Nanetti, R. Y. (1993). *Making democracy work: Civic traditions in modern Italy*. Princeton: Princeton University Press.
Putnam, R. (2000). *Bowling alone*. New York: Simon and Schuster.
Quesada, J. (2009). The vicissitudes of structural violence: Nicaragua at the turn of the twenty-first century. In B. Rylko-Bauer, L. Whiteford, & P. Farmer (Eds.), *Global health in times of violence* (pp. 157–180). Santa Fe: School for Advanced Research Press.
Ratner, C. (2000). A cultural-psychological analysis of emotions. *Culture & Psychology, 6*, 5–39.
Rawls, J. (1973). *A theory of justice*. Oxford University Press.
Regel, S., & Joseph, S. (2010: 8). *Post-traumatic stress*. Oxford University Press. A full list of the diagnostic criteria for PTSD is provided by the National Centre for PTSD. see http://ncptsd.kattare.com/ncmain/ncdocs/fact_shts/fs_dsm_iv_tr.html
Reiss, S., & McNally, R. J. (1985). Expectancy model of fear. In S. Reiss & R. R. Bootzin (Eds.), *Theoretical issues in behaviour therapy* (pp. 107–121). San Diego: Academic Press.
Renault, E. (2010). A critical theory of social suffering. *Critical Horizons A Journal of Philosophy and Social Theory, 11*(2), 221–241.
Rengifo, G. (1987). *La Agricultura Tradicional en los Andes*. Editorial Horizontal-Lima
Resick, P. A., Nishith, P., Weaver, T. L., Astin, M. C., & Feuer, C. A. (2002). A comparison of cognitive-processing therapy with prolonged exposure and a waiting condition for the treatment of chronic posttraumatic stress disorder in female rape victims. *Journal of Consulting and Clinical Psychology, 70*, 867–879.
Revilla, V., Teresa, A., & Jorge Price, M. (1992). *La administración de la justicia informal: Posibilidades de integración*. Lima: Fundación M.J. Bustamante De la Fuente.
Ricoeur, P. (1995a). *Figuring the sacred: Religion, narrative, and imagination* (M. I. Wallace, Ed., D. Pellauer, Trans.). Minneapolis: Fortress Press, 1995a.
Ricoeur, P. (1995b). *Critique and conviction* (B. Kathleen, Trans.). New York: Columbia University Press, 1998 (1995).
Rifkin, J. (2010). *The empathic civilization: The race to global consciousness in a world in crisis*. Cambridge: Polity cited in Krznaric, R., (2014: 15). *A handbook for Revolution: Empathy* Rider Books Ebury Publishing.
Rivers, J. J., & Josephs, R. A. (2010). Dominance and health: The role of social rank in physiology and illness. In A. Guinote & T. Vescio (Eds.), *The social psychology of power*. New York: The Guilford Press.
Roberts, D. (2009). *Global governance and biopolitics: Regulating human security*. London: Zed Books.
Rodriguez-Pereyra, G. (2008). Nominalism in Metaphysics. In N. Z. Edward (Ed.), *The stanford encyclopaedia of philosophy*.
Romer, P. (1986). Increasing returns and long run growth. *Journal of Political Economy, 94*, 1002–1037.
Root, R. (2012). *Transitional justice in Peru*. New York: Palgrave Macmillan.

Rosner, R., & Poswell, S. (2006). Posttraumatic Growth after War. In L. G. Calhoun & R. Tedeschi (2009). (Eds.), *Handbook of post-traumatic growth: Research and practice*. Psychology Press: Taylor and Francis Group.

Ross, L., & Nisbett, R. E. (1991). *The person and the situation: Perspectives of social psychology*. New York: McGraw-Hill.

Rozynko, V., & Dondershine, H. E. (1991). Trauma focus group therapy for Vietnam veterans with PTSD. *Psychotherapy, 28*(1), 157–161.

Russell, A. M., & Fiske, S. T. (2010). Power and social perception. In A. Guinote & T. Vescio (Eds.), *The social psychology of power* (p. 10012). New York: The Guilford Press.

Rylko-Bauer, B., & Farmer, P. (2016). Structural violence, poverty, and social suffering. In D. Brady & L. M. Burton (Eds.), *The Oxford handbook of the social science of poverty* (pp. 47–75). Oxford: Oxford University Press.

Rylko-Bauer, B. & Singer, M. (2010). "Political violence, war, and medical anthropology." Pp. 219–249, in A companion to medical anthropology, by Merrill Singer and Pamela I. Erickson. Malden: Wiley-Blackwell.

Rylko-Bauer, B., Whiteford, L., & Farmer, P. (2009). Prologue: Coming to terms with global violence and health. In B. Rylko-Bauer, L. Whiteford, & P. Farmer (Eds.), *Global health in times of violence* (pp. 3–16). Santa Fe: School for Advanced Research Press.

Saakvitne, K. W., Gamble, S., Pearlman, L., & Lev, B. (2000). *Risking connection: A training curriculum for working with survivors of childhood abuse*. Lutherville: Sidran Press.

Sabatini Scalmati, A. (2000). *Memorie congelate memorie evitate a proposito della relazione terapeutica con le vittime di tortura*. Rome, October 1–3 1999. Third European Conference on Child and Adolescent Psychoanalytic Psychotherapy.

Salomon, G., & Nevo, B. (Eds.). *Peace education: The concept, principle and practice around the world*. Mahwah: Erlbaum London.

Sandin, I. (1995). Values in nurse education – A historical review. *Nordic Journal of Nordic Research, 15*(1)

Santner, E. (1990). *Stranded objects: Mourning, memory and film in postwar Germany*. Ithaca: Cornell University Press.

Saona, M. (2014). *Memory matters in transitional Peru*. London: Palgrave Macmillan Memory Studies.

Savelsberg, J. (2017). Intergenerational criminal law. In R. E. Anderson (Ed.), *Alleviating world suffering*. Cham: Springer.

Schattschneider, E. E. (1960). *The semi-sovereign people: A realist's view of democracy in America*. Fort Worth: Harcourt Brace College Publishers.

Scarry, E. (1985). *The body in pain: The making and unmaking of the world*. New York: Oxford University Press.

Scheff, T. J. (1988). Shame and conformity: The deference emotion system. *American Sociological Review, 53*(3), 395–406.

Scheff, T. J., Retzinger, S., & Ryan, M. (1989). Crime, violence and self-esteem. In A. Mecca, N. Smelser, & J. Vasconcellos (Eds.), *The social importance of self-esteem*. Berkeley: University of California Press.

Schlebusch, L. (1998). Social support, self-efficacy and assertiveness as mediators of study stress in *Psychology* (Savannah, GA.), *34*(3), 61–69.

Scheper-Hughes, N. (1992). *Death without weeping: The violence of everyday life in Brazil*. Berkeley: University of California Press.

Scheper-Hughes, N. (1998). Undoing: Social suffering and the politics of Remorse in the New South Africa. *Social Justice, 25*(4), 114–142.

Schmid, A. (2011). *The routledge handbook of terrorism research*. London: Taylor & Francis.

Schmidt am Busch, H.-C., & Zurn, C. F. (Eds.). (2010). *The philosophy of recognition – Historical and contemporary perspectives*. Maryland: Lexington Books.

Schreuder, B., Kleijn, W., & Rooijmans, H. (2000). Nocturnal re-experiencing more than forty years after war trauma. *Journal of Traumatic Stress, 13*, 453–463.

Schreuder, B., et al. (2001). Intrusive re-experiencing of chronic strife of war. *Advances in Psychiatric Treatment, 7*, 102–108.
Schuster, E., & Boschert-Kimmig, R. (1999). *Hope against hope: Johann Baptist Metz and Elie Wiesel speak out on the Holocaust* (p. 90). New Jersey: Paulist Press 07430.
Schwab, G. (2010). *Haunting legacies: Violent histories and transgenerational trauma*. New York: Columbia University Press.
Schwartz, W. (2002). From passivity to competence: A conceptualization of knowledge, skill, tolerance, and empathy. *Psychiatry, 65*(4), 338–345.
Schwartz, W. (2013). The parameters of empathy: Core considerations for psychotherapy and supervision. *Advances in Descriptive Psychology* 10.
Scott, J. (1990). *Domination and the arts of resistance*. New Haven: Yale University Press.
Scott Peck, M. (1983). *People of the Lie: The hope for healing human evil*. New York: Simon & Schuster.
Sebald, W. G. (2004). *On the natural history of destruction*. London: Penguin Books.
Sedikides, C. (1995). Central and peripheral self conceptions are differentially influenced by mood: Tests of the differential sensitivity hypothesis. *Journal of Personality and Social Psychology, 69*, 757–777.
Seeburger, F. (2012 September, 14). *The open wound: Trauma, identity and community*. CreateSpace Independent Publishing Platform.
Seligman, M. E. P. (1975). *On depression, development and death*. New York: W.H. Freeman.
Sen, A. (1998). "*Mortality as an Indicator of Economic Success and Failure*." (Text of the *Innocenti* Lecture of UNICEF, Florence, Italy, March 1995.). *Economic Journal, 108*(446), 1–25.
Sennet, R. (2012). *Together: The rituals, pleasures and politics of cooperation*. London: Allen Lane.
Shapiro, F., & Silk Forrest, M. S. (1997). *EMDR: The breakthrough therapy for overcoming anxiety, stress, and trauma*. New York: Basic Books.
Shaw, K. L. (1996). An empirical analysis of risk aversion and income growth. *Journal of Labour Economics, 34*(3), 275–291.
Sheer, M. K., & Smith-Caroff, K. (2002). Traumatic loss and the syndrome of complicated grief. *PTSD Research Quarterly, 13*, 1–7.
Silverman, K. (1996). *The threshold of the visible world*. New York: Routledge.
Silvetti, F., & Cáceres, D. (1998). Una perspectiva sociohistórica de las estrategias de reproducción social de pequeños productores del Noroeste de Córdoba. *Debate Agrario, 28*, 103–127.
Simon, B., & Klandermans, B. (2001). Politicised collective identity. *American Psychologist, 56*, 319–331.
Singer, M., & Hodge, G. D. (Eds.). (2010). *The war machine and global health*. Lanham: AltaMira.
Singer, M., & Erickson, P. I. (2011). As the future explodes into the present: Emergent issues and the tomorrow of medical anthropology. In M. Singer & P. I. Erickson (Eds.), *A companion to medical anthropology* (pp. 515–532). Malden: Wiley-Blackwell.
Skaar, E., Malca Gianella, C., & Eide, T. (2015). *After violence: Transitional justice, peace, and democracy*. London: Routledge.
Skar, H. O. (1982). *The warm valley people: Duality and land reform among the Quechua Indians of highland Peru*. Oslo: Universitetsforlaget.
Skultans, V. (1998). *The testimony of lives: Narrative and memory in Post-Soviet Latvia*. London: Routledge.
Sloan, P. (1988). Post-traumatic stress in survivors of an airplane crash-landing: A clinical and exploratory research intervention. *Journal of Traumatic Stress, 1*, 211–229.
Smart, D., Sanson, A., Da Silva, L., & Toumbourou, J. (2000). The development of civic mindedness. *Family Matters, 57*, 4–10.
Smith-Nonini, S. (2010). *Healing the body politic: El Salvador's popular struggle for health rights from civil war to Neoliberal peace*. New Brunswick: Rutgers University Press.
Smith, T. P. (2006). With one heart *Instituto Lingüístico de Verano*. Lima 100, Perú.

Snyder, S. (2009). The roots and repercussions of educational inequality on the indigenous populations of Peru. *Stanford Journal of International Relations, 10*(1), 52–59.

Soares, Y. S. D., Sviatschi, M., Andrade R., & Montenegro, J. (2010). *The impact of improving access to justice on conflict resolution evidence from Peru*. Inter-American Development Bank.

Sontag, S. (2003). *Regarding the pain of others*. Hamish Hamilton.

Spargo, R. C. (2006). *Vigilant memory: Emmanuel Levinas, the Holocaust, and the unjust death*. Baltimore: The Johns Hopkins University Press.

Spelman, E. V. (1997). *Fruits of sorrow: Framing our attention to suffering*. Beacon Press.

Srinisvasa Murthy, R., & Lakshminayaranah, R. (2006). Mental health consequences of war: A brief research of findings. *World Psychiatry, 5*(1), 25–30.

Starn, O. (1991). Missing the revolution: Anthropologists and the war in Peru. *Cultural Anthropology, 6*(1), 63–91.

Starn, O. (1999). *Nightwatch: The politics of protest in the Andes*. Durham: Duke University Press.

Starn, O., Degregori, C. I., & Kirk, R. (1995). *The Peru reader: History, culture, politics*. Durham: Duke University Press.

Scott Palmer, D. (1992). *Shining path of Peru*. London: Hurst & Co.

Staub, E. (1989). *The roots of evil. The origins of genocide and other group violence*. New York: Cambridge University Press.

Staub, E. (1996a). Breaking the cycle of violence: Helping victims of genocidal violence heal. *Journal of Personal and Interpersonal Loss, 1*, 191–197.

Staub, E. (1996b). Preventing genocide: Activating bystanders, helping victims and the creation of caring. *Peace and Conflict: Journal of Peace Psychology, 2*, 189–201.

Staub, E. (1999a). Predicting collective violence: The psychological and cultural roots of turning against others. In C. Summers, & D. Markussen (Eds.), *Collective violence: Harmful behaviour in groups and governments*. Rowman and Littlefield publishers.

Staub, E. (1999b). The origins and prevention of genocide, mass killing, and other collective violence peace and conflict. *Journal of Peace Psychology, 5*(4), 303–336.

Staub, E. (1999c). Preventing genocide: Activating bystanders, helping victims heal, helping groups overcome hostility. In L. Chorbajian, & G. Shirinian (Eds.), *Studies in comparative genocide*. London/New York: MacMillan Press/St. Martin's Press.

Staub, E. (1999d). Genocide. In *The Oxford encyclopaedia of military history*. New York: Oxford University Press.

Staub, E. (1999e). The origins and prevention of genocide, mass killing and other collective violence. *Peace and Conflict: Journal of Peace Psychology, 5*, 303–337 (Lead article, followed by commentaries).

Staub, E. (1999f). The roots of evil: personality, social conditions, culture and basic human needs. *Personality and Social Psychology Review, 3*, 179–192 (Lead article in special issue on violence/evil).

Staub, E. (2003). *The psychology of good and evil: why children, adults, and groups help and harm others*. Cambridge: Cambridge University Press.

Staub, E. (2012). *The roots and prevention of genocide and related mass violence*. Chapter 2 in M. Anstey, P. Meerts, & I. W. Zartman (Eds.), *The slippery slope to genocide: Reducing identity conflicts and preventing mass murder*. New York: Oxford University Press.

Staub, E., Pearlman, L. A., Gubin, A., & Hagengimana, A. (2005). Healing, reconciliation, forgiving and the prevention of violence after genocide or mass killing: An intervention and its experimental evaluation in Rwanda. *Journal of Social and Clinical Psychology, 24*(3), 297–334.

Stauffer, C., & Mariluz, O. (2012 June, 6). Peru's Humala touts rebel capture after deadly protest. *Reuters*. Available at http://www.reuters.com/article/2012/07/06/peru-politics-humalaidUSL2E8I6A7P20120706.

Steel, G., & Zoomers, A. (2009). Social mobility in the Central Andes of Peru and Bolivia: towards a more dynamic and multi-local vision of poverty alleviation. *International Development Planning Review, 31*, 377–396.

Steiner, G. (1967). *Language and silence: Essays 1958–1966*. London: Faber and Faber.

Stern, S. J. (1998). *Shining and other paths: War and society in Peru, 1980–1995 (Latin America Otherwise)*. Durham: Duke University Press.
Stølen, K. A. (2007). *Guatemalans in the aftermath of violence: The refugees' return*. Philadelphia: University of Pennsylvania Press.
Suarez, E. (2013). *Resilience and post-traumatic responses: Lessons of courage from marginalized indigenous women in post-conflict ayacucho (Peru)*. The Society for Social Work and Research, Annual Conference, 2013.
Summerfield, D. (1999). A critique of seven assumptions behind psychological trauma programmes in war-affected areas. *Social Science and Medicine, 48*(10), 1449–1462.
Summerfield, D. (1995). Psychological responses to war and atrocity: The limitations of current concepts. *Social Science & Medicine, 40*(8), 1073–1082.
Summerfield, D. (1997). *The impact of war and atrocity on civilian populations, in Psychological trauma: A developmental approach*. In D. Black, J. Newman, J. Harris-Hendricks, & G. Mezey (Eds.) (pp. 148–155). Glasgow: Royal College of Psychiatrists.
Sumner, L. W. (1996). *Welfare, happiness and ethics*. New York: Oxford University Press.
Tapia, C. (1995). *Auto defensa armada del campesinado*. Lima: *Centro de Estudios para el Desarrollo y la Participación*.
Tarazona-Sevillano, G. (1992). The organization of shining path. In D. S. Palmer (Ed.), *Shining path of Peru* (p. 181). New York: St. Martin's Press.
Tarazona-Sevillano, G. (1990). *Sendero Luminoso and the Threat of Narcoterrorism* (Praeger Series in Political Communication). (Praeger Series in Political Communication.
Taylor, C. (1991). *The ethics of authenticity*. Cambridge: Harvard University Press.
Taylor, C. (1992). *Multiculturalism and the politics of recognition* (p. 1992). New Jersey: Princeton.
Taylor, L. (2006). *Shining path: Guerrilla war in Peru's Northern Highlands, 1980–1997*. Liverpool: Liverpool University Press.
Tester, K. (1994). *Media, culture and morality*. London: Routledge New York and London.
Tester, K. (1999). The moral consequentiality of television. *European Journal of Social Theory, 2*(4), 469–483.
Tester, K. (2001). *Compassion, morality and the media*. Buckingham: Open University Press.
Tiedens, L. Z., & Fragale, A. R. (2003). Power moves: Complementarity in dominant and submissive nonverbal behaviour. *Journal of Personality and Social Psychology, 84*, 558–568.
Theidon, K. (2013). *Intimate memories: Violence and reconciliation in Peru*. Philadelphia: University of Pennsylvania Press.
Theidon, K. (2000). How we learned to kill our brother: Memory, morality, and reconciliation in Peru. *Bulletin of the French Institute of Andean Studies, 29*(3), 539–554. http://www.ifeanet.org/publicaciones/boletines/29%283%29/539.pdf
Thoits, P. (1995). Stress coping and social support process: Where are we, what next? *Journal of Health and Social Behaviour* (Extra Issue). 53–79
Tilly, C. (1985). War Making and State Making as Organized Crime. In P. Evans, D. Rueschemeyer, & T. Skocpol (Eds.), *Bringing the state back* (p. 170). Cambridge: Cambridge University Press.
Towle, M. S., & Lende, D. (2008). Community approaches to preventing mother-to-child HIV transmission: perspectives from rural Lesotho. African journal of AIDS research.
Truth and Reconciliation Commission, Final Report. (2003). Lima: Truth and Reconciliation Commission.
Tracy, J. L., & Robins, R. W. (2003). Death of a (Narcissistic) salesman: An integrative model of fragile self-esteem: Comment. *Psychological Inquiry, 14*, 57–62.
Tshopik, H. (1951). The Aymara of Chucuito, Peru: 1, magic. *Anthropological Papers of the American Museum of Natural History, 44*(part 2), 133–308 New York.
Tulchin, J., & Bland, G. (1994). *Peru in crisis: Dictatorship or democracy?* London: Lynne Rienner Publishers.
Turiel, E. (2002). *The culture of morality: Social development, context, and conflict*. Cambridge: Cambridge University Press.

Ullman, S. E., Filipas, H. H., Townsend, S. M., & Starzynski, L. L. (2007). Psychosocial correlates of PTSD symptom severity in sexual assault survivors. *Journal of Traumatic Stress, 20*(5), 821–831.

Ullman, S. E., & Filipas, H. H. (2001). Predictors of PTSD symptom severity and social reactions in sexual assault victims. *Journal of Traumatic Stress, 14*, 369–389.

United States Department of State. (2005). *Country reports on human rights practices: Peru.*

Uvin, P. (1999). Development aid and structural violence: The case of Rwanda. *Development, 42*(3), 49–56.

Valente, R. V. (2010). *Gender risk, poverty and vulnerability in Peru: A case study of the JUNTOS programme*. ODI.

Van de Poel, E., O'Donnell, O., & van Doorslaer, E. (2007). *Are urban children really healthier? Evidence from 47 developing countries*. Tinbergen Institute Discussion Paper TI 2007-035/3.

Van der Kolk, B. A. (2014). *The body keeps the score: Mind, brain and body in the transformation of trauma*. London: Penguin Books.

Van der Kolk, B. A., & Fisler, R. (1995). Dissociation and the fragmentary nature of traumatic memories: Review and experimental confirmation. *Journal of Traumatic Stress, 8*(1995), 505–525.

Vasquez Villanueva, A. (1993). *Los desafios del agroen la decada del noventa.* Lima: Ministerio de Agricultura.

Vescio, T. K., & Guinote, A. (2010). Power: New understandings and future directions. In A. Guinote & T. K. Vescio (Eds.), *The social psychology of power*. New York: Guilford Press.

Vescio, T. K., Gervais, S., Snyder, M., & Hoover, A. (2005). Power and the creation of patronizing environments: The stereotype-based behaviours of the powerful and their effects on female performance in masculine domains. *Journal of Personality and Social Psychology, 88*, 658–672.

Vetlesen, A. J. (1994). *Perception, empathy, and judgment: An inquiry into the preconditions of moral performance*. Pennsylvania: Pennsylvania State University Press.

Volf, M. (2006). *The end of memory: Remembering rightly in a violent world.* Grand Rapids/Cambridge: Wm. B. Eerdmans Publishing Co.

Volkan, V. (2018). From earthquakes to ethnic cleansing: Massive trauma and its individualized and societal consequences. In A. Hamburger (Ed.), *Trauma, trust and memory: Social trauma and reconciliation in psychoanalysis, psychotherapy and cultural memory* (pp. 5–13). London: Routledge.

Wadsworth, M. E. (2012). Working with low-income families: Lessons learned from basic and applied research on coping with poverty-related stress. *Journal of Contemporary Psychotherapy, 42*(1), 17–25.

Walker, M. U. (2006). *Moral repair: Reconstructing moral relations after wrongdoing*. New York: Cambridge University Press.

Wall, P. (1999). *Pain: The science of suffering*. London: Weidenfeld & Nicolson.

Waller, J. (2002). *Becoming evil: How ordinary people commit genocide and mass killing*. New York: Oxford University Press.

Walter, N., Bourgois, P., & Margarita Loinaz, H. (2004). Masculinity and undocumented labour migration: Injured latino day-laborers in San Francisco. *Social Science & Medicine, 59*(6), 1159–1168.

Wardi, D. (1993). *Le candele della memoria*. Milan: Sansoni.

Watkins, M., & Shulman, H. (2008). *Toward psychologies of liberation*. Basingstoke: Palgrave MacMillan.

Watters, R. F. (1994). *Poverty and peasantry in Peru's Southern Andes, 1963–90*. New York: Macmillan.

Weary, et al. (1993). Depression, control motivation and the processing of information about others. In G. Weary, F. Gleicher, & K. L. Marsh (Eds.), *Control motivation and social cognition* (pp. 255–287). New York: Springer-Verlag.

Webb, R. (2013). *Conexión y Despegue Rural*. Lima: Instituto del Perú, Universidad San Martín de Porres.

Weicke, M., & Guinote, A. (2008, June). When subjective experiences matter: power increases reliance on the ease of retrieval. *Journal of Personality and Social Psychology, 94*(6), 956–970.
Weil, S. (2002). *The need for roots: Prelude to a declaration of duties towards mankind* Routledge Classics, 11 New Fetter Lane, London EC4P 4EE.
Weil, S. (2005). *Simone Weil*. Maryknoll: Orbis Books.
Weine, S. M., Becker, D. F., McGlashan, T. H., Laub, D., Lazrove, S., Voivoda, D., & Hyman, L. (1995). Psychiatric consequences of "ethnic cleansing": Clinical assessments and trauma testimonies of newly resettled Bosnian refugees. *The American Journal of Psychiatry, 152*(4), 536–542.
Weine, S., et al. (1998). Testimony psychotherapy in Bosnian refugees: a pilot study. *American Journal of Psychiatry, 155*, 1720–1726.
Weinreich, P., & Saunderson, W. (Eds.). (2003). *Analyzing identity: Cross-cultural, societal and clinical contexts*. London: Routledge.
Weissmark, M. S. (2004). *Justice matters: Legacies of the Holocaust and World War II*. Oxford: Oxford University Press.
Wessells, M. G., & Monteiro, C. (2004a). Healing the wounds following protracted conflict in Angola. In U. P. Gielen, J. Fish, & J. G. Draguns (Eds.), *Handbook of culture, therapy, and healing* (pp. 321–341). Mahwah: Erlbaum.
Wessells, M. G., & Monteiro, C. (2004b). Psychosocial assistance to internally displaced people in Angola. In K. Miller & L. Rasco (Eds.), *The mental health of refugees* (Vol. 70, pp. 67–94). Upper Saddle River: Erlbaum.
Whiteford, L., & Whiteford, S. (2005). In L. Whiteford & S. Whiteford (Eds.), *Paradigm change in globalization in water and health*. Santa Fe: School of American Research.
Wickham-Crowley, T. P. (1992). *Guerrillas and revolution in Latin America*. Princeton: Princeton University Press.
Wiesel, E. (1960). *Night*. New York: Hill & Lang.
Wiesel, E. (1990). *From the kingdom of Memory: Reminiscences*. New York: Summit.
Wilkinson, R. G. (1996). *Unhealthy societies: The afflictions of inequality*. London: Routledge.
Wilkinson, I. (2001). Thinking with suffering. *Cultural Values, 5*(4), 421–444.
Wilkinson, I. (2004). The problem of 'social suffering': The challenge to social science. *Health Sociology Review, 13*(2), 113–121.
Wilkinson, I. (2005a). *Suffering: A sociological introduction*. Cambridge: Polity.
Wilkinson, R. G. (2005b). *The impact of inequality: How to make sick societies healthier*. New York: The New Press.
Wilkinson, I. (2006). Health, risk and 'social suffering. *Health, Risk & Society, 8*(1), 1–8.
Williams, M., & Bebbington, A. (2008). Water and mining conflicts in Peru. *Mountain Research and Development, 28*(3/4). available at http://snobear.colorado.edu/Markw/Research/08_peru.pdf.
Wilson, F. (2013). *Citizenship and political violence in Peru: An Andean Town, 1870s–1970s* (Studies of the Americas). Palgrave Macmillan.
Winter, D. D. N., & Leighton, D. C. (2001). Structural violence: Introduction. In D. J. Christie, R. V. Wagner, & D. D. N. Winter (Eds.), *Peace, conflict, and violence: Peace psychology for the 21st century* (pp. 99–101). Upper Saddle River: Prentice Hall.
Wiseman, H., Metzl, E., & Barber, J. P. (2006). Anger, guilt, and intergenerational communication of trauma in the interpersonal narratives of second generation Holocaust survivors. *American Journal of Orthopsychiatry, 76*(2), 176–184.
Wolf, E. (1955). Types of Latin American peasantry: A preliminary discussion. *American Anthropologist, 57*(3) Part 1, 452–471.
Wolf, E. (1957). Closed corporate communities in Mesoamerica and Java. *Southwestern Journal of Anthropology, 13*(1), 1–18.
World Bank. (1999). *Peru: Improving health care for the poor*. Washington, DC: World Bank.

Yamawaki, N., Darby, R., & Queiroz, A. (2007). The moderating role of ambivalent sexism: The influence of power status on perception of rape victim and rapist. *The Journal of Social Psychology, 147*(1), 4–56.

Young, I. M. (2000). Five faces of oppression. In M. Adams (Ed.), *Readings for diversity and social justice* (pp. 35–49). New York: Routledge.

Yuval-Davis, N. (1997). *Gender & nation*. London: Sage.

Zayfert, C., & DeViva, J. (2005). Residual insomnia following cognitive behavioral therapy for PTSD. *Journal of Traumatic Stress, 17*(1), 69–73 pages 69–73, February 2004.

Zurn, C. F. (Ed.). (2010). *The philosophy of recognition – Historical and contemporary perspectives*. Maryland: Lexington Books.

Zimbardo, P. G. (1969). The human choice: Individuation, reason, and order vs. deindividuation, impulse, and chaos. In W. J. Arnold & D. Levine (Eds.), *Nebraska symposium on motivation* (pp. 237–307). Lincoln: University of Nebraska Press.

Zoellner, L. A., & Bittenger, J. N. (2004). In G. M. Rosen (Ed.), *On the uniqueness of trauma memories in PTSD, in Post-traumatic stress disorder: Issues and controversies*. New York: Wiley.

Zolkos, M. (2007). Jean Amery's concept of resentment at the crossroads of ethics and politics. *The European Legacy, 12*(1), 23–38.

Zolkos, M. (2011). *Reconciling community and subjective life: Trauma testimony as political theorizing in the work of Jean Améry and Imre Kertész*. London: Continuum Press.

Author Index

T. J. Bowyer, *Beyond Suffering and Reparation*,
https://doi.org/10.1007/978-3-319-98983-9

Subject Index

T. J. Bowyer, *Beyond Suffering and Reparation*,
https://doi.org/10.1007/978-3-319-98983-9

D

MIX
Papier aus verantwortungsvollen Quellen
Paper from responsible sources
FSC® C105338

If you have any concerns about our products,
you can contact us on
ProductSafety@springernature.com

In case Publisher is established outside the EU,
the EU authorized representative is:
Springer Nature Customer Service Center GmbH
Europaplatz 3, 69115 Heidelberg, Germany

Printed by Libri Plureos GmbH
in Hamburg, Germany